MEDICAL IMAGING:
A CONCISE TEXTBOOK

MEDICAL IMAGING:
A CONCISE TEXTBOOK

EUGENE R. JACOBS, M.D., F.A.C.R.

Associate Professor
General Diagnostic Radiology Section
The George Washington University Medical Center
Washington, D.C.

IGAKU-SHOIN NEW YORK•TOKYO

Interior Design by M 'N O Production Services, Inc.
Cover Design by M 'N O Production Services, Inc.
Typesetting by Progressive Typographers Inc.
Printing and Binding by Arcata Graphics/Halliday

Published and distributed by
IGAKU-SHOIN Medical Publishers, Inc.
1140 Avenue of the Americas, New York, N.Y. 10036

IGAKU-SHOIN Ltd.,
5-24-3 Hongo, Bunkyo-ku, Tokyo

Library of Congress Cataloging-in-Publication Data

Medical imaging.

   Includes index.
   1. Diagnostic imaging.   I. Jacobs, Eugene.
II. Title. [DNLM: 1. Radiography. WN 200 M489]
RC78.7.D53M425   1987   616.07'54   87-2644
ISBN 0-89640-126-X

ISBN: 0-89640-126-X (New York)
ISBN: 4-260-14126-0 (Tokyo)

Printed and bound in U.S.A.

10 9 8 7 6 5 4 3 2 1

PREFACE

There is considerable discussion in the field of diagnostic imaging as to how imaging departments should be structured. Some departments are divided according to organ systems such as musculoskeletal or gastrointestinal, while other departments are structured according to diagnostic modalities such as ultrasound or MRI. Some departments are inconsistent in their structure and others have gradually changing structures. The divisions in this book have been chosen on the basis of comfort and convenience for the contributors and readers, and they tend to follow a path that is intermediate between the organ system and modality approach. While many people in the field of imaging have very strong feelings about the proper way to structure imaging departments, there appear to be as many philosophies as there are philosophers.

It will be apparent to the reader that the approach of each of the contributors in this volume is quite different. Each author was encouraged to use a structure and style which he felt most appropriate for the subject matter and most comfortable for his own writing style. Certain organ systems are best approached by considerations of imaging modalities, others by clinical case descriptions, and yet others by analysis of image patterns or clues. We are consciously giving up the convenience of uniformity for the advantages of spontaneity and didactic philosophy. It is hoped that this natural diversity of approach may demonstrate to the reader the multiple ways of reaching the same goal; namely, learning the many rational approaches to understanding the various areas of imaging.

E.R.J.

Affectionately dedicated
to my dear wife
Janet

FOREWORD

Most textbooks of Radiology these days are written for radiology practitioners or residents midway through their training. They are frequently very subspecialized, technical, and often out of date by the time they are published. Very few books are written to appeal to the medical student, first year resident, or general medical practitioner who desires to get a thorough and basic introduction of the specialty to Radiology. Dr. Jacobs and his colleagues at the George Washington University Medical Center have beautifully organized and written this latter kind of text.

Over the past several years, Dr. Jacobs, who is Associate Professor of Radiology at George Washington University, has headed up a very active medical student program in Radiology. Teaching techniques and information imparted to our students are constantly being updated and revised, and the program is highly regarded. Reviews by our students are glowing. Dr. Jacobs has utilized techniques developed in this aggressive medical student program in the writing of this wonderful book. Discussions of imaging modalities, clinical cases, and methods of image pattern analysis are used by the authors to explain "the rational approaches to understanding the various areas of imaging." In today's changing health care environment, the specialty of medical imaging is changing, perhaps faster than others. Clinicians can no longer order tests and examinations in a "shot gun" fashion. Indications for examinations and proper sequencing of examinations must be thoroughly understood and appreciated by the clinician to ensure optimum health care. Dr. Jacobs' text promotes this approach.

Initial chapters discuss the physics of modern day radiology and imaging, positioning for examinations, and issues of cost. These chapters, beautifully written by Dr. Jacobs himself, are extremely informative and easy to understand. Subsequent chapters, written by Dr. Jacobs and his coauthors, cover in detail the various subspecialties in Radiology, including musculoskeletal radiology, chest radiology, gastrointestinal radiology, genitourinary radiology, ultrasonography, neuroradiology, interventional radiology, and nuclear medicine. A final chapter speculates on the future of imaging. In the subspecialty sections the basic imaging approach to the organ system or modality is stressed. Chapters flow logically and information is well-organized and thoroughly up to date.

Dr. Jacobs should be congratulated for organizing and writing with his colleagues this excellent book which is sorely needed. Medical students, young radiology residents, and medical practitioners will find this a welcome addition to their libraries, and Radiology will be aided in general by having a more informed consumer.

William W. Olmsted, M.D.
Professor and Director
Division of Diagnostic Radiology
The George Washington University Medical Center
Washington, D.C.

CONTRIBUTORS

DAVID J. CURTIS, M.D., F.A.C.R.
Professor
Head, General Diagnostic Radiology Section
Department of Radiology
The George Washington University Medical Center
901 23rd Street, N.W.
Washington, D.C. 20037

THOMAS S. DINA, M.D.
Associate Professor
Neuroradiology Section
Diagnostic Radiology Division
The George Washington University Medical Center
901 23rd Street, N.W.
Washington, D.C. 20037

EDWARD M. DRUY, M.D.
Professor
Head, Interventional and Vascular Radiology Section
Division of Diagnostic Radiology
Department of Radiology
The George Washington University Medical Center
901 23rd Street, N.W.
Washington, D.C. 20037

CONTRIBUTORS

DAVID S. FEIGIN, M.D.
Associate Professor
Department of Radiology (V-114)
University of California, San Diego
La Jolla, California 92093
Assistant Chief of Radiology
Veterans Administration Medical Center
San Diego, California

MICHAEL C. HILL, M.B.
Professor
Head, Body Cross-Sectional Imaging Section (US/CT)
Division of Diagnostic Radiology
Department of Radiology
The George Washington University Medical Center
901 23rd Street, N.W.
Washington, D.C. 20037

EUGENE R. JACOBS, M.D., F.A.C.R.
Associate Professor
General Diagnostic Radiology Section
Chief, Musculoskeletal Radiology Service
The George Washington University Medical Center
901 23rd Street, N.W.
Washington, D.C. 20037

EDUARD V. KOTLYAROV, M.D., P.H.D.
Associate Clinical Professor
Divisions of Nuclear Medicine and Diagnostic Radiology
Department of Radiology
The George Washington University Medical Center
901 23rd Street, N.W.
Washington, D.C. 20037

RICHARD C. REBA, M.D.
Professor of Radiology and Medicine
Director, Division of Nuclear Medicine
Department of Radiology
The George Washington University Medical Center
901 23rd Street, N.W.
Washington, D.C. 20037

CONTENTS

x i

CHAPTER 1

INTRODUCTION

Eugene R. Jacobs

Until recent years, a reasonable goal governing the choice and performance of medical imaging procedures was to obtain the most useful, relevant information with the least patient discomfort, short term risk, and long term radiation burden.

Today, that is not enough! Since our society now seems to have decided that it must put a finite limit on health care expenditures, the choice and performance of imaging procedures must be modified to consider absolute and relative costs and impact on hospital length of stay.

IMAGING IN MEDICINE

Medicine has now reached a stage in its development where we must change our vocabulary to keep up with and reinforce our changing philosophies. We must abandon the phrase "ordering an x-ray" and instead consider requesting an "imaging consultation." This simple change will lead to more caring examinations tailored to the individual patient's needs with less discomfort, risk, radiation burden, and less ultimate cost.

Because of the remarkable technologic advances in medical imaging, we are seeing exploratory surgical procedures being performed less often since we can now image soft tissue structures with the aid of sonography, computed tomography (CT), and magnetic resonance imaging (MRI). Even now, examinations previously requiring ionizing radiation are being supplanted by ultrasound and MRI. MRI promises spectral analysis of tissues in the future.

Imaging-directed percutaneous needle biopsy is replacing some open surgical proce-

1

dures. Diagnostic and therapeutic catheter procedures directed by imaging techniques are making great strides in finding and treating hemorrhage as well as occlusive vascular problems.

Quantitative computed tomography (QCT) is providing evaluation of spinal trabecular bone density in milligrams of calcium per cubic centimeter volume without an invasive bone biopsy.

Nuclear medicine studies are providing more specific information with much smaller radiation dosages than in years past.

THE PHYSICIAN'S ROLE IN REQUESTING AN IMAGING CONSULTATION

You must approach each imaging study with care. As when setting up a scientific experiment, you must ask yourself the following questions:

1. What information am I seeking?
2. Will a positive or negative result materially alter therapy and ultimate outcome?
3. Can the same information be obtained by other means which may be safer, faster, less uncomfortable for the patient, less costly, or may entail less radiation burden?
4. Will the performance of this exam interfere with the ability to do a subsequent study (e.g., a barium study could obscure the lumbar spine)?
5. Have I first checked to obtain any previous imaging studies which may already exist and which may either answer my questions or materially contribute to the meaningful interpretation of the anticipated new study?
6. Would it be more appropriate to state the problem to an imaging specialist (radiologist) and ask for advice as to the most appropriate modified examination to meet the needs of this particular patient?
7. Have I assembled all currently available relevant history, physical examination findings, and laboratory findings and transmitted them to the radiologist to aid in the optimal performance and optimal interpretation of the imaging study finally decided upon?

THE FINAL FIT

Just as it is necessary to fit the choice of imaging study to the patient, the meaningful "results" of the study must fit the patient. All too often we try to fit the patient into an imaging diagnosis that is incongruous with the history and physical findings and with other available data. At times it may be necessary to rethink the entire problem. If the shoes you just bought seem too small, the answer is not to cut off your toes, but to try a different size. Remember that even with our very sophisticated technologies, even when we do everything "right," there are still false negatives and false positives. When *my* bone hurts with exquisite point tenderness and the "x-ray" is negative, I protect the part and then reevaluate if the clinical symptoms persist.

CHAPTER 2

IMAGING MODALITIES
(As described for the Nonphysicist and Nonmathematician)

Eugene R. Jacobs

To the reader (nonphysicist and nonmathematician): I commend you for resisting the natural urge to skip this chapter! I assume that you bring with you a basic knowledge of anatomy and physiology as well as pathology. Unfortunately, that is not quite enough. You must understand the broad basic concepts of how images are obtained in order to even begin to evaluate them. Much but not all of what follows may not be new to you. Nevertheless, I will proceed as though we are starting from the very beginning.

CONVENTIONAL RADIOGRAPHY

PRODUCTION OF THE RADIATION

A vaccum tube including a cathode at one end and an anode at the other is used. The cathode filament is heated and a cloud of electrons is "boiled off" from the cathode. These electrons are attracted by the positively charged target of the anode. When the high voltage circuit is completed and an exposure is made, the cathode electrons are accelerated in the direction of the anode and hit the target of the anode at a great speed. The electrons are stopped, losing their energy, to produce a great deal of heat and a relatively small amount of radiation (Fig. 2-1).

Assume that the radiation is arising from what is essentially a point source, the size of the point varying with the construction of the unit. From that point, divergent rays go out in *all* directions. These rays are all attenuated by the lead in the tube housing, and a mechanical collimator is used to control the size and shape of the divergent beam of x-rays which leave the collimator aperture.

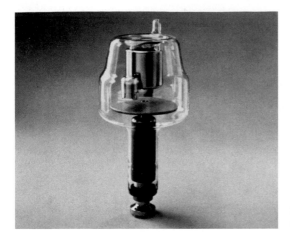

Figure 2-1. Modern x-ray tube. (Courtesy of General Electric Company, U.S.A.)

The closer the part of the patient being imaged is to the x-ray tube, the more it is geometrically distorted by the divergence of the rays.

The amount of radiation leaving the collimator is affected by the amount (milliamperage) of current flowing from the cathode to the anode, the potential difference (kilovoltage) between the cathode and the anode, and the duration of the time (exposure time) that the current flows.

Milliampere-seconds (mAs) is the product of the tube current and exposure time. If the kilovoltage remains fixed, an increase in the tube's mAs will result in a proportional increase in the amount of radiation produced. A 100mA current flowing for a 1sec exposure is the equivalent of a 1000mA current flowing for $\frac{1}{10}$ sec, or 500mA for $\frac{2}{10}$ sec, or 50mA for 2sec. For each case, the total mAs will be 100 and the total amount of radiation will be the same.

A short exposure is important in situations where there is motion of the patient. The problem with short exposures, however, is that with a high milliamperage and a short exposure, one must be concerned about dissipating the heat from the target of the anode rapidly so that the target will not overheat and possibly melt.

The kilovoltage or kV, sometimes written as kVp, contributes to the quality or penetrability of the radiation as well as to the quantity. The higher the kV, the shorter the wavelength of the radiation and the greater its ability to penetrate tissues.

When using radiographic contrast, it is necessary to keep in mind that the differential absorption of various elements is quite different at different kV levels. For example, there is a greater difference between the ability of iodine-based contrast materials to stop radiation and the ability of soft tissues to stop radiation at the 70kV level than there is at the 90kV level.

Because of the divergence of the x-rays arising from a point source, the exposure diminishes with the square of the distance from the radiation source (inverse square law). Thus, the radiation exposure is a function of mA, time, kV, and distance from the source. Please note that the exposure in roentgens does not depend on field size, but rather on the area of the patient exposed.

Because of some of these considerations noted above, the kV and mAs can be adjusted by the radiologic technologist to produce the optimal image to solve the imaging problem at hand.

CONSIDERATIONS AFFECTING IMAGE PRODUCTION

RADIATION AND THE PATIENT

Once the radiation reaches the patient, some may be scattered, producing "fog" (meaningless darkening of the film), some may be transmitted essentially unchanged, and some may be absorbed. Obviously the transmitted radiation will darken the film and the absorbed radiation will not reach the film.

The radiation leaving the patient has a pattern of radiation intensity corresponding to the pattern of absorption and transmission within the patient. In order to enhance the image, the film is generally placed between intensifying screens.

INTENSIFYING SCREENS

Intensifying screens are made of tiny crystals which emit light when excited by radiation. This light contributes more to the darkening of the film than does the radiation directly. Intensifying screens are described as detail, par, and high speed. The higher the speed, the more light produced per unit of radiation. With increasing speed there is generally some loss of fine detail. So-called detail screens provide very fine images at the expense of higher radiation dosage to the patient.

A new generation of screens, referred to as "rare-earth" screens, are more efficient in absorbing x-rays and convert that energy to light. Although rare-earth screens typically require less radiation exposure to produce an adequate density film, image detail is maintained.

GRIDS

When we radiograph a finger, radiation that scatters from the finger is not a serious problem. With a thick body part like the abdomen, the amount of scatter can seriously compromise contrast. Grids are used to cut down scatter. Grids are composed of parallel strips of thin lead with radiolucent spacing material between the strips. The strips are arranged to permit the passage of x-rays that are aligned with the radiation leaving the x-ray tube, but they will not permit the scattered radiation to pass. By filtering out the scattered or deflected rays, the grid provides a cleaner picture. The grid is installed in an x-ray table between the patient and the film cassette, or on the front of what is called a grid cassette. The grid has the disadvantage of requiring greater x-ray exposure since it absorbs some signal as well as scatter.

Because of the lead strips we will sometimes see very fine stripes on the film called grid lines. The grid lines can be avoided by using ultrafineline grids whose lines can be appreciated only with a magnifying lens but are not usually seen with the naked eye.

BUCKY

Another solution to the grid line problem is the Bucky grid. This is a grid which is moving throughout the exposure time so that the lines and spaces cancel out and we see a uniform picture without stripes. Occasionally even the best technologist will neglect to push the Bucky button and the Bucky "malfunctions," producing grid lines. Most thick part x-rays are made with either a fine line grid or a Bucky.

MAGNIFICATION

As noted above, the x-rays producing an image are divergent rays arising from an almost point source. Because of this divergence, the further an object is from the film, the greater the magnification of that object. Some practical examples of this include the following:

> If a chest x-ray is done with the patient facing the film so that the sternum and heart are near the film and the x-rays enter from behind, then the heart is only slightly magnified, since it is close to the film. With the patient facing in the opposite direction, with his back to the film, the heart is more significantly magnified.
> If a patient has a fracture of the right temporal region of the skull and an image is made with the right side adjacent to the film, the fracture will be sharply defined and only very slightly magnified. If a second exposure is made with the fracture side away from the film, the fracture will appear wider but somewhat less sharply defined.

We sometimes view x-ray images which are intentionally magnified by moving the object closer to the x-ray tube and thus further from the film. All of us have experimented with this as children as we made animal images on the wall by the shadows of our hands. We found that the images became less sharp with increasing magnification and that they were really good images only if we had a single point source of light.

TARGET SIZE

The sharpness of x-ray images is highly dependent on the size of the source of the radiation. Obviously a $0.3mm^2$ source more closely approximates a "point" source than a $1.0mm^2$ or $2.0mm^2$ source. The larger the source and the closer the object to the source, the less sharp the image.

Practically, it is difficult to dissipate heat from a small source and, since a melted x-ray tube is of little use, a compromise must be made between the ideal of a true point source and a feasible small source. All tubes, therefore, have sources of small but finite size, so there are varying degrees of unsharpness. It would seem that in physics, as elsewhere, you can't get something for nothing. This explains why some magnification techniques increase the size of an object but do not necessarily increase meaningful information about it.

One further comment on the problems of magnification relates to the total target film distance. When a chest x-ray is done at the patient's bedside with portable equipment, the distance between the source of the radiation and the film will generally be less than the 6 foot distance usually used in the x-ray rooms. Thus the x-rays will be relatively more divergent with the short distance and the magnification will be increased, making comparison more difficult than if the films were exposed with identical geometric factors.

ROTATION

If we view a translucent model of a three-dimensional object as it rotates about an axis, we will readily see that portions of the model in front of the axis will all move in the same direction, while structures behind the axis will move in the opposite direction. Furthermore, the greater the distance that an object is from the axis of rotation in any direction, the greater the displacement of the image on the film will be as the body part is rotated. For example, the patella is anteriorly placed, and the head of the fibula is more posteriorly placed, in relation to the rotational axis of the knee.

Let us assume that there is a patient with a small fragment of metal somewhere in the knee region. With only one projection, a single anterior view, if there were no lateral, we could not evaluate the location of the metal fragment with respect to how far anterior or posterior it might be. If we then added an oblique view and noted that the position of the fragment appeared to be displaced laterally by an amount about equal to the amount that the patella was displaced medially, then we would know that the metal fragment must be about as far posterior to the axis of rotation as the patella is anterior to the axis of rotation.

If a calcification in the right upper lung field seems to be displaced about the same amount and direction as the right sternoclavicular joint, it most likely lies in the far anterior portion of the lung. Using similar reasoning, if a film of the chest is obtained with the patient's back to the film, and the central ray coming from the x-ray tube is tilted slightly upward toward the head, then the anterior structures, like the anterior ribs and clavicles, would appear higher than the posterior structures.

Because human beings are irregularly contoured, it is obvious that it is extremely difficult to get precisely comparable projections for comparison with each other. It is difficult to obtain entirely comparable depth of respiration, size of swallow, rate of peristalsis, etc. It is also difficult to get comparable precision in terms of exposure, developer temperature, developer chemistry, and illumination of adjacent viewboxes.

We are dealing with dynamic systems and attempting to characterize them by a few fleeting glances from varying vantage points. Considering all the problems, imaging does very well, but we must recognize the limitations.

CONTRAST

Contrast is the difference in image intensity that permits us to differentiate adjacent portions of an image. It is based in part on the differential absorption of the radiation by the tissues.

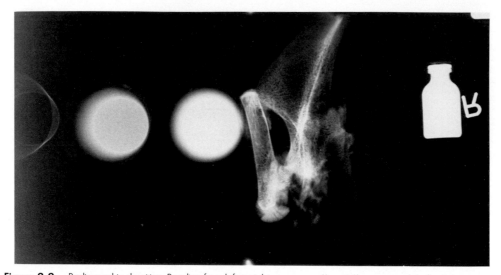

Figure 2-2. Radiographic densities. Reading from left to right, we see an "empty" paper cup (air density), a paper cup of salad oil (fat density), a paper cup of water (water density), a turkey bone (bone density), a small bottle of iodinated contrast material (iodine density), and a lead marker (heavy metal density).

Listed below are substances we may encounter on radiographs in order of their increasing ability to absorb radiation. The substances near the top of the list are referred to as radiolucent, while those near the bottom of the list are referred to as radioopaque (Fig. 2-2).

> Air
> Fat
> Water, (Blood, Muscle, Tendons, and Other Nonfatty Soft Tissues)
> Calcification and Bone
> Iodinated Contrast Materials
> Heavy Metal: (Barium, Lead, Iron, etc.)

It must be remembered that not only the nature of a substance but its thickness will affect its apparent radiographic density. An immense soft tissue mass may obscure a very thin metallic density. A high concentration of iodine may be more dense than bone, but a very low concentration of iodine in the renal pelvis may be less dense than bone. Therefore, we must consider both the physical properties of a material and its thickness.

In addition, as noted earlier, we must be aware of the differential absorptive abilities of the elements at different wavelengths of radiation. The spectrum of wavelengths is dependent upon the kV chosen by the technologist. While the interactions of kV range, film screen combinations, development time and temperature, and developer chemistries all contribute to the appearance of the film, they are beyond the scope of this volume and generally beyond the control of the nonradiologist.

OTHER IMAGING METHODS AND MODALITIES

BODY SECTION RADIOGRAPHY—TOMOGRAPHY

Conventional or noncomputerized (mechanical) body section radiography is also referred to as tomography or laminography. In its simplest form, linear body section radiography, we have the following elements: x-ray tube, patient, and film. With the patient lying motionless on the table, the x-ray tube moves in one direction while the film moves in the opposite direction at the same speed as if both were attached by a lever arm (Fig. 2-3). In the plane of the fulcrum of the lever arm, its axis of rotation, there is no blurring of the image, but in all other planes of the patient, there is blurring which increases as the distance of the plane from the fulcrum increases.

Thus, if we are interested in seeing a depressed fracture in the central portion of the medial tibial plateau, we can see it to greater advantage by blurring out the overlying and

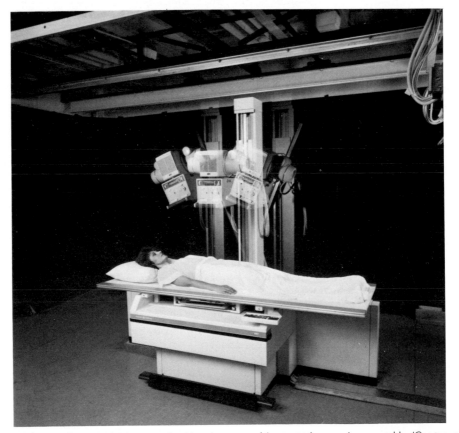

Figure 2-3.   Conventional linear tomography. Note the motion of the x-ray tube over the x-ray table. (Courtesy of General Electric Company, U.S.A.)

underlying bony structures. Similarly, we might see the radiolucent nidus in an area of bone sclerosis in an osteoid osteoma. This radiolucent nidus might otherwise be obscured by the overlying and underlying sclerotic bone on a conventional film without the aid of the tomography.

Through the years we have been able to get more efficient blurring with less streaking by substituting more complex motions, e.g., hypocycloidal motion, for the simple linear motion. With refinements in instrumentation, we can now precisely choose planes of sharp focus, and, by varying the arcs of motion, we can get planes of varying thickness appropriate to the diagnostic problem at hand.

It should be noted that conventional tomography can often answer a question as well as computed tomography (CT) at less than half the cost.

STEREOSCOPIC VIEWS

With all of the new modalities that have become popular in recent years, stereoscopic radiology has become far less utilized, but may again come into vogue because of its simplicity and cost effectiveness. Stereoscopic views are obtained in an ingenious, but straight-forward manner. The patient is first positioned in the usual manner for a conventional x-ray exposure, with the central ray centered over the center of the film at a 40-inch target distance. Before the exposure is made, the tube is moved two inches to the left of center and an exposure is then made from that vantage point. Then the film cassette is removed and a new cassette is placed in the precise position as the previous cassette, and the x-ray tube is moved 2 inches to the right of the center before the second exposure is made. The two films are then viewed with the aid of a stereoscopic viewer at a distance of 10 times the interpupillary distance, with the left eye viewing the left film and the right eye viewing the right film.

With just a little practice, one can "see" a single three-dimensional image which allows us to get a better feel for the interrelationships between the anatomical structures visualized. This is often very useful in gaining information otherwise available only with the aid of CT or a very great number of conventional oblique projections. There are some people who can cross their eyes at will and have no difficulty seeing stereoscopic images without the need of a stereoviewer. (Those of us who can neither cross our eyes nor wiggle our ears are often awed by the demonstrations.)

Stereoscopic shifts may be up-and-down or right-to-left, with one being somewhat more helpful than the other depending on the problem at hand. The use of stereoscopic views in learning radiographic anatomy is often of great value, since it allows the viewer to see the three-dimensional picture and gain a realistic concept of the anatomical relationships.

FLUOROSCOPY

Fluoroscopy provides us with the ability to watch dynamic processes such as respiration, heart beat, and peristalsis. Through the use of fluoroscopy we can observe contrast material as it passes along a sinus tract or moves about within a joint space. Further, we can follow the advancing position of a nasogastric tube or an opaque catheter within a vascular structure. Fluoroscopy allows us to position our patients more precisely to obtain the exact films we desire.

The radiation exposure for modern fluoroscopy is much less than that in past decades because of the electronic image intensifier tube. This tube enormously brightens the fluoroscopic image permitting good visualization without excessive radiation exposure. Nevertheless, the careful fluoroscopist will make every effort to minimize fluoroscopy time and thus minimize patient and personnel exposure. The image intensifier screen can be viewed directly by optical systems, but it is most often viewed by a high-resolution television camera and projected on a television monitor. Then the dynamic images can be recorded by a video recorder and studied in more detail at a later date.

In addition, the image screen can also be viewed by cinecamera with very rapid exposures to allow such things as slow motion study of swallows. Documentation of the fluoroscopic image can also be obtained with the 105mm roll film camera which can photograph the image intensifier screen, or by conventional x-ray cassette spot films that bypass the image intensifier tube.

While fluoroscopy is of great value in positioning for exposures and viewing "anatomy in action," we must not stare at the TV endlessly while action progresses and radiation exposure builds up. One can meditate over a conventional x-ray film for hours without increasing the radiation dosage to the patient, but every effort must be made to avoid permitting ourselves the dubious luxury of meditating with our foot on the fluoroscopy switch. With the exception of necessary dynamic studies, fluoroscopy can often be avoided. You can save your patient additional radiation and cost by judiciously choosing a few proper projections to tailor a nonfluoroscopic study to the patient's needs.

XERORADIOGRAPHY

Conventional radiography, like conventional photography, is a photochemical process with light producing a photochemical reaction that blackens the film. In the case of conventional radiography, the visible light is emitted from the intensifying screens and produces far more blackening than the amount caused by the direct action of the radiation on the silver compounds in the film emulsion.

Xeroradiography is based on a physicoelectrical process, specifically, an electrostatic process. The reusable Xerox plate consists of a thin selenium layer affixed to a rigid aluminum support. A uniform electrostatic charge is deposited on the plate, which is then automatically placed in a light-tight cassette shortly before the patient examination. The cassette is used as one would use a conventional x-ray cassette. An x-ray exposure is then made using appropriate exposure factors for the body part involved. The exposure factors are generally greater, i.e., require more radiation exposure than for a conventional radiograph of that body part. The peak sensitivity is in the 40 to 50kV range, which is lower than is usually used in conventional radiography.

During the time of the x-ray exposure, the plate is partially discharged according to the pattern of radiation reaching the plate after passing through the patient. This produces a latent image of varying amounts of static electricity distributed over the plate. The cassette is then returned to the Xeroradiographic processor and exposed to an atmosphere of air containing electrostatically charged particles of blue developer powder. The charged particles of blue powder are attracted to the surface of the selenium plate, turning the latent image into a real image in shades of blue. The powder is then transferred to a plastic-covered paper. The plastic is heated and the image is incorporated into the plastic.

Why bother? Why have a separate processor, separate cassette, and separate technique charts? Why accept the higher radiation dose? Why deal with nontransparent films that you read on a table and not on a view box? Why deal with the blue powder that rubs off films and gets on your fingers and your white coat? These questions are hotly argued, but there are some real advantages in selected situations.

The principal advantage of Xeroradiography is edge enhancement (Fig. 2-4). Distinct lines can be seen at transition zones between areas of different density. This is because at the zone of transition between a highly charged and a less charged area, the peak charge of the highly charged area accumulates near the edge of that area and then precipitously decreases. The powder distribution then follows the charge distribution and edges are accentuated in an almost unnatural, ultravivid fashion. The edge enhancement is reminiscent of the appearance of colored comic strips with the lines about the margins of all of the figures.

On the Xeroradiograph each edge is demarcated by a line of extra powder buildup adjacent to a white, almost powder-free zone. The prominence of the dark/light interface

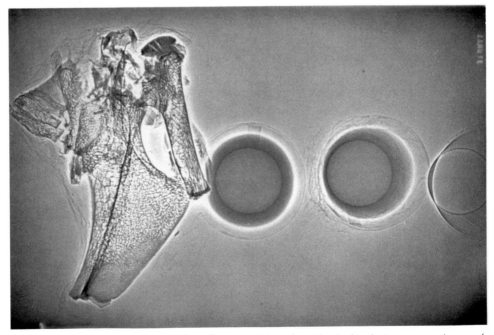

Figure 2-4.   Xeroradiograph. Note the edge enhancement. You can see the ultrathin plastic wrap over the cup of salad oil. The presence of this wrap was far less apparent in Figure 2-2 with a conventional radiograph of the same items. Compare the bony trabeculation in the xeroradiograph with that seen in Figure 2-2.

varies with the degree of dissimilarity of the radiographic density of the adjacent tissues. Because of this advantage there is unfortunately an accompanying disadvantage. A very fine structure lying close to one of these exaggerated interfaces, e.g., cortical bone vs. soft tissue, could be totally lost. This is referred to as "extinction phenomenon."

The use of Xeroradiography has waxed and waned. Xeromammography is quite common, despite the added radiation exposure because of the advantages of edge enhancement. Xeroradiography is useful in the musculoskeletal area because of the excellent visualization of soft tissue planes which might be disrupted by tumor, trauma, or infection. In addition, it is often of very great value in attempting to identify foreign bodies whose density may be very close to that of surrounding tissues, e.g., glass, splinters, etc. It is also felt by many to be valuable in demonstrating the soft tissues of the anterior cervical region. I would certainly advise consultation with the radiologist before requesting nonmammography Xeroradiographic studies so that a study tailored to the patients problem can be performed.

NONSCREEN FILM STUDIES

In some very limited situations, such as the visualization of foreign bodies in soft tissues, one may wish to use conventional x-ray film without intensifying screens to avoid the possible unsharpness or artifacts produced by the intensifying screens. In this case, the photochemical changes in the emulsion are produced only by the x-rays without the aid of light from the screens. This consequently requires a greater radiation exposure to the patient but may be of value in exceptional situations. This should be done only with prior consultation with a radiologist.

COMPUTED TOMOGRAPHY

Computed tomography (CT) is a marriage between an expensive, complicated x-ray machine and an expensive, complicated computer. This extremely complex union provides us with some relatively simple cross-sectional x-ray images of the human body which have had a dramatic effect on the practice of medicine. We have seen a decrease in hospital stays because of more rapid accurate diagnoses, and because of a decrease in otherwise unavoidable exploratory procedures. Radiologists who practiced before the days when CT's became commonplace never cease to be amazed at the clear-cut findings on CT which were only hinted at or not at all visible on conventional plain film studies.

The CT unit includes a special automated table for the patient to allow precise positioning to a fraction of a millimeter in both vertical and horizontal planes. The table is fitted into a gantry which surrounds the table and the area of interest in the patient. The gantry includes an x-ray tube to produce radiation and arrangements of x-ray detectors to quantitate the radiation that has passed through the patient. There is also the usual high voltage generating equipment, electronic connections between the detectors and the computer, and a viewing console with TV monitors and controls to position the patient, control the slice thickness, control the angle of plane of the slice, adjust the contrast, and generally control the multiple functions of the unit (Fig. 2-5A,B).

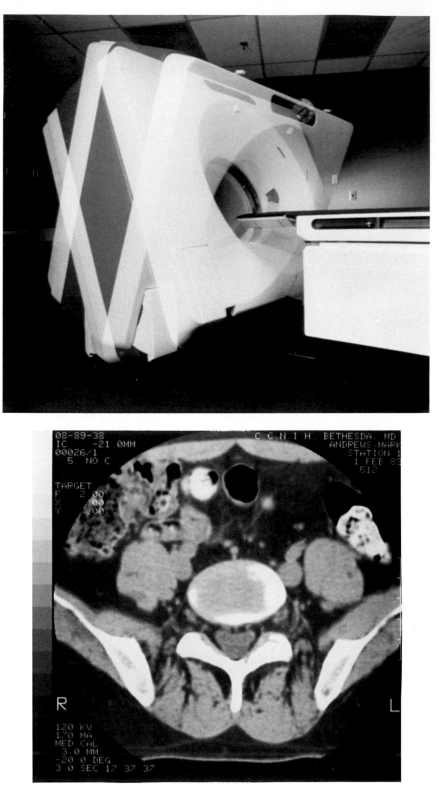

Figure 2-5. **A:** CT scanner with gantry at various tilt angles. **B:** CT scan of pelvis. (Courtesy of General Electric Company, U.S.A.)

After many highly collimated beams of radiation have passed through the area of interest at many different angles, the intensity of radiation sequentially perceived by the array of detectors is gathered and correlated by the computer to reconstruct the radiographic density of the structures in the plane of interest. The detectors are of varying design but generally have crystals such as calcium fluoride or sodium iodide which detect the radiation.

The more individual determinations made, the more precise the reconstruction can be, but the greater will be the patient exposure to radiation and the greater will be the acquisition time for the information. As acquisition time increases, the image is subjected to increasing degradation by such patient motion as respiration, heart beat, and peristalsis. In addition, we must consider the problem of voluntary patient motion. It is difficult to be perfectly still for prolonged periods, and this is even more of a problem in sick or disoriented patients.

Still another factor which must be considered is that the total examination time for any one patient decreases the availability of the CT scanner for use by other patients. Today in most institutions there are many patients who need CT studies, and efforts must be made to utilize such expensive equipment cost-effectively.

There are some terms in the jargon of CT to which you should be exposed. Every CT picture you look at is a matrix of dots of varying intensity. If the matrix measures 256 dots in each direction, there would be a total of 256^2 dots of varying intensity in a square field. Since circular fields are used, the number of dots is less (πr^2). Each dot is called a *pixel* or picture element and corresponds to a thin volume element or *voxel*. The Houndsfield or CT number (H) for specific tissues or for a group of pixels of interest is arrived at by the following equation:

$$H = 1000 \left(\frac{\text{Attenuation Coefficient of Tissue}}{\text{Attenuation Coefficient of Water}} - 1 \right)$$

By this formula, which you may now forget, the CT number for water is established at 0. Positive numbers denote an attenuation of radiation by the substance greater than the attenuation of radiation by water, and negative numbers denote an attenuation less than that of water. CT numbers will vary for the same substance at different kV levels. They will also vary because the spectrum of x-ray wave lengths from a beam of a specific kV will be altered as it passes through different tissues before it gets to and after it leaves the area of interest.

After the CT image is obtained, it may be altered as to contrast, and varying windows or narrow contrast bands may be studied. Let us assume that we are looking at a CT of the ankle. There will be some ranges of contrast which will best display variations in the cortical bone density, and other contrast ranges or "windows" which will allow us to see the soft tissue structures such as muscle bundles and tendons. One of the truly great advantages of CT is the ability to differentiate between densities which are similar but very slightly different.

After the optimal CT images are obtained on the monitor screen, they can be put on film by the mere press of a button to make the images available for easy viewing at a site distant from the scanner room. Thus, a permanent record or "hard copy" can be made from the stored electronic images.

With the aid of advanced computer technologies, it is also possible to reconstruct computerized images into planes other than those in which the information was acquired. This is only possible, however, if the information originally acquired was obtained in a format suitable for reconstruction. If you suspect that you may need a reconstructed image, be sure to consult with the radiologist in advance so that this can be planned for before the initial study is performed.

ULTRASOUND

If you have ever shouted and heard an echo you have already been exposed to the theory of ultrasound. The rest is a matter of technical refinements, imaging, and anatomical considerations.

Audible sound is generally in the range of 20 to 20,000 cycles per second. Since Hertz (Hz) equals 1 cycle per second, audible sound may be defined as 20 to 20,000Hz. 1KHz equals 1000Hz; 1MHz equals 1,000,000Hz. The frequencies used in most medical applications of ultrasound are generally in the range of 1 to 10MHz. The 2 and 3.5MHz ranges are most useful for the more common applications of ultrasound.

Sound travels through a substance as a mechanical disturbance in that substance in the form of a wave motion. The speed of sound through different substances is different depending on such factors as the elasticity and density of the medium. While sound travels in a straight line in a homogeneous medium, it is reflected and refracted (bent or deviated) when it reaches an interface separating two substances having different sonic properties.

GENERATION OF ULTRASOUND AND THE PIEZOELECTRIC EFFECT

Ultrasound waves are produced by the piezoelectric effect. There are crystals which can convert electrical energy to mechanical energy and mechanical energy to electrical energy. These piezoelectric crystals are called transducers. When an electric current is applied to the crystal, the crystal structure is deformed and the electrical impulse is converted to a mechanical impulse. By controlling the current, one can control the ultrasound waves emitted. Similarly, when the same transducer crystal is serving as a detector of sound waves, the ultrasound echoes reaching the crystal produce measurable electric current. When a current is applied to the transducer it will resonate at a frequency whose wavelength is equal to one-half of the thickness of the crystal.

In calculating the depth of tissue from which an echo originates, the computer must consider the time elapsed between the original signal emitted by the crystal and the arrival of the echo back at the crystal surface, as well as the speed of sound in the tissue of interest. A two-dimensional image can be produced through processing the angles and coordinates provided by the mechanical arm holding the transducer and assigning appropriate gray values to the returned ultrasound pulses (B-mode scanning). The information thus received can be displayed on a cathode ray tube (CRT) screen and can be displayed on a film for a permanent record. Many ultrasound systems consist of an array of transducers pulsing in a

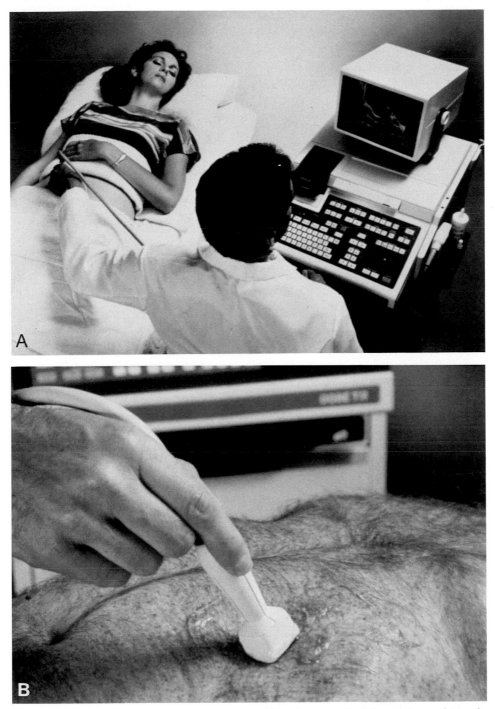

Figure 2-6. **A:** Patient undergoing ultrasound examination of the pelvic region. **B:** Abdominal ultrasound. Note the gel between the transducer and the skin. (Courtesy of General Electric Company, U.S.A.)

sequential manner, thus providing a dynamic image on the CRT screen. This realtime ultrasound is rapidly displacing the static images of the older B-mode scanners.

During the examination there is no discomfort for the patient and no risk has been demonstrated at the usual diagnostic power levels. In order to allow for transmission of the sound from the transducer to the patient's skin, a thin layer of oil is placed on the skin to provide a satisfactory coupling medium. It is important that this oil be maintained throughout the examination to avoid artifacts due to inadequate quantities of the coupling medium (Fig. 2-6A,B).

MAGNETIC RESONANCE IMAGING

Magnetic resonance imaging (MRI) is an exceedingly complex field. The physics involved would require a volume many times this size to explain. A knowledge of physics beyond that usually encountered among physicians would be necessary to fully understand it. This does not mean that a general qualitative, nonmathematical understanding cannot be rapidly acquired, permitting sufficient understanding to be comfortable with the anatomy as portrayed on the MRI studies and to be comfortable with the jargon of MRI. It is with this goal that we will procede.

Atomic nuclei with an odd number of protons and neutrons, such as hydrogen, have a property called spin. The nucleus spins on its axis like a child's top. Since the nuclei have a charge and are in motion they have a "magnetic moment"; that is, a vector force having a direction and strength or intensity. Thus, each spinning nucleus acts like a miniature bar magnet with a north and south pole. Under usual conditions there is a random orientation of the spins and, thus, the magnetic moments so that they all cancel each other out and there is no net measurable magnetic moment of the body. When the body is placed in a strong magnetic field, many of the previously randomly oriented spins tend to line up with the direction of the field of the strong magnet in either a parallel or antiparallel manner. Rather than precisely line up in the direction of the field, the spins, much like a wobbling top, tend to precess around the axis of the magnetic field. The protons (hydrogen ions) whose spins are parallel to the magnetic field are at a lower energy state than those that are antiparallel. The transition between energy states is referred to as *resonance*.

If, while many of the hydrogen nuclei are "lined up" with the strong external magnetic field, an appropriate radiofrequency field (RF) is applied at 90° to the direction of the magnetic field for an appropriate duration of time, the spins will be reoriented to 90° from their positions before the RF pulse. When the RF pulse is completed, the spins will gradually resume their prepulse positions. The combined magnetic moments of all of the protons which were altered by the RF pulse will cause an induced voltage in a receiver coil in a plane at 90° to the plane of the strong magnetic field.

As time passes, the magnitude of the magnetic moment in the transverse plane decays, and the amount of current induced in the coil decreases. This process is described as *free induction decay*. The time required to return to the equilibrium state with the external magnetic field after the RF pulse is turned off is called the *relaxation time*. The longitudinal relaxation time constant in the plane of the external magnet is termed T1. The time to reach magnetic equilibrium in the plane at $90°$ to the applied magnetic field is the transverse relaxation time constant, T2.

If appropriate RF pulses are used to excite hydrogen nuclei, then stronger signals will be received from those areas of the body where hydrogen is in greater concentration and lesser signals from those areas in the body where there is less available hydrogen. In order to image a volume of interest, it would be necessary to localize the source of the signals received. This is done by imposing a small linear gradient on the external magnetic field, so that the resonance frequency of the signal coming from each region would be slightly different.

These frequencies are all superimposed and are received from differently placed coils. All the data are readily sorted out by a mathematical process called *Fourier transformation*. The Fourier transformation process performed by the computer sorts the frequencies and their amplitudes to provide a picture which is bright in proportion to the available hydrogen ions at each location. While this is complex, it is the least we should expect for the million dollars we have spent for the machine.

SPIN-LATTICE RELAXATION TIME, T1

In actual practice, instead of using a single RF pulse and awaiting the complete relaxation following the pulse, a series of closely spaced pulses are used. If the pulse interval is very short with respect to relatively long T1, the signal returning to the coil will be very significantly diminished; but if the T1 is short, the signal will not be significantly diminished by the short pulse interval. An example is the contrast between brain and cerebrospinal fluid. Cerebrospinal fluid (CSF) has a longer relaxation time (T1) than the soft tissue of the brain. Thus, as the RF pulse repetition time is shortened, the signal from the CSF will diminish more rapidly than the signal from the brain, so that the CSF will appear more black (low signal) than the soft tissue which will appear lighter (high signal).

The above example is just one way that factors may be altered to change the apparent contrast between anatomical structures which may be only slightly different in actual proton density. Through such mechanisms as inversion recovery, utilizing a sequence of a $180°$ pulse following a $90°$ pulse, and choosing various pulse intervals, still other apparent contrast alterations may be effected.

SPIN-ECHO IMAGES

Still another approach is to evaluate the T2 (transverse relaxation times) of the tissues in the area of interest. This can be done by the use of a $90°$ pulse in the transverse plane followed by a $180°$ pulse in the same transverse plane to compensate for the partial dephasing of the magnetization. This method is called *spin-echo*. When evaluating T2 transverse recovery times by spin-echo, the signals from a substance with a short T2 will be more attenuated than the signals from a substance with a long T2. Since the T2 of CSF is longer than the T2 of brain, CSF will appear to have a stronger (whiter) image than brain which, having a weaker signal, will appear more gray on the picture. Note that with this method of imaging, the CSF/brain contrast is the *reverse* of that described with T1 imaging.

In general, small molecules, such as unbound water, have long T1 and T2 times, and large complex molecules and protein-bound water have shorter relaxation times.

I would not be surprised if you got lost somewhere in the last few pages. It is enough to understand that by varying the RF pulse sequences, the operator of the MRI device can significantly alter the apparent contrast of adjacent tissues and alter black and white values. By the time this book goes to print, it is hoped that new sequences will be developed which will supplement and perhaps replace those in current use. We are at the very frontier of a new imaging technique which should provide progressively improved ways to characterize tissue by its magnetic properties.

FLOW PHENOMENA

Because of flow phenomena, one can visualize vessels with surprising clarity. Let us assume that at the time of the first RF pulse, the blood in the aorta in the plane of interest is excited by the pulse. By the time the return signal is being detected from that plane of interest, the excited blood has moved on down the aorta and is no longer in that plane. It should be possible to devise signal sequences to evaluate the rate of flow with considerable accuracy.

By now I am sure you are anxious to visit the nearest MRI unit and see it in action. By all

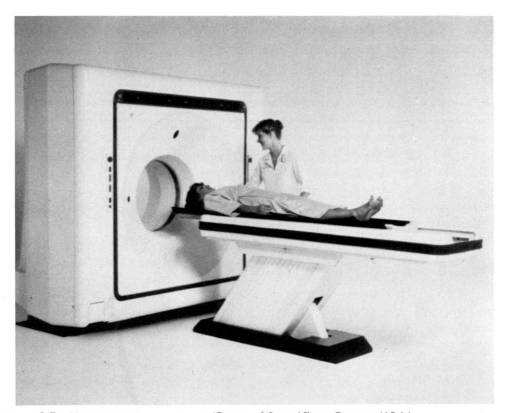

Figure 2-7.   Magnetic resonance imaging unit. (Courtesy of General Electric Company, U.S.A.)

means, do, but please leave your credit cards and all other magnetic material at home since they may be wiped out if you get too close to the magnet (Fig. 2-7).

THERMOGRAPHY

In learning the rudiments of physical diagnosis, we have all assessed the circulation to the lower extremities by touching the surface of the feet to note if they are unduly cold or to note if there is a significant difference between the right and left foot. We have all assessed the temperature of the skin over an area of suspected underlying infection in order to add one more parameter to our evaluation. Thus, we have all been using primitive thermography as have generations of physicians before us.

LIQUID CRYSTAL THERMOGRAPHY

Liquid crystals are substances which appear to change color with changes in temperature. If such crystals are incorporated in a flexible plate which can be closely approximated to a body surface, a pattern of color is seen which corresponds to the surface temperature of the skin, assuming that the surface temperature is not significantly altered by the pressure of the plate.

INFRARED THERMOGRAPHY

Infrared thermography is far more convenient to use than the liquid crystal method noted above. An infrared thermography unit collects heat radiated from a defined area of skin surface and focuses it on detectors of various design which convert the infrared radiation into electric impulses that are proportional to heat emitted from the skin.

Whatever technology is used by various manufacturers, the image, basically a surface temperature map of the skin, is generally displayed on a TV image tube with various colors representing various temperature ranges, or the image may be displayed in various intensities of black and white. The final image can be photographed for a permanent record (Fig. 2-8).

Thermography requires a cool, draft-free, constant temperature environment. The patient, after disrobing, should lie quietly for about 15 minutes to adjust to the room temperature. The skin must be clean and free from cosmetics, creams, perspiration, etc.

While thermography is not new, modern scientific advances have allowed more accurate mapping of skin temperature with varying degrees of accuracy and with displays of varying degrees of elegance. Without a doubt, there are some areas where thermography has its place. Unfortunately, there are many who have been swept up by the attractive technology and oversold the usefulness of the method. In some cases, utilizing thermography to obtain information which may not be valuable, or which may duplicate information from other studies, has tended to tarnish those areas of thermography which could be useful in making or confirming diagnoses.

It is the impression of many that thermography appears to be more useful in determining the extent of known disease and following its course than in discovering unknown disease in a

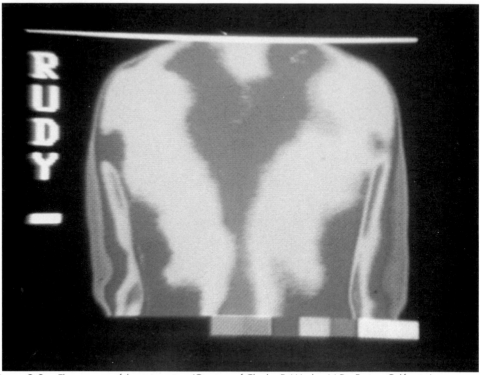

Figure 2-8.   Thermogram of thoracic region. (Courtesy of Charles E. Wexler, M.D., Encino, California.)

definitive manner. While attempts have been made to detect breast cancer with thermography, there have been too many false positives and false negatives to make thermography a really dependable diagnostic study for this purpose.

NUCLEAR MEDICINE IMAGING

After the administration of the appropriate radionuclide for the planned examination and the elapse of the appropriate amount of time for the nuclide to reach the area to be imaged, the patient is examined by an imaging device. The images record activity from the side of the patient facing the detector. Thus, both anterior and posterior views may be obtained, and both right and left lateral views may be required.

SCANNERS

Linear scanners are composed of a scintillation detector protected by a collimator and connected to a photomultiplier tube. When gamma rays from the patient reach the scintillation crystal, light is emitted from the crystal and detected and amplified by the photomultiplier tube. The electrical impulses from the tube are then recorded as dots on paper or on transparent x-ray film. The scanner mechanically moves back and forth across that portion of the patient being imaged until a finished map of radiation density is obtained.

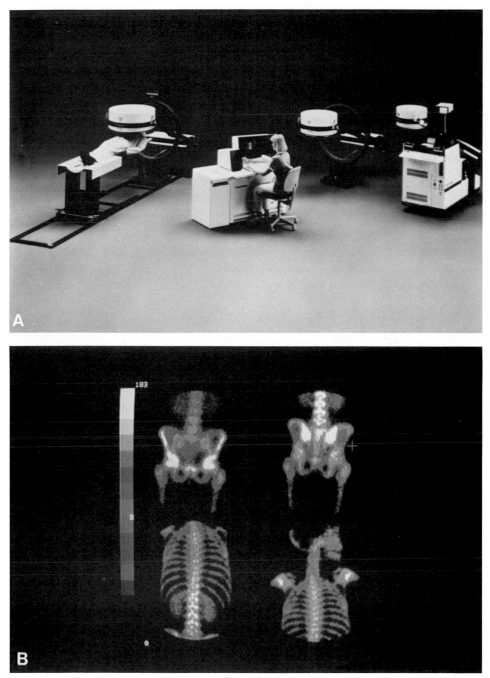

Figure 2-9. **A:** Modern gamma camera. **B:** Image from a gamma camera displayed in color. Note the color scale adjacent to the image. (Courtesy of General Electric Company, U.S.A.)

GAMMA CAMERAS

A gamma camera is a fixed radiation detector which does not mechanically "scan" the patient (Fig. 2-9A). The detector, which is protected by a collimator, is a very large scintillation crystal which "sees" the whole field of interest. The crystal is connected to photomultiplier tubes, and the image may be displayed on a TV screen and may be photographed for a hard copy permanent record (Fig. 2-9B).

SUBTRACTION TECHNIQUES

In order to better visualize the distribution of injected contrast material, subtraction techniques may be utilized. First, an initial plain film of the area of interest is obtained. Then, the contrast material is introduced. Next, a new film is obtained with precisely identical positioning without moving the x-ray tube or the patient and without changing the position of the x-ray cassette.

An intermediate film which is a positive or reversed image of the initial film is then exposed in the darkroom. This film, called the mask, is black where the initial film was white, and white where the initial film was black. The mask film is then carefully superimposed on the contrast film and the combination copied. The result is that almost all that is the same on the initial film and on the contrast film is subtracted or cancelled out, leaving only the things that are different between the two films, namely the injected contrast material (Fig. 2-10).

DIGITAL RADIOGRAPHY

Digital radiography is a means of acquiring, storing, and manipulating images electronically. The information is stored not in an analog fashion with a smooth response as we expect from the minute hand on a clock, but in the form of fixed numerical values as numbers change on a digital watch. Once the numbers are recorded, they are less susceptible to degradation by electronic noise than with analog storage. Because of the speed with which digital images can be manipulated, very small contrast differences can be accentuated by electronic digital subtraction. While there is some loss of spatial resolution, the increased brightness or contrast resolution permits visualizing iodinated contrast material in relatively dilute concentration in the aorta, carotid arteries, femoral arteries, or pulmonary vasculature after an injection through a catheter placed in the vena cava, rather than an intraarterial injection (Fig. 2-11).

QUANTITATIVE CT

Quantitative CT is used to determine the amount of calcium in spongy bone without the necessity of an invasive biopsy. The patient is placed in a conventional CT unit with a patented phantom placed beneath the patient's back. This phantom contains solutions of known density including ethanol, glycerol, water, and dipotassium hydrogen phosphate. Slices of known thickness are taken through predetermined areas in the upper lumbar

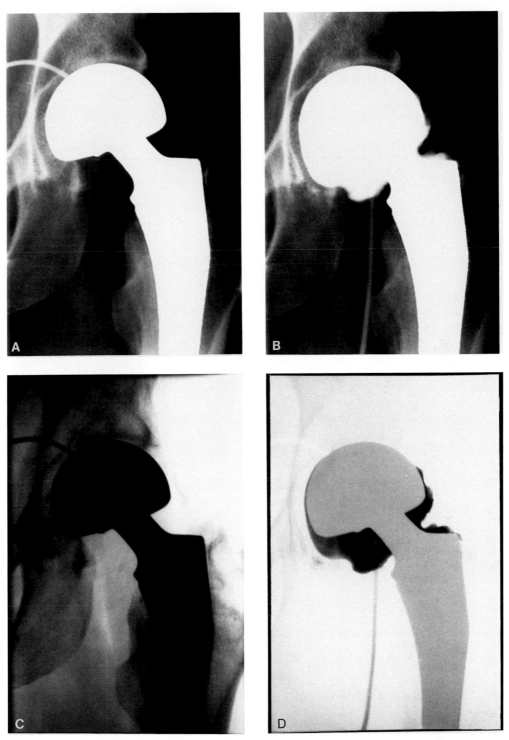

Figure 2-10. **A:** Hip arthrogram. Preliminary film after needle placement but before the introduction of contrast material. **B:** Film exposed immediately after the introduction of contrast material. **C:** Reversal film made from film shown in Figure 2-10A. **D:** Subtracted image film demonstrating the injected contrast material. Do you see a problem?

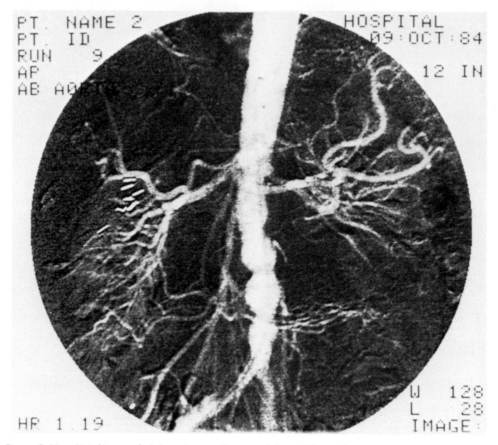

Figure 2-11. Digital image of abdominal aorta. (Courtesy of General Electric Company, U.S.A.)

vertebral bodies. These areas are chosen not to include cortical bone. The volumes of the samples are calculated and their average radiographic density compared with the recordings made of the density of the various parts of the phantom described above (Fig. 2-12). The recordings are made at the time of each exposure so that they are relatively independent of the possible drift of the machine between exposures. A patented software package permits rapid calculation of the calcium content per cubic centimeter of spongy bone.

Figure 2-12. **A:** Preliminary lateral film of spine with cursors demonstrating planes of interest through the vertebral bodies. **B:** Cross-sectional image through the patient and phantom at the levels shown in Figure 2-13A demonstrating the known densities in the phantom and the density of the selected volume of trabecular bone in the vertebral bodies imaged. (Courtesy of Image Analysis, Inc.)

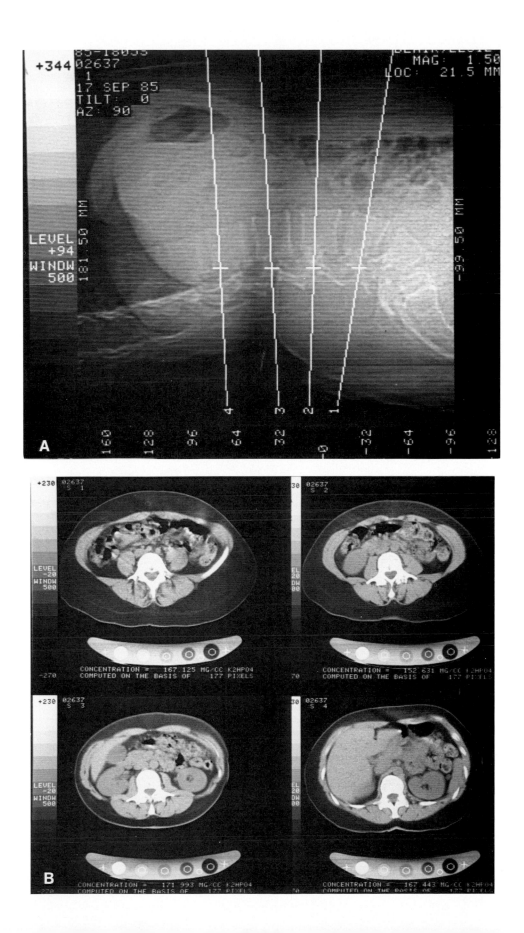

POSITIONING FOR THE NONRADIOLOGIST
SPECIAL CONSIDERATIONS, SPECIFIC EXAMPLES, AND PITFALLS

Eugene R. Jacobs

There are many standard texts devoted entirely to x-ray positioning. Some are directed almost completely to the x-ray technologist and deal with the most minute details of positioning for routine and more obscure x-ray projections. These are excellent reference books which can be used to learn how to do an uncommon projection which may be unfamiliar to the average diagnostic technologist. These reference books also include examples of how the radiograph for every particular projection should look and often have comments as to the specific advantages of the particular special view. These books are generally available at every x-ray department library and it is not intended to duplicate them here. It is advised that you browse through some of them to become aware of their scope so you can use them as a reference when needed.

There are also many books on x-ray positioning for the radiologist. These usually include a more superficial explanation as to how patients are positioned, and generally include radiographs and labeled anatomic diagrams.

I strongly recommend reading one of these because, under the guise of positioning books, they painlessly and interestingly teach the reader the anatomy which is basic to the understanding of radiology. Further, they serve as excellent reference books to identify the various bumps, grooves, and dimples which may puzzle even the more experienced x-ray viewer.

PROJECTIONS HAVE NAMES

Projections have names which are sometimes very revealing and essentially describe the basic facts defining the projection, as in the case of left lateral view of the skull. Projections also may have people's names, as Ferguson view or Waters projection. In the case of such projections, the names may refer to the person who devised them or popularized them. The "proper names" may not be universally accepted at different institutions or in different geographical areas. Occasionally, different names may connote minor variations of the same basic view.

Superimposed on all of the above are the names of views which are institution-specific. If Dr. Barebones is Chief of Orthopedics at University General Hospital and has a pet view to demonstrate the sesamoids plantar to the first metatarsal, he will order it frequently and specifically. Soon, it will be known at University General Hospital as the Barebones view. Residents, interns, and students trained at UGH will be surprised at the blank expressions they receive from technologists and others when they request Barebones views at a hospital in another city. Newcomers to UGH who are perfectly competent to order and interpret a sesamoid view may seem dull if they have to ask, "What is a Barebones view?"

UNDERSTANDING NAMES OF PROJECTIONS

Following is a list of some rules which should be helpful in understanding names of projections:

A. Rules are not always followed.

B. Projections are often named by the direction the central ray travels through the patient's body on its way to the film.

   1. *PA Chest: Posteroanterior View of the Chest.* The patient's anterior chest wall is near the film and the patient's back faces the x-ray tube. Thus, the heart is not as magnified as in the AP view of the chest.

   2. *AP Chest: Anteroposterior View of the Chest.* The patient's back is close to the film and the patient faces the x-ray tube. Thus, the heart, being farther from the film, is magnified more than in the PA.

   3. *Dorsal-Plantar View of the Foot.* The plantar surface of the foot faces the film and the dorsum of the foot faces the x-ray tube. (This is often called an AP view of the foot. While this is technically erroneous, it is fully accepted nomenclature.)

   4. *PA of the Hand.* The palm of the hand is on the film cassette and the dorsum of the hand faces the x-ray tube.

   5. *AP of the Hand.* This theoretically means the dorsum of the hand is flat on the film cassette with the palm facing up toward the x-ray tube. This can be done, but in actual practice it is ignored, and when an AP of the hand is ordered, it is done as a PA. Hardly anyone knows; hardly anyone cares; and no one complains. Most patients find the PA projection, or more properly, the dorsal-palmar projection, far more comfortable and natural than an AP view.

6. *AP of the Forearms.* This must be done as a true AP. The volar surface is up, facing the x-ray tube, and the posterior surface is facing the film cassette. If attempted with the radius rotated, a film is produced which is very difficult to interpret since the radius and ulna appear to cross each other.

C. Projections are also named by the part of the patient closest to the film.

1. *Left Lateral of the Skull.* The left ear is near the film and the right ear faces the x-ray tube.

2. *Left Posterior Oblique.* The left posterior part of the area in question is closest to the film. This terminology is generally used with chest, abdomen, or spine films.

3. *Left Anterior Oblique.* The left anterior part of the body is closest to the film. This terminology is generally used with chest, abdomen, or spine films.

D. Extremity films are also named by the direction of motion of the extremity with respect to the classically accepted anatomical position of the body.

1. *Internal Rotation Oblique.* For hips, knees, and ankles, the patient is lying on his back with the toes turned part-way toward the midline of the body. The lateral malleolus, the head of the fibula, and the greater trochanter all move away from the film.

2. *External Rotation Oblique.* For hips, knees, and ankles, the toes point out part-way laterally, so that the medial malleolus, the medial femoral condyle, and the lesser trochanter move away from the film.

   See Figure 3-1 (A – D) for these views of the ankle. Please note that while lower extremity examples are given, the same sort of considerations apply to the upper extremities.

E. Views are also named according to the direction in which the body parts are bending away from the classically accepted anatomical position.

1. *Erect Right Lateral Bending View of the Lumbar Spine.* The patient is standing in an AP position and bending the torso to the right. This view would usually be accompanied by a left lateral bending view to complete the picture.

2. *Flexion View of the Cervical Spine.* The patient is in a lateral position with the head tilted forward. This is usually accompanied by a companion view, the extension lateral, with the head tilted back.

3. *Ulnar Deviation View of the Wrist.* The patient's wrist is in a PA projection with the hand pointed to the ulnar side. This may be contrasted with a radial deviation view of the wrist.

4. *Flexion and Extension Lateral Views.* Flexion and extension lateral views of the wrist should be apparent as are dorsiflexion (toes up) and plantar flexion (toes down) lateral views of the foot and ankle.

5. *Adduction and Abduction Views.* Adduction and abduction views of shoulders and hips should be apparent.

F. Views are sometimes defined by the angle made by the central ray when the central ray is not perpendicular to the film. These may be described in such terms as 30-degree uptilt, 30-degree cephalically, or 30-, 45-, and

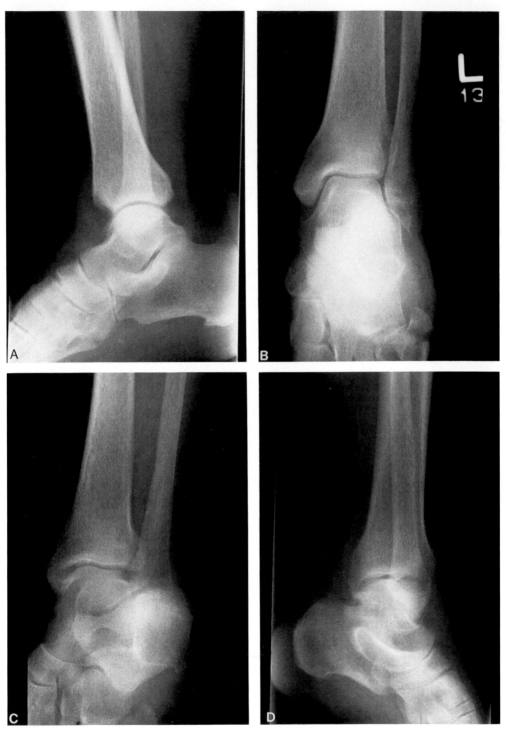

Figure 3-1. In the following views of the ankle, note the way the fibula changes position with respect to the tibia between internal and external rotation. Note also that while the malleoli are intact, there is a fracture of the proximal tip of the fifth metatarsal. **A:** Lateral view of the ankle. **B:** AP view of the ankle. **C:** Internal rotation oblique view of the ankle. **D:** External rotation oblique view of the ankle.

3 2

60-degree views of the patella, or perhaps as tangential views of a bump on the head.

G. Stress views are made with mechanical stress applied in an attempt to determine if there is abnormal laxity of a joint. Examples include inversion and eversion stress applied to the ankle and weight-bearing views of the acromioclavicular joints.

A more subtle type of stress view is the standing view or weight-bearing view of the knee. This can be very deceptive if not properly done. There is a real difference between standing on one foot and bearing weight, and standing seemingly on both feet, but bearing weight only on the right side, while radiographing the painful left side. It is vitally important that weight-bearing views really be weight-bearing.

IDENTIFICATION MARKERS

Identification markers may be found near a corner of the radiograph and should state the institution or office where the film was exposed. The patient's name should be clearly visible as well as the examination date. The markers also frequently include patient identification numbers and date of birth and/or age. An erudite interpretation of the wrong patient's films or the right patient's films taken on the wrong date is of no value and can lead to very serious error. Always check the marker.

Since x-ray films are transparent, one can read the marker from either side of the film. On one side the printing will read like the printing on this page, while on the other side the printing will look like a mirror image. In some x-ray departments, identification markers will be "right-reading," so that if you look at the side of the film which faced the x-ray tube during the exposure (called the tube side of the film), you can readily read the identification markers. In other departments you will see the mirror image printing on the tube side of the film, and the easily read regular printing on the opposite side of the film.

Once you learn the local ground rules, you are ready to solve positioning problems through some simple reasoning. Let us say the problem is an unmarked, or possibly incorrectly marked, posteroanterior view of the hand. If you know that in your x-ray department you can read the identification rectangle on the tube side of the film, then put up the film so that the label is easily read, and if the thumb points to your left as you read the film, it is a right hand. Fit your own right hand over the picture and you can see that this is correct.

Let us now assume that you know that the films in your particular department are flashed so that the printing is a mirror image on the tube side of the film. You can now take a dorsal-plantar view of the foot (often called an AP of the foot) and put that film up so that the identification label appears as a mirror image rather than as normal printing. If the big toe lies on your right, and the small toe lies on your left as you view the film, you are viewing a left foot.

If you don't know how the films are marked at a particular institution, you can ask the local radiologist or work backward from films you know are correctly marked or from known films such as an erect PA chest. (The chances of situs inversus are small but that possibility cannot be entirely excluded.) Please note that the entire identification marker problem as discussed above does not apply to pasted on identification labels which are only as reliable as the person who pasted them on. Serious medical decisions should not be based solely on pasted-on labels.

CHAPTER 4

COSTS OF IMAGING PROCEDURES

Eugene R. Jacobs

Costs of imaging procedures may be defined from many standpoints. We may simply look at the price of the procedure. The price may include a *surgical component*, as in the case of the lumbar puncture required to do a myelogram. The *professional component* is the radiologist's fee for interpretation of the imaging study. The *technical component* is the cost of performing the technical procedure. The technical component includes the costs of operating the building, paying for the equipment and supplies, and the salaries of technologists, file clerks, receptionists, and others necessary to the function of an imaging department.

Costs must also be evaluated in the light of how much the patient's length of hospital stay will be increased or decreased by the imaging study. We must also consider whether we may be avoiding a costly and perhaps dangerous surgical exploration. Costs must also be evaluated on the basis of patient discomfort and risk, including the risk of a contrast reaction and the radiation burden of the examination. Compare an oral cholecystogram with an ultrasound study of the gallbladder! Or compare a CT scan of the chest with a lung biopsy! Have *you* had a barium enema lately?

It is unfortunate that many medical students and young physicians who frequently order imaging studies seem to be very insulated from the costs of the various alternatives available to them. Costs are different in various settings: urban or rural, university hospitals, small community hospitals, or private offices. Costs vary with inflation and with the effect of government control. Costs may vary from East to Midwest to West and from North to South. They frequently vary from 19th Street to 22nd Street to 23rd Street.

With the aid of a Medicare intermediary,[1] I have obtained a list of selected imaging studies

---

[1] The information for Medicare selected prevailing profiles for surgery, professional component fees, and technical component fees were obtained on written request for the purpose of this book from Pennsylvania Blue Shield for the District of Columbia Metropolitan Area, dated June 25, 1985. (Report No. CPRP9300-003 Run date 06/25/85) Sample total prevailing costs.

TABLE 4-1. MEDICARE SELECTED PREVAILING FEE PROFILES (1985)

EXAMINATION	TOTAL COST*
Skull	$ 86.00
Cervical Spine — 2 views	80.00
Cervical Spine — 4 views	95.00
Thoracic Spine — 2 views	60.00
Lumbosacral Spine — 2 views	82.00
Lumbosacral Spine — 5 views	87.00
Chest — 1 view	34.00
Chest — 2 views	49.00
Pelvis — 1 view	56.00
Hip — 2 views — unilateral	58.00
Hip — 2 views — bilateral	86.00
Knee — 2 views	51.00
Knee — 4 views	74.00
Ankle — 2 views	44.00
Ankle — 4 views	62.00
Foot — 2 views	47.00
Foot — 3 views	55.00
Shoulder — 2 or more views	39.00
Elbow — 3 or more views	58.00
Wrist — 3 or more views	62.00
Hand — 3 views	57.00
Abdomen — 1 view	45.00
Abdomen — complete	77.00
CT Head — without contrast material	375.00
CT Head — with contrast material	385.00
CT Head — with and without contrast material	528.00
CT Chest — with contrast material	575.00
CT Abdomen — with contrast material	575.00
CT Extremity — without contrast material	402.00
Lumbar Myelogram	372.00
Arthrogram — Shoulder	270.00
Arthrogram — Knee	263.00
Upper GI Series	138.00
Upper GI Series — with air contrast	210.00
Upper GI Series and Small Bowel Follow-Through	237.00
Small Bowel Study Alone	97.00
Barium Enema — air contrast	169.00

* Total cost including professional component, technical component, and (where appropriate) surgical component

TABLE 4-1. *(Continued)*

EXAMINATION	TOTAL COST*
Oral Cholecystogram	88.00
Ultrasound Examination of the Gallbladder	208.00
Intravenous Pyelogram	167.00
Intravenous Pyelogram with Drip Infusion and Nephrotomography	205.00
Abdominal Aortography	495.00
Bilateral Carotid Arteriograms	1103.00
Venography of Extremity	162.00
Mammography — bilateral	110.00
Tomography (Conventional Noncomputer Assisted)	148.00
Ultrasound of Pelvis — Realtime	193.00
Nuclear Medicine — thyroid imaging	146.00
Nuclear Medicine — liver imaging	225.00
Nuclear Medicine — brain imaging	251.00
Nuclear Medicine — bone imaging	305.00

* Total cost including professional component, technical component, and (where appropriate) surgical component

and the prevailing fee paid for the surgical, professional, and technical components in a large East Coast metropolitan area at the end of July 1985. The components obtained were totaled and fractional dollars rounded out for the following sample procedures. The dollar values listed are the total costs of all components. Although there do seem to be some inconsistencies, there has been very little change in these payments since that time.

CASE STUDIES

CASE 1

Matthew Mason is 94 years old, has had two major myocardial infarctions, and has been in and out of cardiac failure. He has a well-established diagnosis of inoperable bronchogenic carcinoma and he has several areas of known metastasis. There are days when he is quite lucid and fairly comfortable and there are days when he is quite disoriented.

For reasons that are not entirely clear, someone ordered a stool guaiac and this was reported as mildly positive. He currently does not have any complaints referrable to his gastrointestinal tract and would not be considered a candidate for a surgical procedure because of his cardiac status. Does he need a plain film of the abdomen, an abdominal ultrasound study, a colonoscopy, or a barium enema as the initial procedure of choice?

Though neither the plain film of the abdomen nor the abdominal ultrasound are very unpleasant from the standpoint of the patient, it is exceedingly unlikely that either will explain the positive guaiac. It is further exceedingly unlikely that either of these examinations will provide information which will alter Mr. Mason's therapy or clinical course. While it is possible that either or both the barium enema and colonoscopy might explain the positive stool guaiac, both procedures are, to say the least, very unpleasant and debilitating. It is unlikely that any of the examinations will enhance the quality of Mr. Mason's remaining life.

CASE 2

Mary Carpenter is a 64-year-old female, whose pneumonia has been followed with a portable chest x-ray every other day. On Tuesday she is going down to the x-ray department for an intravenous pyelogram. Wouldn't it be worthwhile substituting a chest x-ray in the x-ray department for the portable examination scheduled that day? Mary would get a better study in the department and be saved a fee for a portable examination.

CASE 3

Harry Walters is a 45-year-old male who appears to have some problem related to his elbow. At this time, we do not know precisely what the nature of that problem is. It is assumed that the person requesting the imaging examination has a valid reason for requesting the elbow study and some expectation as to the nature of pertinent information which may be gleaned from the examination.

Unfortunately, the person requesting the examination sometimes assumes that the reason for the study and the pertinent history will be magically transmitted to the radiologist charged with the interpretation of the examination. This information is important to the radiologist; as an accurate diagnosis can be compromised if vital information is omitted. No rational person can philosophically deny the logic that good medicine requires an informed radiologist.

A recent x-ray consult form read "x-ray right elbow — impotence work-up." I hesitate to comment further on this issue or make any provocative conjectures. The elbow fortunately had an entirely normal radiographic appearance and there was no further clinical follow-up as to the precise reason for the examination.

CASE 4

Charles Baker has been having complaints that suggest the need for an intravenous pyelogram. In reviewing his history, we find that he had an intravenous pyelogram at Elsewhere Community Clinic last month. It is acknowledged that the studies at Our Place General are more elegant than Elsewhere, but is it worth the added risk of a contrast reaction, added radiation exposure, added cost, and added discomfort to the patient to repeat the study rather than send for the old films?

CURRENT FISCAL CONSIDERATIONS

As scientists, we are trained to learn all there is to know about how the body works. In the past, we were taught to spare no expense to that end. With the expansion of the horizons of knowledge and the expansion of expensive technology, the scope of what we can know and what we can do is fantastic. If there were no fiscal constraints, the costs could bankrupt society. Finding appropriate priorities is a very difficult bioethical and political question, well beyond the scope of this book.

At the very least, we should avoid duplication of procedures and we should avoid procedures whose yield is unlikely to influence the course of treatment, improve the quality of life, or alter the final outcome.

CHAPTER 5

MUSCULOSKELETAL RADIOLOGY

Eugene R. Jacobs

AN APPROACH TO MUSCULOSKELETAL RADIOLOGY

After thoroughly studying a radiograph and noting all of the pertinent "negative" findings, one must look for certain clues or "positive" findings. Having found one or more clues, we try to integrate them with each other and with the information from the patient's history we have already brought to the examination in order to find a solution. It is unfortunate that most textbooks, in describing a disease, will tell the reader what clues are frequently associated with this disease process, but very rarely do these texts explain what these clues look like.

Frequently, the coexistence of several clues with a particular patient history will neatly "wrap up" the diagnosis. But first, we must recognize the clues. In the first part of this chapter we will demonstrate some of the more common clues and their appearance will be discussed. After you have learned to recognize these clues, you will be given an opportunity to look at radiographs and relate these clues to specific disease processes. It is hoped that you will be able to build on the information you have seen and, much like a detective, be able to add together the history, the facts, and the clues to come up with a solution or diagnosis.

ALTERATIONS IN THE APPEARANCE OF BONE

Despite the complexity of interpretation of musculoskeletal radiographs, bone is really limited in the manner in which it can alter its roentgen appearance. The radiographs are two-dimensional representations of three-dimensional structures in various shades of black

41

and white. The *more* calcium present, the *whiter* that part of the radiograph. The *less* calcium present, the *blacker* that part of the radiograph. While it is an oversimplification, we can remember that more bone equals white, still more bone equals whiter, less bone equals gray, and still less bone equals black. The clues that follow will amplify the above statement.

The following tables list some of the more common clues which you will encounter in musculoskeletal radiology. Listed along with each clue are examples of conditions where the clue may be evident. This is not to be considered an encyclopedic list, but rather a beginning to provide you with a rough matrix on which to hang further information as you learn. Consider this a bookcase with labeled shelves and examples which you can, through the years, fill out and rearrange. The illustrations that follow this list should serve to translate the word images into more meaningful real images. After reviewing the lists, compare the clues with the illustrations that follow.

TABLE 5-1. DECREASED BONE DENSITY

CLUES	EXAMPLES
Osteopenia (diminished bone density—diminished bone)	Osteoporosis (decrease in osteoid formation)
	Senile
	Endocrine
	Osteomalacia (decreased mineralization of the osteoid)
	Nutritional
	Endocrine
	Renal, etc.
Regional decrease in bone density	Hyperemia
	Disuse atrophy
	Reflex sympathetic dystrophy (spotty demineralization)
Local diffuse demineralization	Early osteomyelitis
	Hyperemic change
	Early metastatic lesions
	Early primary bone tumor
Localized loss of bone—permeative pattern	Round cell tumors
	Primary matrix-producing tumors
	Secondary malignancies (metastases)
	Osteomyelitis
Localized loss of bone with sharply defined margins	Fresh surgical lesions
	Histiocytosis
	Gout (punched-out overhanging edges)
	Myeloma

TABLE 5-1. (Continued)

CLUES	EXAMPLES
Lucent lesion with fine sclerotic margin	Benign cortical defect
	Bone cysts
	Healed bone graft donor site
Lucent lesion with cortical thinning	Fibroxanthoma
	Chondromyxoidfibroma
Lucent lesion with cortical expansion (Please note: The cortex does *not* expand; it is destroyed on the inside and rebuilt on the outside in a constant process that gives the impression of expansion, but it is really a process of inner destruction and outer rebuilding.)	Giant cell tumor
	Unicameral bone cyst
	brown tumor
Lucent lesion with cortical breakthrough (pathologic fracture)	Aggressive benign tumor
	Malignant tumor
	Infection
Lucent defect with thick sclerotic margin. (The sclerotic margin may predominate.)	Osteoid osteoma
	Old chronic, low-grade infection

TABLE 5-2. INCREASED BONE DENSITY

CLUES	EXAMPLES
Widespread increased bone density	Osteopetrosis
	Myelosclerosis
	Fluorosis
	Hypervitaminosis (A & D)
Scattered areas of spotty increased density	Bone infarct
	Chondroma with calcified matrix
	Multiple osteoblastic metastases
Very local increase in bone density	Bone islands (one or more)
Nonlucent lesion simulating lucent lesion	Fibrous dysplasia
Areas of mixed increase and decrease in density	Paget's disease
	Metastases
	Chronic osteomyelitis
	Old trauma
Bony callous formation	Postfracture healing
	Posttraumatic soft tissue ossification
Tumor bone (malignant tumor cells producing bone)	Osteosarcoma

TABLE 5-3. MISCELLANEOUS BONE FINDINGS

CLUES	EXAMPLES
Degenerative cysts	Osteoarthritis
	Posttraumatic degenerative arthritis
Erosion	Rheumatoid arthritis
	Seronegative spondylarthropathy
	Pigmented villonodular synovitis
Periosteal reaction	Trauma
	Infection
	Neoplasm
	Venous insufficiency

TABLE 5-4. MISCELLANEOUS CARTILAGE FINDINGS

CLUES	EXAMPLES
Chondrocalcinosis (cartilage calcification)	Calcium pyrophosphate dihydrate deposition disease (CPPD)
	Hemochromatosis
	Hyperparathyroidism
	Asymptomatic aged individuals
Joint space narrowing (cartilage destruction)	Degenerative arthritis
	Rheumatoid arthritis
	Acute or old septic arthritis

TABLE 5-5. SOFT TISSUE CHANGES

CLUES	EXAMPLES
Soft tissue calcification	Myositis ossificans
	Injection granuloma
Soft tissue swelling	Well-defined soft tissue swelling (lipoma)
	Posttraumatic swelling (edema, hematoma)

TABLE 5-6. POSTTRAUMATIC BONE CHANGES

CLUES	EXAMPLES
Posttraumatic changes	Linear fracture
	Buckle fracture
	Impacted fracture
	Stress fracture

At this point, compare the illustrations #1 through #19 with the text material so far presented in Chapter 5, including the tables listing clues and examples. Many of the clues will be further amplified in the legends accompanying the illustrations.

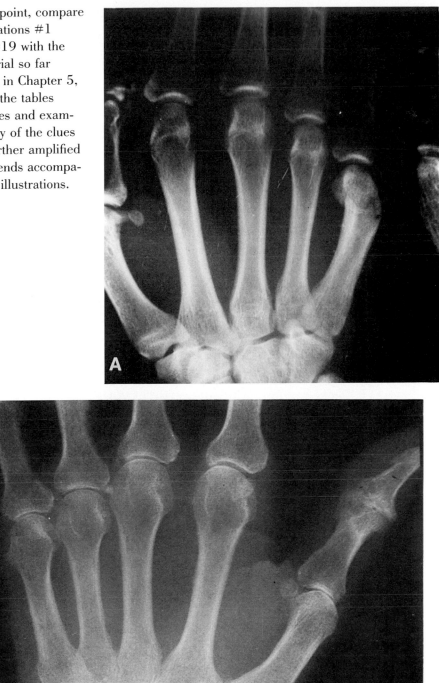

Figure 5-1. **A:** Normally mineralized bone. Note the normal thickness of the cortex and normal appearing medullary cavity in the midshaft region of the second metacarpal. Incidental note is made of a recent fracture of the extreme distal shaft region of the fifth metacarpal, with some lateral angulation of the distal end of the distal fragment with respect to the proximal fragment. **B:** Osteoporosis. Contrast the ratio of cortex to medullary cavity in the midshaft of the second metacarpal with that seen in normal bone in Figure 5-1A.

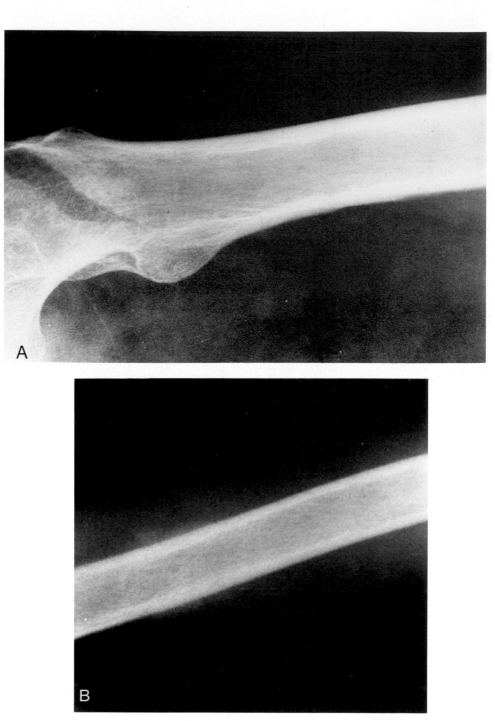

Figure 5-2. **A:** Normal bony architecture in a long bone which incidentally has a recent fracture. Note the sharply outlined cortical margins and the delicate trabecular pattern, without evidence of interruptions in the pattern except at the fracture site. **B:** Long bone demonstrating periosteal new bone formation and a permeative lesion disturbing the trabecular pattern with very fine areas of radiolucency scattered through the area of involvement. This patient happens to have leukemia. However, there could be many other clinical reasons for periosteal reaction and for a permeative-appearing lesion. Contrast this with the appearance of a normal long bone in Figure 5-2A.

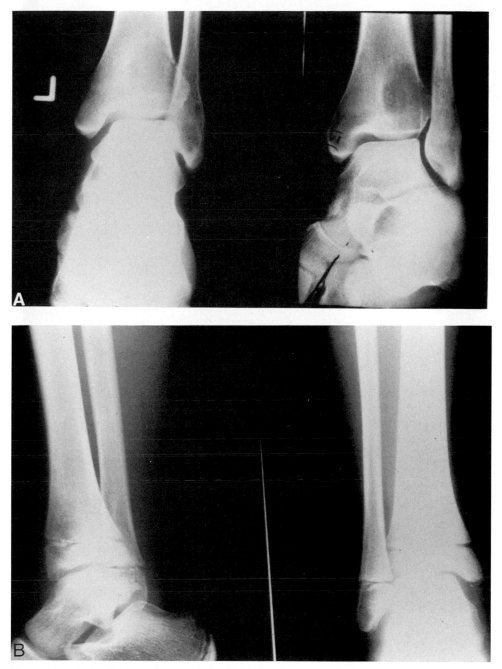

Figure 5-3. **A:** Localized loss of bone with sharply demarcated margins but little, if any, surrounding reactive bone. Note the very well-defined lesion in the distal lateral portion of the tibia, extending down to the region of the distal articular surface. This lesion is a giant cell tumor. **B:** Local diffuse loss of bone. Note the ill-defined localized area of decreased bony density in the anterior portion of the distal metaphyseal region of the tibia. It is difficult to draw a definite line at the edge of the area of bone loss; rather, there is a gradual fall-off between the area of lucency and the area of normal bone. This particular lesion represents osteomyelitis. Contrast this local diffuse loss of bone with the local sharply defined lesion seen in Figure 5-3A.

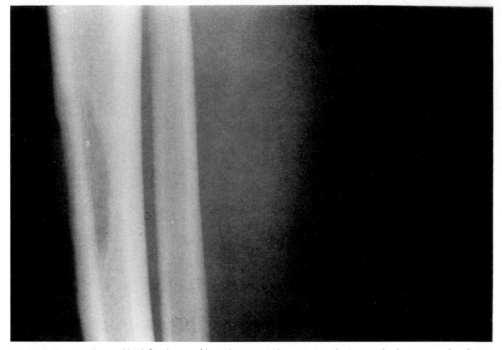

Figure 5-4.   Local smoothly defined area of bone loss. Note the very smooth corticated edges surrounding the area of radiolucency in the anterior portion of the tibial shaft. The lesion seen is a healed surgical defect, in this case, a bone graft donor site. The smooth margins of the defect resemble the smooth margins along the edges of normal bone.

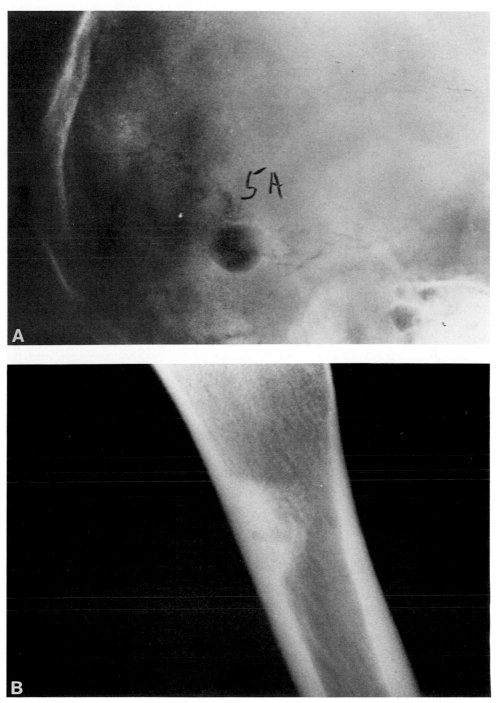

Figure 5-5. **A:** Localized bone loss with a fine sclerotic margin. Note that surrounding the area of lucency there is a very fine white rim which clearly separates the lucent area from the surrounding normal bone. The lesion seen here is an epidermoid inclusion cyst of the calvarium. **B:** This is a radiolucent area surrounded by a very thick sclerotic margin. When we first see the lesion, our eye is caught by the thick sclerotic margin. However, as we study it closely, there is a tiny radiolucent nidus seen in the central portion of the area of sclerosis. This lesion is an osteoid osteoma. The thick sclerotic area represents host reaction to the underlying radiolucent lesion.

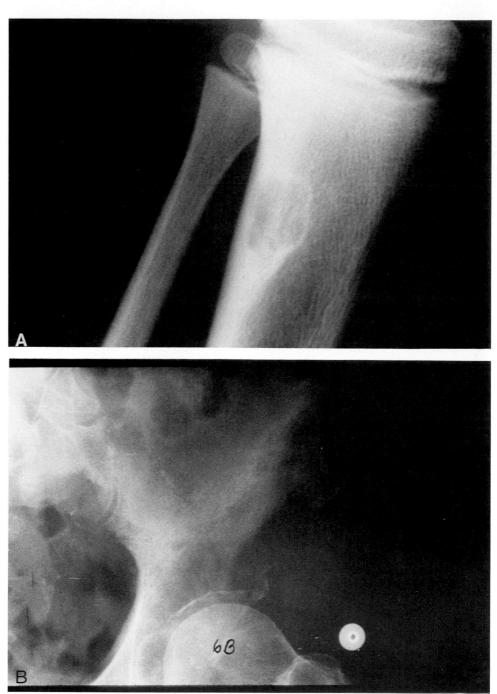

Figure 5-6. **A:** Cortical thinning without expansion. If we study the lucent lesion in the posterior portion of the proximal metaphyseal region of the tibia near its junction with the tibial shaft, we can see that there is slight narrowing of the posterior cortex in the region of the upper portion of the radiolucent lesion. While there is cortical narrowing, there is no evidence of breakthrough or "expansion" of the cortex. This lesion is a large benign cortical defect. **B:** Cortical breakthrough. There is a radiolucent lesion lying in the left ilium just above the acetabular joint. The lesion has thinned the usually dense thick cortex of the acetabular roof and appears to imperceptibly blend with the normal ilium medial and superior to it. Further, it has broken out through the lateral cortex of the ilium into the adjacent soft tissues. This is an excellent example of cortical breakthrough by a very aggressive lesion which, in this case, represents a metastatic malignancy. Contrast this breakthrough with the mere cortical thinning seen in Figure 5-6A.

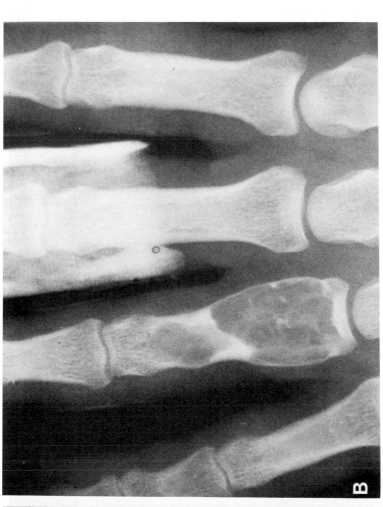

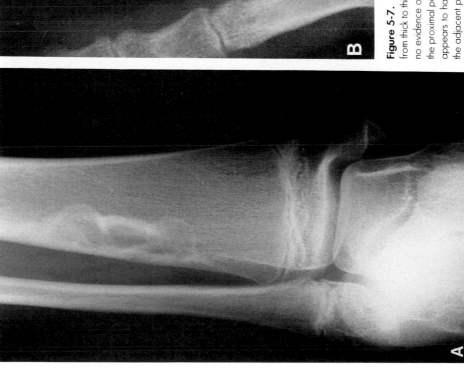

Figure 5-7. **A:** No significant cortical expansion. Here we see a radiolucent lesion with a sclerotic margin that varies from thick to thin. It appears to very slightly thin the lateral cortex of the distal tibia. There is no significant expansion and no evidence of breakthrough. This represents a benign lesion, a fibroxanthoma. **B:** Cortical expansion. If we observe the proximal portion of the proximal phalanx of the left ring finger, we can see that there is a radiolucent lesion which appears to have "expanded" the medial and lateral cortex of the proximal phalanx so that it is no longer shaped like the adjacent phalanges, but is convex where it was previously concave. It has not only thinned the cortex, but it has changed the apparent contour of the cortex. Note also that within this rather well-defined lucent lesion, there are some very faint white spots. These white spots represent small areas of calcified cartilage. The lesion is benign; it is an enchondroma. This is a very classical appearance of an enchondroma in a phalanx. Contrast this with Figure 5-7A.

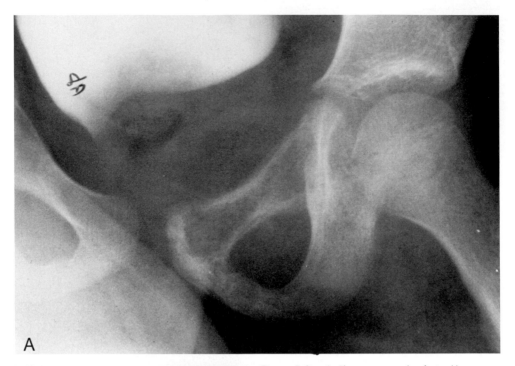

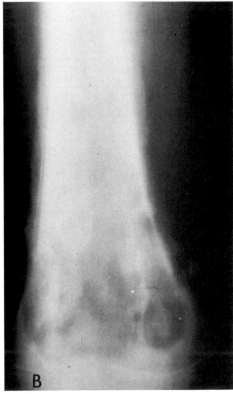

Figure 5-8. **A:** This is an example of mixed bone destruction and bone production. If we direct our attention to the left pubic bone and superior pubic ramus, we can see that there is a considerable amount of bone destruction with increased lucency. There is also some evidence of new bone production about the periphery of this region, with what appears to be periosteal new bone seen along the edges of the pubic ramus, both superiorly and inferiorly. In addition, we can see that the contrast-filled bladder is deformed and displaced by a soft tissue mass, presumably associated with this lesion. This particular lesion represents a Ewing's sarcoma in this 6-year-old child. It is exceedingly difficult, from the roentgen appearance alone, to completely exclude the possibility that this could represent an area of osteomyelitis. **B:** Mixed lucency and sclerosis. This is a tomogram of a distal femur. There are areas of fairly well-defined lucency and areas of less well-defined lucency, as well as evidence of old irregular periosteal thickening. This patient had a long history of chronic osteomyelitis. In the face of this much chronic change, it is exceedingly difficult to definitely rule in or rule out the possibility of current activity. Contrast this with Figure 5-8A. It is very difficult in many cases to distinguish between osteomyelitis and malignant neoplasia.

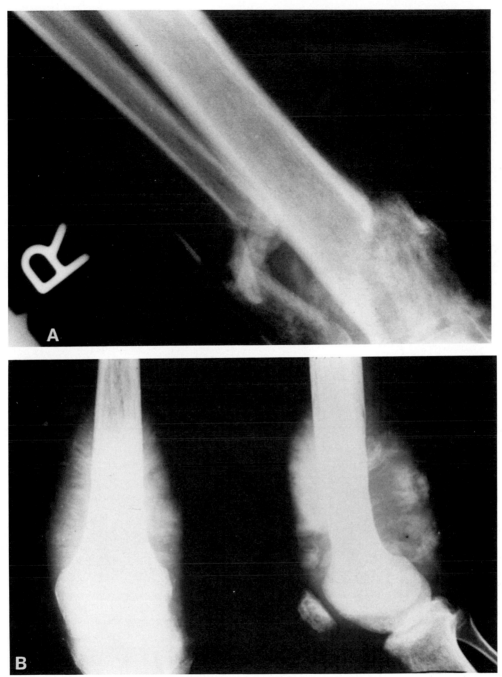

Figure 5-9. **A:** Bone callus. This illustrates a healing comminuted fracture of the distal tibia and fibula. Note the ill-defined new bone produced as part of the healing process. The new bone is not as well organized as mature bone and has many characteristics suggestive of an aggressive lesion. This is not only the case on radiographs, but would be the case on histologic examination. **B:** Tumor bone. This illustration shows an anterior and lateral view of the distal femur. One can see the classic sunburst appearance of new bone production by this osteoblastic osteosarcoma. Contrast this with Figure 5-9A.

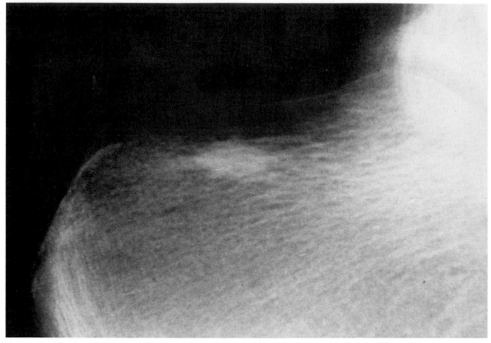

Figure 5-10. Localized area of increased bone density. Observe the magnified view of the upper margin of the posterior portion of the os calcis. Here we can see a localized area of normal-appearing bone of increased density. This represents a bone island. It is of no real clinical importance. It may occur in any bone and merely represents a localized area of compact bone in an area where one would not usually expect to find compact bone.

Figure 5-11. **A:** Generalized increased bone density. Note the stark white appearance of the bones, resembling ivory. There is a loss of delineation of the medullary cavity, so that the bones look almost uniformly white. This represents osteopetrosis. This is very different from the white bones of an underexposed film where one can still see the normal ratio of medullary cavity to cortex. **B:** Generalized decrease in bone density. In this patient, we can see that not only is there a loss of bone density with thinning of the cortices, but there is also destruction of the bone in the region of the shafts of the distal phalanges. There is destruction of the midshaft region of the distal phalanx of each index finger and in the midshaft region of the distal phalanx of each thumb. Note also how the distal phalanges of the fifth fingers, particularly on the right, tend to appear to be sharpened, coming to a point distally. Further, if we examine the middle phalanx of each index finger, it can be seen that the cortical margins laterally (on the thumb side) appear very fuzzy due to active osteoclastic activity. This is an example of renal osteodystrophy. Can you find similar changes elsewhere on these films which are perhaps less dramatic than those described, but similar in nature? Contrast the appearance of these demineralized hands with Figure 5-11A.

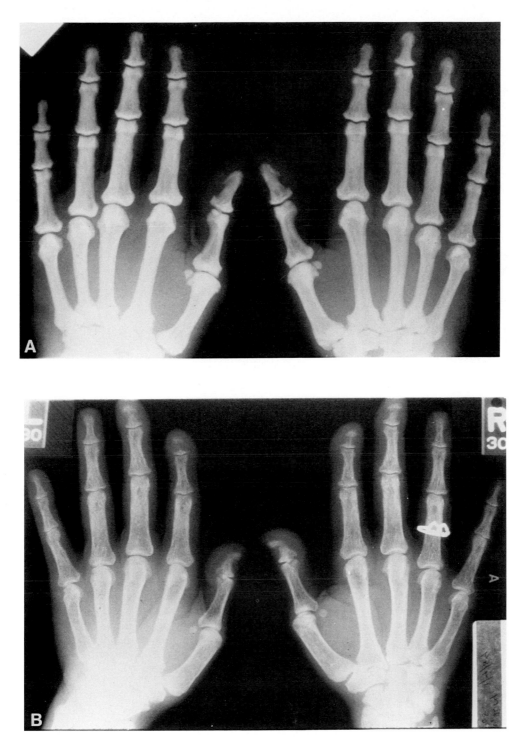

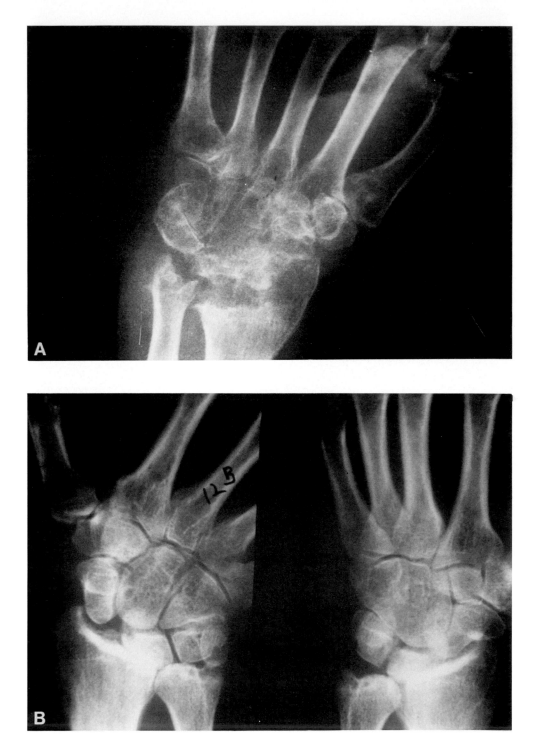

Figure 5-12.   A: Erosion. In the region about the styloid process of the ulna, note how the styloid process appears to be eroded with loss of its cortex and loss of its normal boundaries. It has a "chewed-up" appearance. Note also the region of the inferior radioulnar junction where we can see erosions on both sides of the joint, with bone destruction producing varying degrees of sharpness of the margins of destruction. This is a classical appearance of erosions in the ulnar styloid region. Note also the soft tissue swelling about the distal ulna, the narrowing and destruction of the radiocarpal joint, the marked narrowing and destruction of many of the intercarpal joints, and the destruction of much of the navicular and lunate. Note also the juxtaarticular distribution of demineralization in the visualized bony structures. This is a patient with rheumatoid arthritis. **B:** Degenerative cysts. In studying the region of the styloid process of the ulna, it can be seen that the outer margins and contours of this process are reasonably preserved. There are radiolucent cystic lesions with fine to thick sclerotic margins that are very well defined from the surrounding normal bone. These lucent lesions with sclerotic margins represent degenerative cysts. This patient has osteoarthritis. Note the narrowing of the radiocarpal joint between the radius and the lunate. Incidentally, note also the widening of the space between the scaphoid and the lunate. One would certainly suspect that this patient may have a torn scapholunate ligament. Note also the degenerative cyst in the proximal lateral portion of the capitate. It is a lucent area with a fine sclerotic margin. These are classic degenerative cysts. Contrast them with the erosions noted in Figure 5-12A.

←——

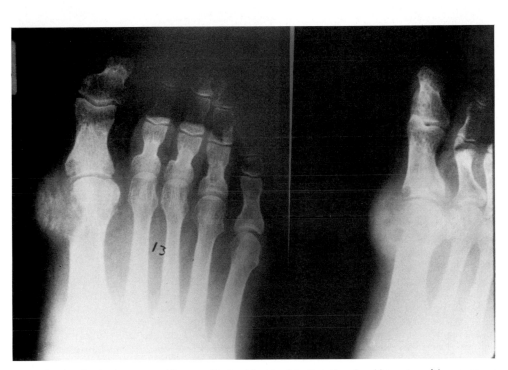

Figure 5-13. Punched-out areas of lucency. On the right side of the illustration, the oblique view of the great toe, in the region of the medial portion of the proximal phalanx, just immediately distal to the first metatarsal-phalangeal joint, one can see a very sharply defined, punched-out area of radiolucency. In addition to having a punched-out appearance, it is noted to have an undercut appearance, as though there were a small entry-way made and then a larger excavation so that we see undercutting of the edges. This patient's bones are *normally* mineralized. There is an adjacent punched-out lesion of the distal medial portion of the first metatarsal. Note the soft tissue swelling and the increased density of the soft tissue, caused by the deposition of calcium urate. This is a classic appearance of gout. Please note that the most common x-ray findings in early gout are entirely normal x-rays or possibly some minimal swelling of the soft tissues without bony changes. Incidentally, have you wondered why the proximal phalanges of the second and third toes look so short? This foreshortening is due to hyperextension of the toes with respect to their metatarsals.

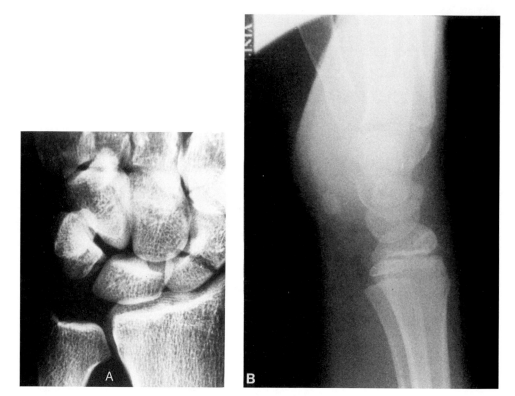

Figure 5-14.   A: Linear fracture through the waist of the carpal navicular. Note that the bony margins along the radiolucent fracture line are not corticated the way the other edges of the bone are corticated. Rather, we are looking at a raw sharp broken edge, similar to what would be seen if one broke a leg of a piece of furniture, revealing the jagged splintered edges of the broken wood as contrasted with the well-finished surfaces in other areas. **B:** Buckle fractures. Buckle fractures occur in children whose bones are still somewhat malleable, being not as brittle as the bones of an adult. Rather than seeing a radiolucent fracture line, one can see a buckle similar to the type of deformity one would see in a dented fender. At the posterior margin of the distal metaphyseal region of the radius, there is a small bump extending posteriorly where there would normally be a slight degree of concavity as can be seen on the volar surface of the radius. The posterior bump represents a buckling of the bone secondary to a mechanical stress. Note the soft tissue swelling about the region of the fracture site. These fractures are hard to see unless one is familiar with the normal anatomy of the part. They are certainly less obvious than the fracture seen in Figure 5-14A.

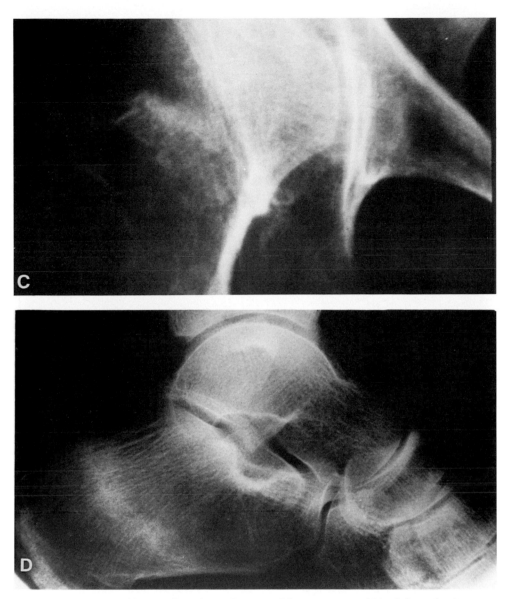

Figure 5-14. **C:** Impacted fracture. If we observe the region of the upper portion of the right femoral neck, we can see the changes associated with impacted fractures. Instead of there being a radiolucent fracture line, there has been a telescoping of the bone into itself, so that in one area there is twice as much bone as there would normally be, since two segments of the bone are now essentially occupying the same space. Therefore, instead of the lucent line, we see a zone of increased bone density representing the impacted bone. The bone density extends from the lateral portion of the femoral neck obliquely, inferiorly, and medially. Further, it can be seen that there is minimal offset of both the medial cortical margin and the lateral cortical margin in approximately the same plane as the area of increased bone density. This is the classic appearance of an impacted fracture of the femoral neck. **D:** Stress fracture. In this lateral view of the os calcis, there is a clearly seen, though ill-defined, zone of increased density at about the junction between the posterior one-third and the anterior two-thirds of the os calcis, extending in a plane parallel with the normally dense posterior margin of the os calcis. This represents a healing stress fracture. A stress fracture may not be seen at the time of the patient's initial complaints; however, as healing progresses, the area of increased bone density becomes more apparent. Long before the healing is radiographically apparent, the stress fracture can be diagnosed by nuclear medicine studies. Contrast the stress fracture with the impacted fracture in Figure 5-14C, and note that in the case of the stress fracture, there does not have to be any deformity of the bony contours. No "offsets" of the cortical margins are necessarily seen, though there may be some alteration of the bony contour on the basis of periosteal new bone.

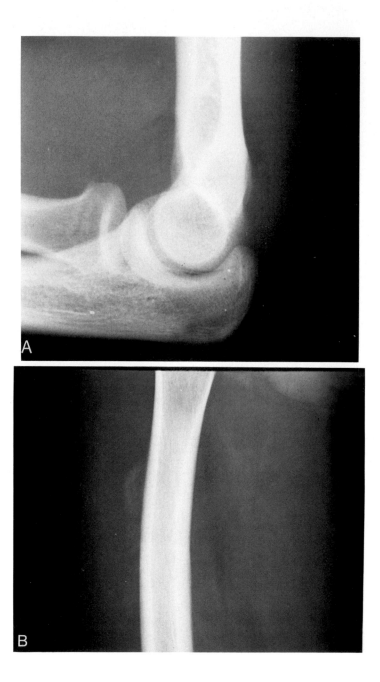

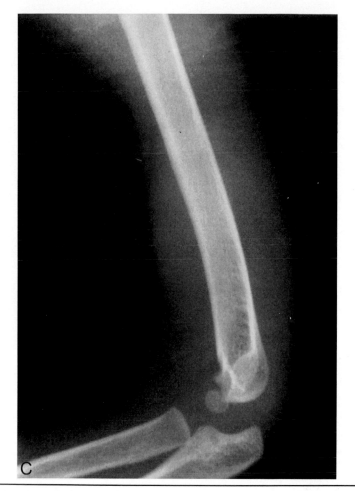

Figure 5-15. **A:** Posterior displacement of the posterior fat pad of the distal humerus. In the normal anatomy of the region of the olecranon fossa on the posterior margin of the distal humerus, there is a fat pad which lies within the olecranon fossa. It is usually not seen on a normal lateral view of the elbow because the surrounding bone making up the walls of the fossa obscures the fat pad within it. If, however, there is either bleeding into the joint capsule or effusion into the joint capsule, then the expanding joint capsule will displace the fat pad posteriorly beyond the bony margins, so that it can be readily visualized as the fat contrasts with the slightly more dense water densities of soft tissues. When we see a displaced fat pad, we must strongly suspect the possibility of bleeding into the joint capsule caused by an occult fracture. Frequently, this is an occult fracture of the radial head or neck which will bleed into the capsule and produce the changes noted. Even if the fracture is not readily seen, one should treat such a patient as having a possible fracture and obtain follow-up films if clinical symptoms persist. Note that there is also some anterior displacement of the anterior fat pad; however, this is a much less reliable sign. **B:** Posttraumatic soft tissue calcification. Observe the region just lateral (to your left) to the upper portion of the femoral shaft. This calcification appeared approximately 10 to 12 days after the patient sustained blunt trauma to this region. This is an example of posttraumatic heterotopic bone formation. **C:** This is an example of artifactual soft tissue swelling and soft tissue constriction. This patient sustained a minor injury to the elbow region, and the radiograph reveals what appears to be some constriction of the soft tissues in the upper humeral shaft region and some slight swelling of the soft tissues in the lower humeral shaft region. The swelling is not due to the patient's injury. The technician, instead of removing the patient's shirt, pulled the elasticized sleeve up from the wrist to the upper arm region where it was very tight and constricted the tissues. Since the tissues were constricted above, they tended to bunch up below. One must always be cautious not to see abnormalities where there are none, and one must always caution technicians not to pull up sleeves or trousers and produce spurious areas of soft tissue swelling. A similar problem can be produced by pulling tight jeans above the knee so that there appears to be suprapatellar soft tissue swelling. We are fortunate here that we can see the area of constriction. Sometimes the area of constriction is not on the film, and all we can see is the area of pseudo-swelling.

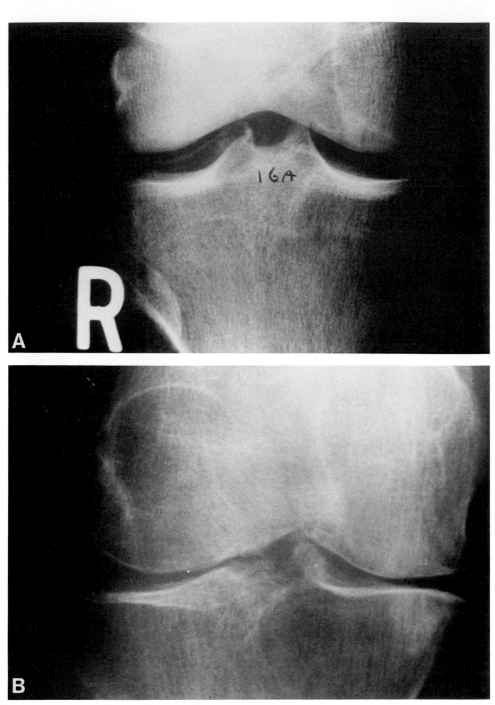

Figure 5-16. **A:** Cartilage calcification. In this close-up view of the knee joint, there is evidence of some sharpening or roughening of the margins of the tibial spines, but there is no evidence of significant narrowing of either the medial or lateral compartment. It can be seen, however, that there is some faint calcification of the surface of the articular cartilage which is here best seen in the region of the lateral compartment. This is an example of chondrocalcinosis, which is merely an expression of the presence of calcification in cartilage; it is not an etiologic diagnosis, as there are many causes for chondrocalcinosis. **B:** Joint space narrowing. In this patient there is moderate to marked narrowing of the joint cartilage spaces, both in the medial compartment and, to a slightly lesser extent in the lateral compartment. Contrast this joint space narrowing with the normal-width joint spaces seen in Figure 5-16A. Narrowing of the joint space is really an abbreviation for the concept of destruction of the joint cartilage which composes the joint *cartilage* space.

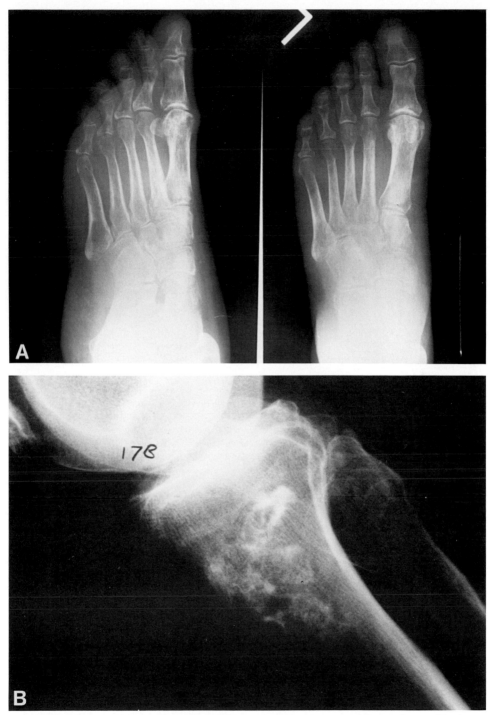

Figure 5-17. **A:** Spotty decreased bone density. There are multiple spotty areas of demineralization diffusely distributed over a region involving many individual bones in the distal tarsal region, the metatarsal region, and the region of the toes. This type of spotty demineralization frequently has a neurovascular cause and can be described as reflex sympathetic dystrophy. Another term for this same condition is Sudeck's atrophy. It generally occurs following a relatively minor trauma. There is a disproportionate amount of pain for the amount of trauma, it persists for a disproportionately long time considering the extent of the trauma, and it is frequently associated with shiny red skin in the overlying area. **B:** Spotty increased density in a localized area. The presence of spotty increased density within the medullary cavity of the bone in a localized area suggests either an old, healed, calcified bone infarct or an old, calcified, "burnt-out" enchondroma. The differential diagnosis between these two is often very difficult. Fortunately, neither require specific care. The details of the differentiation are unfortunately sometimes controversial.

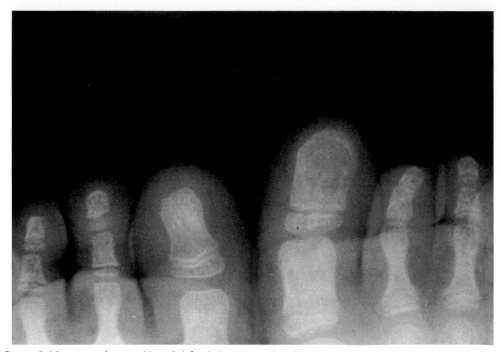

Figure 5-18.   Area of reasonably well-defined alteration in trabecular pattern without true alteration in bone density. Contrast the appearance of the distal phalanx of the left great toe with the right great toe. If you look at the normal left great toe, you can see a normal pattern of trabeculation throughout the medullary cavity of the distal phalanx; while on the right, there is a large central area where there is a loss of trabecular architecture and a more ground-glass appearance, yet the actual degree of density on the white/black scale is not significantly different from the normal left side. The area of homogeneity without true mature trabeculation is variously well-defined and less well-defined from the surrounding normal bone. It has obviously caused an alteration in the size and contour of the bone, and it is not as black as a truly lucent lesion. This represents fibrous dysplasia. The bone involved is fiber bone and does not have the maturity of fully developed bone, as seen on the contralateral side.

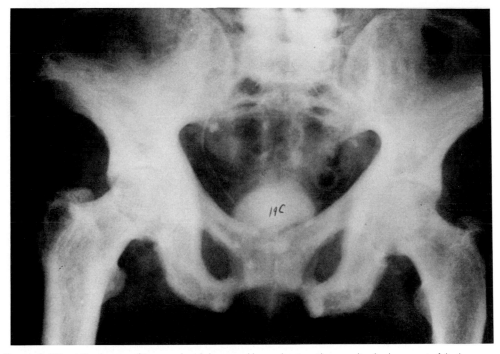

Figure 5-19. Mixed areas of increased and decreased bone density with generalized enlargement of the bony structures involved. As we view this particular radiograph, we can see that there is contrast material in the ureters and bladder from a recent intravenous pyelogram. The bony structures are enlarged as we may best appreciate by looking at the obturator foramina which appear smaller than usual because their surrounding bones have enlarged in all directions, leaving less space for the foramina. In addition to the enlargement of the bones, we can see that there is a disturbed pattern of trabeculation in the involved areas. Part of the density increase may be due to the enlargement of the bones and part may be due to the trabecular alterations. This patient has Paget's disease.

NORMAL AND VARIATIONS OF NORMAL

Undoubtedly the most difficult diagnosis in radiology is "normal." Even if we are thoroughly familiar with the classic roentgen appearance of an area of the body, there are countless variations which may occur which are of little or no pathologic significance. It is important to recognize these variants so that they will not be falsely considered to be the cause of a patient's current symptoms. Failure to recognize a normal variant for what it is could trigger unnecessary surgery, unnecessary immobilization, or perhaps a series of unnecessary diagnostic studies. To attempt to list or describe all or even many variants would be far beyond the scope of this book. Instead, we will describe some broad groups of variants.

ACCESSORY CENTERS OF OSSIFICATION AND SESAMOID BONES

These separate bony densities are most common in the region of the foot and ankle and in the region of the hand and wrist. An accessory center of ossification generally lies adjacent to the major ossification center of the otherwise unremarkable bone. A sesamoid lies in a predictable location in a tendon. Sesamoids themselves may be bipartite or multipartite. While there are some special cases where an accessory bone may be troublesome to the patient, for the most part, it is important to know that they are not recent fractures.

In addition to having a characteristic location, accessory bones and sesamoids are bounded by well-defined cortical margins and not by jagged edges of uncorticated spongy bone. In the case of small fractures, one can usually, but not always, find the jagged edge of the larger bone from which the small piece in question became separated (Fig. 5-20).

The presence of soft tissue swelling always suggests a fracture, but the coincidental presence of swelling near a smoothly contoured, well-corticated accessory bone or sesamoid

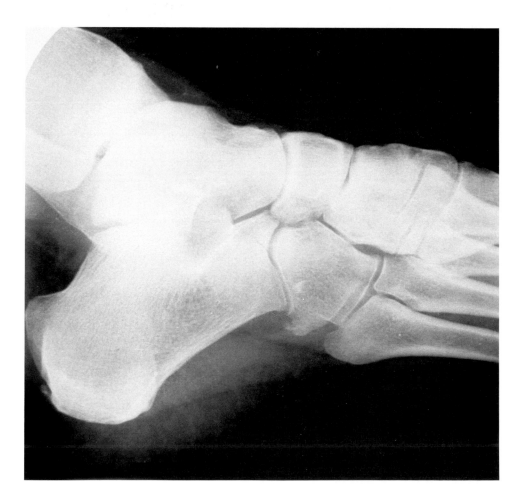

does not make a diagnosis of fracture. It is more difficult to differentiate between an old ununited fracture which is now well corticated and an accessory bone or sesamoid; however, that differential is rarely of real clinical importance.

EPIPHYSEAL AND APOPHYSEAL LINES AND PSEUDOEPIPHYSES

Still another group of problems is the differentiation of as yet unfused secondary epiphyseal and apophyseal centers from remnants of old epiphyseal and apophyseal lines at ossification centers which are already fused. These problems can be resolved by consulting standard charts or comparing the part with the contralateral side. Epiphyseal or apophyseal lines may be irregular, but are always smooth and not jagged or sharp like a fracture line (see Fig. 5-3B). Note the epiphyseal lines of the distal tibia and fibula and the apophysis of the os calcis. Can you find an accessory bone, the os trigonum, lying just behind the talus on the lateral projection?

NUTRIENT VESSELS

Perforating arteries generally coming from the direction of the heart (that is, the more proximal portion of the bone as opposed to the more distal end of the bone) will pass through the cortex of the shaft of the bone at a rather acute angle with the long axis of the bone, so that the nutrient vessel will appear to be almost parallel with the cortex. The walls of the nutrient vascular channel are very smooth and parallel to each other and are surrounded by cortical bone (Fig. 5-21).

ENTHESES

At areas of muscular, tendinous, or ligamentous junction with bone, there are frequently variable degrees of deformity of the bony contours due to the pulls exerted by these soft tissue structures. These varying degrees of alteration in the bony contour must be recognized

---

Figure 5-20. Contrast fracture fragment with sesamoid. There is a fine linear fracture in the region of the anterior horn of the os calcis. Note that the margins of this linear fracture are not corticated. If they were corticated, one might think that this either represented an old ununited fracture or an os calcaneus secundarius, an accessory bone which can exist in that precise location.

The os peroneum is a sesamoid bone in the peroneus longus tendon. We see a portion of an os peroneum peeking out from the superimposed shadow of the cuboid. The margins of the os peroneum which are seen free of the overlying shadow of the cuboid are noted to be sharply defined and corticated as opposed to the uncorticated margins of the fracture line. This os peroneum is not a chip or avulsion fracture from the cuboid. It is important to be able to differentiate sesamoid bones and accessory centers of ossification from fresh fractures. It is more difficult to differentiate these structures from ununited fractures. Standard reference books will list the locations, variations in appearance, and names of accessory ossification centers and sesamoid bones. Do you know the name of the largest sesamoid bone? Surely you are familiar with that bone, but you may not think of it as a sesamoid bone which it truly is, the patella.

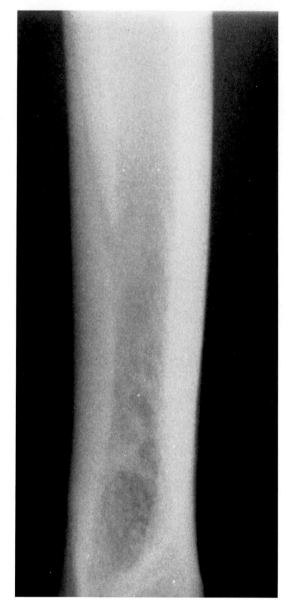

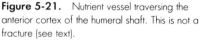
Figure 5-21.   Nutrient vessel traversing the
anterior cortex of the humeral shaft. This is not a
fracture (see text).

for what they are. They may be accentuated in very muscular individuals. (Note the
irregularities at the insertion of the Achilles tendon into the os calcis posteriorly in Figure
5-20.)

MISCELLANEOUS AND ASSORTED BUMPS AND DIMPLES

There are many miscellaneous and assorted bumps and dimples which can be seen relatively
rarely in normal individuals. Some of these are either not recognized or seen and ignored.

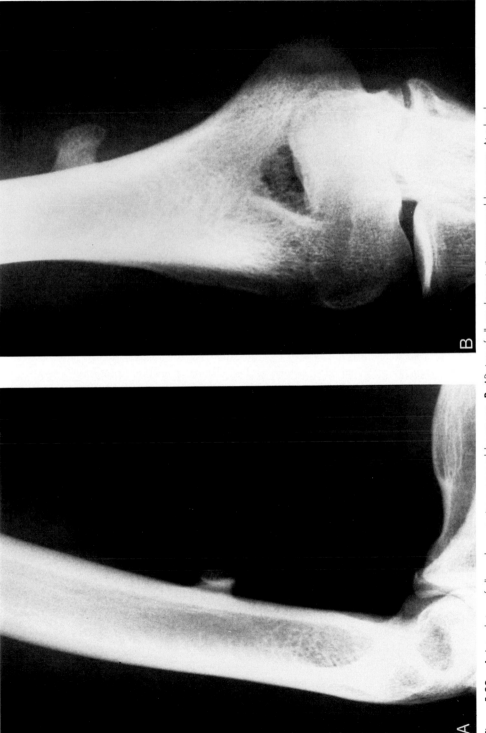

Figure 5-22.   **A:** Lateral view of elbow demonstrating supracondylar process. **B:** AP view of elbow demonstrating supracondylar process. At a level described as a hand's breadth above the elbow joint, one can occasionally find a large exostosis-like outgrowth from the anterior margin of the distal humeral shaft directed distally anteriorly and medially. This is seen routinely in some varieties of apes. A fibrous band extends between the distal end of the supracondylar process and the medial epicondyle of the humerus. Despite the similarity in appearance, the supracondylar process is not an osteochondroma.

Occasionally, there are some which are so prominent that they demand our attention. An example of this would be the supracondylar process of the distal humerus, seen in a very small percentage of patients (Figs. 5-22A,B). Interestingly, this is standard in cats and some varieties of apes. If one were not aware of its existence as a genetic variant, one might suspect that it represented an osteochondroma.

TRAUMA

By far, the majority of bone films are exposed because of a history of trauma. In evaluating these films, one is aided by a precise clinical history, including the location of point tenderness.

SOFT TISSUE

In viewing the trauma film, first look for soft tissue swelling or foreign bodies. If the foreign bodies are more dense (more radiopaque) than soft tissues (e.g., metal fragments or gravel), they will be readily visualized. If they are less dense (e.g., gas), they will be seen only with close observation. Most exposures will probably require a bright light to evaluate the soft tissues properly. Remember, if a foreign body cannot be seen, it must not be excluded, since we will not be able to see foreign bodies of approximately soft tissue density. This would include many types of glass, wood splinters, and small bits of plastic. Sometimes, Xerora-diographs (described in Chapter 2) will permit visualization of foreign bodies not definitely seen on conventional roentgenograms.

Soft tissue swelling may be discerned not just by the apparent increase in the soft tissues, but by the interruption of normal fat planes. If subcutaneous fat or fat between muscle planes is infiltrated by edema (water density), the fat will no longer sharply contrast with adjacent muscles, tendons, and other structures of water density.

Remember that soft tissue swelling may not be due to trauma, but could represent infection or edema due to venous or lymphatic blockage, or edema due to systemic causes. The 85-year-old patient with an old ununited chip fracture and swollen ankle due to congestive heart failure does not necessarily have a recent fracture, despite the presence of the swelling.

FRACTURES

There are many ways of classifying fractures. We will leave the more complex classification to the orthopedic surgeons. We will, however, provide you with some simple definitions which should enable you to look at an x-ray film and describe the findings in a readily understandable fashion.

A *linear fracture* is a radiolucent fracture line traversing a bone. If the fracture line extends only partway through the bone, it is an *incomplete fracture*. If the fracture line extends all the way from one cortex to another, it is a *complete fracture*. It is assumed that if the fracture is not described as *incomplete,* then it is *complete* and need not be described specifically as being complete (see Fig. 5-14A).

If the fracture consists of a single line separating two fragments, it is a *simple fracture.* If there are more than two fragments at the fracture site, it is considered to be a *comminuted fracture.* In a simple fracture, there is a *proximal fragment* (closest to the center of the body) and a *distal fragment* (farthest from the center of the body). In a comminuted fracture, there may be a *principal proximal fragment,* a *principal distal fragment,* and an *intermediate fragment.*

An *open fracture* is one in which there is an open wound associated with the fracture site. A fracture not associated with an open wound is a *closed fracture.* Fractures are considered to be closed and not generally specifically described as closed unless they are being contrasted with *open fractures.*

The term *compound fracture* is a "no, no." It has no medical meaning and should *not* be used.

A fracture through a joint surface is called an *articular fracture.* When a fracture line crosses a joint surface, that fact should be mentioned, as in the statement, "There is a comminuted articular fracture of the distal phalanx of the right thumb."

Buckle or *greenstick fractures* are seen only in children. Rather than a fracture line, there is a buckle or bend in the bone. In order to recognize such fractures, one must be very familiar with the normal anatomy (see Fig. 5-14B).

Another special type of fracture seen in children is an *epiphyseal separation.* This is a fracture through the physis or epiphyseal plate. There may be only minimal widening of the plate or considerable displacement of the epiphysis from the metaphysis. Epiphyseal separations may be very subtle, especially in young children, where only a portion of the epiphyseal ossification center is ossified.

Impacted fractures present with an area of increased density rather than a radiolucent fracture line. This is because the proximal and distal fragments have telescoped into each other and, for a short distance, the substance of two bony fragments is occupying the "same space" (see Fig. 5-14C).

Stress fractures may occur when a bone is stressed by a level of physical activity well above the patient's usual activity level. Initially, there may be no x-ray findings, but after a few weeks, increased bone density may be seen as healing progresses. Some of the new bone may be spongy bone and some may be periosteal new bone formation (see Fig. 5-14D).

Chip fractures are minute pieces of bone which may be chipped off a bone by trauma. *Avulsion fractures* are small pieces of bone which may be pulled off a larger piece by the forceful pull of a muscle, tendon, or ligament.

A *pathologic fracture* is a fracture through a preexisting bone lesion, frequently a tumor or sometimes an infection or area of aseptic necrosis. The pathologic fracture is characterized by a history of no trauma, or minor trauma not generally anticipated to be sufficient to fracture the bone in question. An example would be: "The patient was typing and felt a crack through the index finger." (See Fig. 5-7B, not fractured *yet.*)

Fractures may be described as *undisplaced* or in anatomical position. If they are not undisplaced, then they are described in terms of the *position* and *alignment* of the fragments.

Even if the proximal fragment of a fracture is relatively small and the distal fragment is more impressive, it assumed that the proximal fragment is where it belongs and the distal fragment has moved away.

If we assume that the fragments of a bone are *not* at an angle with each other, but that their long axes are parallel, then the *displacement* may be described as in the following examples:

1. The distal femoral fragment is displaced medially by one cortical width.
2. The distal femoral fragment is displaced anteriorly by one-half of a shaft width.
3. The distal femoral fragment is displaced posterolaterally by about three-fourths of a shaft width and displaced distally (distracted) by about 2 cm.
4. The distal femoral fragment is displaced medially by more than a full shaft width and displaced proximally (overriding) by about 2.5 cm.

Describing displacement is not as difficult as describing alignment. There are, unfortunately, many approaches to the description of how fragments are aligned. It is hoped that someday there will be universal agreement. In the meantime, here is a way that will be readily understood, if not always followed:

1. The distal end of the distal radial fragment is dorsally angulated. (This is also frequently stated in a shorter form, though a form possibly more apt to be misconstrued: "The distal radial fragment is dorsally angulated.")
2. The distal end of the distal radial fragment is anteriorly (volarly) angulated.
3. The distal end of the distal radial fragment is angulated dorsally and laterally with respect to the proximal fragment.

Next are three ways of saying the same thing about the clavicle. Note that in the clavicle, the distal fragment is the lateral fragment and the proximal fragment is the medial fragment.

1. The distal fragment of the clavicle is inferiorly angulated with respect to the proximal fragment. (My favorite.)
2. The fracture site is angled superiorly.
3. The clavicle is bowed superiorly at the fracture site.

The rules are simple but not everyone goes by the same rules. Good luck!

Refer back to Figure 5-1A and test yourself. Now that you can describe fractures, how do you find them? You look for them! What does this mean? It means that very tediously and thoroughly, in a very organized fashion, you must follow *every* cortical margin on *every* projection and search out the most minute area of irregularity so that you may evaluate it for being a true cortical discontinuity. We cannot expect a fracture to jump out of the film and bite us. It must be very carefully searched for, and even then, some subtle fractures will be missed.

DISLOCATIONS, SUBLUXATIONS, AND NORMAL JOINTS

In the case of each joint, there is a range of normal relationships between the proximal bone and the distal bone. Some joints are rather mobile and have a relatively broad range of normal relationships, as in the case of the temporomandibular joint or the first carpal-metacarpal joint. Other joints may have a more narrow range of normal relationships, as in the case of the joint between the distal humerus and the ulna, or the subtalar joint.

When the range of normal relationships for a particular joint is slightly exceeded, it is called a *subluxation*. When it is grossly exceeded, it is called a *dislocation*. The line separating the two is often arbitrary, but rarely an area of serious conflict. In describing the relationships at a joint, it is always assumed that the more proximal bone is in the correct position and it is the more distal bone that is subluxed or dislocated in the direction observed.

Joint relationships can frequently be evaluated better with the aid of stress films. Stress may be applied either by standing and bearing the patient's weight, weight-bearing by having a patient hold a weight in his hand while evaluating the acromioclavicular joint, or by external stress applied either by the patient or by someone else in an effort to alter the at-rest relationships of a joint. When this is done, one should generally evaluate the similarly stressed contralateral side for comparison.

METABOLIC BONE DISEASE

Metabolic bone disease is one of the most fascinating and complex subjects in radiology. There are many subtle interactions occurring among diverse mechanisms, some of which are not currently understood. This area would take several volumes to cover completely, so here we will only mention the highlights.

Osteoporosis has always been with us, but now that there have been reasonable approaches to quantitating it (see Chapter 2), it is gaining more attention. Osteoporosis results from a problem with the production of osteoid. On conventional films, it is said to require a 40 per cent bone loss before osteoporosis can be recognized.

Senility, endocrine abnormalities (either endogenous or iatrogenic), dietary deficiencies, as well as idiopathic osteoporosis all must be considered in the differential diagnosis. Also remember that multiple myeloma may present with an appearance that is virtually indistinguishable from osteoporosis.

Clinically, the loss of spongy bone in osteoporosis causes a predisposition to fractures, especially compression fractures of the vertebral bodies, fractures of the distal radius, and fractures of the femoral neck and trochanteric region. In addition to the anterior wedging of vertebral bodies, there is increased concavity of the vertebral endplates (Fig. 5-1A,B).

Osteomalacia is the term used to describe inadequate mineralization of the osteoid which is present. In children this presents as rickets, and in adults as osteomalacia. The differential diagnosis includes nutritional deficiency, malabsorption, changes due to anticonvulsive drugs, hereditary vitamin-D-resistant rickets, and disorders of the renal tubules. The classic findings of osteomalacia include decreased bone density, coarsening of the trabecular pattern, and cortical striations, followed by cortical thinning as the disease progresses. A normal roentgenogram does not exclude the presence of early osteomalacia, since considerable histological change may be present before one can perceive the earliest roentgenographic changes.

In the presence of approaching renal failure, we see the changes of *renal osteodystrophy* with superimposed changes of *secondary hyperparathyroidism*. Today, we are seeing increasing numbers of patients with the bony changes of renal osteodystrophy (Fig. 5-11B). This is because the renal failure patient is being kept alive with dialysis and renal transplants. These patients generally have long-standing renal disease, initially due to glomerulonephritis or pyelonephritis. Early in renal failure, we may see secondary hyperparathyroidism related to phosphate retention; later, with more severe failure, the hypocalcemia seems to be the more prominent factor in producing the increased parathyroid activity.

In patients with *secondary hyperparathyroidism,* we see subperiosteal cortical bone resorption. This is best observed along the radial margin of the middle phalanx of the index finger. As the condition progresses, changes become apparent in other fingers and at the terminal tufts. Longitudinal striations of the cortex are due to tunneling of osteoclasts stimulated by the elevated parathormone levels. Endosteal resorption also occurs, producing further cortical thinning and irregularities. Subchondral, subtendinous, and periodontal changes are also seen. *Osteosclerosis* is a poorly understood manifestation of secondary hyperparathyroidism. It may be a result of healing and contributes to the appearance of the "rugger-jersey" spine. *Chondrocalcinosis* is more common in primary than in secondary hyperparathyroidism. Brown tumors, while occasionally seen, are uncommon in secondary hyperparathyroidism. Soft tissue calcification can also be seen.

Primary hyperparathyroidism, frequently caused by a parathyroid adenoma, presents with changes similar to secondary hyperparathyroidism already described above. Brown tumors and chondrocalcinosis are more common in primary hyperparathyroidism than in secondary hyperparathyroidism. Osteosclerosis and soft tissue calcification are less common in primary hyperparathyroidism than in secondary hyperparathyroidism.

Osteopenia and *demineralization* are terms which reflect the physics of the disease processes, not the etiology, physiology, or histopathology. *Osteopenia* describes a decrease in bone density. *Demineralization* is a similar descriptive term which, while alluding to calcium, really is referring to the presence of osteopenia.

INFECTIONS

Osteomyelitis may occur anywhere, as a direct extension of a soft tissue infection or from an open fracture. Hematogenous osteomyelitis usually begins in the metaphyseal region of long bones because of their blood supply. The infectious process may spread through the subperiosteal region, through the marrow cavity, or both.

When the patient first presents with symptoms of osteomyelitis, the roentgenogram may be negative or may show some slight soft tissue swelling. A radioactive bone scan at this time would be positive, however. In attempting to identify early osteomyelitis in a patient with a one-week history of symptoms, compare the cost of an extremity x-ray with the cost of a bone scan (see Chapter 4). After 10 days to 2 weeks, faint demineralization of the area of bone involvement is visible, with progressive changes of a permeative type of demineralization (see Figs. 5-2B and 5-3B). Further, there may be loss of sharpness of the cortical margin and faint periosteal new bone formation. One or more layers of new bone formation may be seen as the infection advances and regresses in degree of activity.

The more active and aggressive the infection, the more bone destruction and, consequently, the more radiolucency will be seen. The periosteal new bone and sclerotic changes relate to the tissue's attempt to reconstruct normal bone (see Fig. 5-8A).

When the increased pressure build-up in bone has caused compromise of the blood supply, there may be a dense, avascular fragment of dead bone called a *sequestrum*. There is generally a fair amount of pus about the area of the sequestrum, and there may also be evidence of sinus tracts. As healing progresses, we may see a peripheral build-up of new bone called an *involucrum*.

If an osteomyelitis becomes chronic, there will be altered architecture with multiple areas of relative lucency surrounded by areas of sclerosis and areas of cortical thickening and cortical irregularity (see Fig. 5-8B). In the case of smoldering infections, there tends to be less radiolucency due to bone destruction and more sclerosis due to tissue reaction to the smoldering infection.

It is often difficult to differentiate a low grade infection or Brodie's abscess from an osteoid osteoma. Tuberculous osteomyelitis tends to involve the adjacent joints and tends to promote joint fusions. The drainage into adjacent soft tissues may produce soft tissue swelling and the resultant "cold" abscess may calcify.

NEOPLASMS

It is postulated that totipotential mesenchymal cells will develop and differentiate into one of the varieties of cells which populate the skeletal system according to the environment in which it finds itself. A mesenchymal cell in the region of the epiphysis may thus become a chondroblast. Were this same mesenchymal cell in the metaphyseal region, it might become an osteoblast, and in the diaphyseal region, it might become a fibroblast or even an undifferentiated round cell. If these cells stray from the path of normal development into the less-controlled growth patterns of neoplastic processes, they still tend to behave in some fashion according to the type of cell that they have become.

The round cell in the diaphyseal marrow cavity may become the Ewing's sarcoma seen in the midshaft region, or perhaps a reticulum sarcoma or a myeloma. The fibrous cell in the metaphyseal region may become a fibroxanthoma, a fibrous cortical defect, or even a fibrosarcoma. The osteoblast in the metaphyseal region may become an osteoblastoma or even an osteosarcoma. The osteoclast in the cut-back zone where the metaphysis is being narrowed to the diameter of the shaft may become a giant cell tumor. The chondrocyte may become an enchondroma or chondrosarcoma. The epiphyseal chondroblast may become a chondroblastoma. These concepts help to explain why different tumors occur in different parts of a bone and why they behave in a somewhat predictable fashion.

Tumors occur with greatest frequency in the areas where the most rapid growth is going on, where there is least stability. This is why the distal femur and proximal tibia are such common locations for primary bone neoplasms. This also explains why osteosarcomas occur in the distal femur so often in children and adolescents. Their next peak time of occurrence is in older adults superimposed on Paget's disease. Again, this is in an area of increased activity or instability.

While round cell tumors and fibrous tumors have no roentgenographically recognizable matrix, cartilage tumors tend to produce a cartilage matrix if they are reasonably well-differentiated. We may see punctate patterns of calcification which are characteristic and we may see overlapping arcuate contours. (See the calcifications and scalloped edges of the enchondroma in Fig. 5-7B.)

Osteoblasts produce bone. While osteosarcomas may be purely osteolytic, they may be osteoblastic and produce bone exuberantly. (See the osteoblastic osteosarcoma in Fig. 5-9B.)

Perhaps the most important thing to determine about a primary bone tumor is whether it is benign or malignant. Generally, benign tumors do not have an aggressive appearance, while malignant tumors tend to appear very aggressive. If a tumor is not aggressive, then its slow growth rate respects local "ground rules" and allows the adjacent normal tissue to "wall it off" from the normal bone. In a nonaggressive lesion, there is a definite "geographic" appearance, well-defined by a thick sclerotic margin, a thin sclerotic margin, or even no sclerosis at the margin, but excellent clear-cut definition of the interface between the lesion and normal bone.

In progressively more aggressive lesions, there is next the geographic lesion with a poorly defined margin, then the so-called "moth-eaten," regionally invasive pattern of bone destruction, and the permeative, or diffusely destructive, lesions. (Contrast the geographic lesion with a fine sclerotic margin in Fig. 5-5A with the geographic lesion with a sharp edge in Fig. 5-3A and with the permeative lesion in Fig. 5-2B.)

The slow-growing, nonaggressive lesion may thin and "expand" cortex. (See the enchondroma of Fig. 5-7B and contrast it with the cortical breakthrough seen in Fig. 5-6B, a metastatic lesion.)

Benign or nonaggressive tumors will tend to conform to the bony architecture, i.e., they may be longer than they are wide in a long bone; while the similarly placed aggressive tumor will tend to take on a more spherical shape and not respect the local "ground rules." Some aggressive tumors will tend to permeate through the cortex and periosteum and have a large soft tissue component, while a benign tumor would be confined to its host bone. (See the Ewing's tumor displacing the bladder in Fig. 5-8A.)

Metastatic lesions to bone are often multiple and often present in a patient with an already known primary malignant tumor elsewhere. Nevertheless, when a solitary, very aggressive lesion with ill-defined margins and perhaps a permeative appearance is seen in an individual who is middle-aged or older, metastatic malignancy must be considered more likely than a primary bone tumor. Most metastatic tumors are osteolytic; however, adenocarcinoma of the prostate is most frequently seen to produce an osteoblastic response. Adenocarcinoma of the breast will sometimes present as a blastic lesion, as will some lymphomas, particularly Hodgkin's disease. An initially osteolytic metastatic lesion may convert to osteoblastic under the influence of radiation therapy, chemotherapy, or hormonal therapy.

A nuclear medicine bone scan is the method of choice in evaluating for the presence of bone metastases in a patient with a "solitary," aggressive, lytic lesion or a known primary, such as a bronchogenic carcinoma or breast carcinoma. The bone scan is more expensive than a conventional x-ray bone survey (see Chapter 4), but as the initial study, it has greater sensitivity, though less specificity, than conventional x-ray studies. The areas which are "hot" on the nuclear medicine study can then be more specifically evaluated with regional, conventional x-ray examinations. Finding an early metastatic lesion may significantly alter the plan of therapy and perhaps save the patient from futile surgery. Everything "hot" on a bone scan is not necessarily a metastatic lesion.

Another group of neoplasms which should be considered here are the lipomas and liposarcomas. They are generally primarily soft tissue tumors, but may involve bone or even arise as intraosseous lesions. Portions of intraosseous lipomas may become necrotic and calcify, presenting a rather characteristic appearance. In soft tissues, the well-differentiated lipoma is sharply outlined from the denser surrounding soft tissue (water density). It presents as a radiolucent area of fat density which can generally be readily visualized.

There are many lesions of bone which are lumped with neoplasms because they tend to look like neoplasms, though their behavior is usually much different. Some are transient developmental changes like a small benign cortical defect. (See Fig. 5-6A which approaches the size of a small fibroxanthoma.) Others are alterations in maturation, like fibrous dysplasia, which begins as a fibrous lytic lesion and matures with the production of immature fiber bone, producing a "ground-glass" appearance as the new osteoid begins to calcify (see Fig. 5-18). Another lesion is the osteoid osteoma, of uncertain cause, but most likely inflammatory (see Fig. 5-5B).

Life is never easy and, in the area of bone tumor diagnosis, the pitfalls are sometimes more numerous than the safe paths. One of the problems is that the general concepts described above work most of the time but not all of the time. Fibrosarcomas and chondrosarcomas, which are both unquestionably malignant lesions, may first present with an appearance which would be classified as nonaggressive and benign by the usual guidelines. They may even have metastasized already while they still have an innocent roentgenographic appearance. The rare chondromixoid fibroma may range in appearance from benign to questionable. Some osteosarcomas appear less aggressive than some giant cell tumors.

How do we know what we are dealing with in the face of all of these variables? We do a very good job; we have a very good batting average, but we don't win them all! It is only by correlation of history, physical examination, and laboratory findings with nuclear medicine studies, roentgen appearance, and histology that an accurate final diagnosis can be made in some cases.

ARTHROPATHIES

OSTEOARTHRITIS (DEGENERATIVE JOINT DISEASE)

Osteoarthritis may be secondary to previous infection or old trauma. In these cases, there is more degenerative change in the particular joint that had been traumatized than may be found in corresponding regions elsewhere in the body.

Primary osteoarthritis tends to involve weight-bearing joints such as the knee, where changes are seen especially in the medial compartment and the patellofemoral compartment. In the hip, changes are seen superolaterally. The tibiotalar joint is rarely significantly involved, except for changes along the anterior margin of the distal articular surface of the tibia; these are most likely posttraumatic in origin.

In the hand, there is typically involvement of the trapezionavicular joint and the first carpal-metacarpal joint. In addition, there is involvement of the distal interphalangeal joints of the fingers and the interphalangeal joint of the thumb, with lesser changes at the proximal interphalangeal joints and at the metacarpal-phalangeal joints.

In the foot, there is often involvement of the first metatarsal-phalangeal joint. In addition to joint space narrowing and subchondral sclerosis, there is subchondral degenerative cyst formation and osteophyte formation along the joint margins. Juxtaarticular osteoporosis is not a feature of osteoarthritis.

In the spine, changes are seen in the facet joints throughout and at the uncovertebral joints (Luschka's joints) in the cervical region. Degenerative disc disease is also seen with associated osteophyte formation. Sacroiliac joint involvement is common. The sclerotic joint margins of the sacroiliac joint are sharply defined as opposed to the changes seen in the inflammatory arthritides. (See Fig. 5-12B and note the degenerative cyst formation in the styloid process of the ulna. The changes at the radiocarpal joint are most likely secondary to trauma. Also see Fig. 5-16B and note the joint space narrowing and marginal osteophyte formation.)

EROSIVE OSTEOARTHRITIS

Distinct from osteoarthritis is erosive osteoarthritis. This entity involves the interphalangeal joints with very rapidly progressing bony changes, and there is associated inflammatory change with considerable soft tissue swelling about the joints. Severe erosive destruction of the subchondral regions is seen. The changes may progress to bony ankylosis.

RHEUMATOID ARTHRITIS

Rheumatoid arthritis may involve any synovial joint. The sacroiliac joints are involved only infrequently. The greatest involvement is in the small joints of the hands and wrists with sparing of the distal interphalangeal joints, and there is also involvement of the small joints of the feet. Initially, there may be only fusiform soft tissue swelling about the fingers and some juxta-articular osteoporosis. The changes at first may be asymmetrical, but soon there is relative, but not necessarily absolute symmetry. Uniform narrowing of the joint cartilage spaces is seen fairly early, and about the same time, there are early erosive changes. These typically occur at the "bare" areas.

In a typical synovial joint, the articular surface is covered by cartilage. However, there is generally a short segment of bone between the cartilage covering and the capsule insertion that is not covered by cartilage or by periosteum but by synovium. This is referred to as the "bare" area where the inflamed synovium has direct access to the bone and where erosions begin. (See Fig. 5-12A and contrast with Fig. 5-12B.)

Involvement of the soft tissues about the joints may lead to ulnar deviation of the fingers at the metacarpal-phalangeal joints. Late in the disease, there may be fusion of the carpal bones and of the tarsal bones. Fusion can occur at the interphalangeal joints, but this is much less common. The cervical spine, especially the C1-C2 junction, is often involved.

Superimposed on all of the above, there are often changes secondary to osteoarthritis.

CHRONIC ARTHRITIS IN CHILDREN

Numerous chronic arthritic disorders occur in children and will not be individually covered here. Sometimes short phalanges are seen, due to premature closure of the epiphyses, and interphalangeal joint fusion is fairly common.

CALCIUM PYROPHOSPHATE DIHYDRATE DEPOSITION DISEASE (CPPD)

In CPPD, crystals of calcium pyrophosphate dihydrate are deposited in the fibrocartilages such as the menisci and, to a lesser extent, in the hyaline cartilages of the joint surfaces. (See Fig. 5-16A. Can you see the thin streak of chondrocalcinosis of the hyaline cartilage?)

The mere presence of chondrocalcinosis (calcification in cartilage) does not establish the diagnosis of CPPD, as other calcium salts can produce a similar x-ray appearance. The calcium pyrophosphate dihydrate crystals may be histologically identified in the cartilage and present in the joint fluid, but not seen on the x-ray.

The x-ray changes of CPPD resemble osteoarthritis. However, there are differences in distribution, such as involvement of the knee in the patellofemoral joint and lateral compartment, but sparing of the medial compartment. In the hand, there may be involvement of the metacarpal-phalangeal joints while sparing the interphalangeal joints. Involvement of the elbow and tibiotalar joints is also seen to a greater degree than in osteoarthritis.

GOUT

The most common x-ray finding in gout is a normal x-ray. With more advanced disease, there is involvement of one of the first metatarsal-phalangeal joints. There is no routinely associated osteoporosis and no particular symmetry of involvement. In addition to soft tissue swelling, urate deposits in the soft tissues may be seen. These deposits may or may not be calcified. Adjacent to the tophi, one sees the punched-out erosions of gout, frequently with an undercut appearance (see Fig. 5-13).

ANKYLOSING SPONDYLITIS

Early in ankylosing spondylitis there is sacroiliac joint involvement with blurring of the joint margins and some reactive sclerosis. The changes may be more apparent on one side, but soon they become symmetrical and progress in the direction of joint fusion. The primary involvement is in the axial skeleton. There is "squaring" of the vertebral bodies and syndesmophyte formation. Osteoporosis is generally prominent. The fibrocartilage joints like the symphysis are frequently involved. In one-half of the patients, the appendicular skeleton is also involved, especially in the shoulders, hips, hands, and feet. The superficial erosions are associated with reactive sclerosis and bone proliferation leading to joint fusions.

PSORIATIC ARTHRITIS

While many of the changes are similar to those seen in rheumatoid arthritis, the changes in psoriatic arthritis are likely not to be symmetrical. Also, there is greater involvement of the distal interphalangeal joints than the proximal interphalangeal joints in the hand. Joint fusion is more common than in rheumatoid arthritis, and destruction of the terminal tufts, especially in the feet, is sometimes seen. Osteoporosis is not a constant finding. There is frequently abundant subperiosteal appositional bone formation. Sacroiliac joint involvement may be unilateral or bilateral. The spinal involvement may be similar to ankylosing spondylitis, or there may be striking asymmetry and skip areas without involvement.

REITER'S SYNDROME

Many of the findings of Reiter's syndrome may be difficult to separate from those of ankylosing spondylitis, rheumatoid arthritis, and psoriatic arthritis. Reiter's syndrome has a greater tendency to involve the feet and lower extremity joints with relative sparing of the upper extremities. The spinal changes are more apt to resemble the asymmetric changes of psoriatic arthritis than the more uniform changes of ankylosing spondylitis.

Favorite sites of involvement are the interphalangeal joint of the great toe and the posterior plantar margin of the os calcis (lover's heel). The metatarsal-phalangeal joints are also often involved. The associated history of urethral and eye complaints helps with this diagnosis.

SEPTIC ARTHRITIS

Septic arthritis may be due to hematogenous spread or direct extension from bone or soft tissue. Traumatic open wounds and joint aspirations or injections may also lead to septic arthritis. In addition to soft tissue swelling and local osteopenia, there is rapid cartilage destruction. There may be initial widening of the joint space due to effusion early in the course of the disease. Rapid diagnosis and rapid treatment are required if any of the articular cartilage is to be saved.

NEUROPATHIC ARTHROPATHY

Neuropathic joints are characterized by soft tissue swelling about the joint, loss of cartilage, fragmentation of the subchondral bone, bone resorption, and formation of large, sometimes unusual-appearing osteophytes. The appearance suggests an osteoarthritis gone wild, with shards of calcified cartilage and bone distributed about the site. There is often no significant osteoporosis and subluxations are common.

INFARCTION AND ASEPTIC NECROSIS

Loss of blood supply to bone may be due to trauma, such as a fracture of the femoral neck or of the waist of the navicular, or perhaps dislocation, as with traumatic dislocation of the hip or treatment of congenital dislocation of the hip. Other causes include obstruction of vessels in sickle cell disease and macroglobulinemia. Vasculitis, as in systemic lupus erythematosis, is another causative factor, as is steroid therapy. In addition, the classical occurrence of caisson disease must be considered.

In the case of infarction of the femoral head, the overlying articular cartilage, which receives its nutrition from the joint fluid, is at first not disturbed by the underlying bone infarction. Since dead bone will not support weight as well as living bone, with time and use, multiple small fractures occur in the infarcted area. Many of these microfractures impact, causing an area of increased bone density and altered architecture. Before long, the x-ray shows a radiolucent cleft which has developed between the immediate subchondral bone and the impacted spongy bone below. This cleft is referred to as the *crescent sign*.

As the disease progresses, with continued loss of underlying support, changes in the articular cartilage are seen as well, with joint space narrowing and secondary osteoarthritic changes.

It must be understood that the x-ray changes of infarction are not due to the infarction itself, but to the postinfarction structural changes and postinfarction reparative changes. The calcific changes in bone infarction relate to calcification of necrotic fat in the marrow cavity.

TOTAL JOINT REPLACEMENT

In order to be called a total joint replacement, it is required that both surfaces of a joint be replaced by artificial material. Most replacements have a metallic component and a component of high-density polyethylene or similar material. These joint replacements are generally maintained in position by methyl methacrylate (bone cement). While methyl methacrylate itself is radiolucent, barium is almost always added to the methacrylate to make it radiopaque and thus visible on the roentgenograms.

The cement is not an adhesive, but when it sets, it fits into the surface irregularities of the bone, metal, or plastic materials with which it interfaces, and thus, serves to affix the prosthesis to the bone. After the methacrylate powder and liquid catalyst are mixed, heat is given off as the cement polymerizes. This heat can cause cell death in the immediately adjacent bone. Because of this, there is often a 1 to 2mm lucent line between the bone and the cement. This line represents the result of the bone destruction by the exothermic reaction.

If the width of the lucent line at the interface between the bone and the cement exceeds 2mm, we must suspect mechanical loosening or infection, or both. A lucent zone between the methyl methacrylate and the prosthesis is usually not seen because of the tight fit. When there is infection at the cement/bone interface, there may be a permeative pattern in the adjacent bone as the infection progresses; but with mechanical loosening, one expects the widened lucent line to be bounded by a thin sclerotic margin. While this seems quite reasonable, it is often impossible to be certain as to the presence or absence of infection when there is more than a 2mm lucent zone.

Arthrography is the method of choice in making this determination (see Figs. 2-11A,B,C,D). The arthrogram of a joint with a total replacement serves two basic functions. A specimen of joint fluid or joint washing is obtained for aerobic and anaerobic cultures and perhaps for Gram stain. The contrast material is then injected through the same site, proving that the specimen actually came from the neocapsule of the artificial joint.

Contrast material entering the cement-bone interface is a sign of loosening. Failure of the contrast material to enter the interface does not exclude loosening, as the lucent zone may be filled with fibrous tissue.

Many surgeons are now using uncemented, porous-coated prostheses. Portions of the metallic stems of these prostheses are covered with a porous metal surface with many small interstices into which it is hoped that the patient's bone will grow, thus affixing itself to the porous surface layer of the metal stem. In these cases, cement is not used. Rarely, due to technical difficulties in seating the prosthesis in soft bone, at the last minute a surgeon may decide to use cement with a porous-coated prosthesis.

CONCLUSIONS

Now that you have learned how bone reacts in a limited number of ways to some very different stimuli, we hope that you will provide the radiologist with sufficient clinical information to make a meaningful diagnosis. You have learned how similar a leukemia and an osteomyelitis may appear. You have learned how there may be a delay before the roentgen changes of some undisplaced fractures and some stress fractures become apparent on radiographs. You are aware of the importance of a clinical history and laboratory data in the differential diagnosis of arthritis.

We hope that you will approach the film as a physician first, and as a pathologist second, remembering that the patient is more important than the film. We hope that you will consult with the radiologist *before* ordering special studies. We hope that you will be mindful of costs and patient comfort and not request a study unless you have first decided how its results may impact on the patient's future care and well-being.

In presenting this introductory approach to bone radiology, there are many important and fascinating areas which we have not been able to include because of the limited space and scope of this textbook. We hope that you will apply the approaches you have learned here as you encounter those areas not specifically addressed.

CHAPTER 6

RADIOLOGY OF THE CHEST

David S. Feigin

BASIC APPROACH

Most physicians view chest radiographs by a search pattern rather than attempting, in random fashion, to detect any specific abnormality. Any search pattern is effective, provided that all the parts of the film are viewed, and the most attention is given to the areas with either the greatest frequency of abnormalities or the greatest difficulty of their visibility. The order of the search thus is not crucial; many students begin with the periphery of the chest and upper abdomen, simply because that is the area that they most fear they will ignore, especially if they have seen an abnormality elsewhere. It is probably preferable to view the periphery last, as the pleural space, bones, and soft tissues often provide information that corroborates or amplifies the meaning of abnormalities seen in the heart, lungs, or mediastinum. It is, however, far better to view the periphery first than to ignore it entirely.

All search patterns should emphasize the most crucial areas of the chest film: lung fields, mediastinum, and lower neck. The lungs may be viewed first from top to bottom or bottom to top, but each portion of the lung fields should then be viewed with a side to side comparison to the opposite lung field. This exercise not only provides a second look at each portion of the lung field but also permits the detection of changes in blood flow, airway shadows, and asymmetric densities which may be masses. It is vital to include the lung field behind the heart shadow (right and left) in both the first and second look at the lung fields.

The mediastinum may be viewed along its entire margin on both sides. Then, however, the interior of the mediastinum should also be viewed with special attention to the airways, including the trachea as far superior as it is visible.

If a lateral film is available it should receive nearly as much attention as the frontal view. The center of a lateral film includes more information regarding the hila, especially the airways and vessels, than does the frontal view. If any abnormality has been viewed on the frontal, it can be corroborated and localized on the lateral view. The spine, diaphragms, upper abdomen, and neck may be viewed on the lateral before these structures are studied on the frontal view.

Before leaving the film, whether or not abnormalities have been detected, it is vital to sit back and "gestalt" the entire film, both frontal and lateral views. This permits the detection of subtle abnormalities that may not be apparent when you study the film too closely. It also permits an overall evaluation of vessels, heart size, bones, especially the shoulders, and soft tissues, especially in the lower neck and above the clavicles.

Be sure to complete your search even if you detect significant abnormalities immediately. It is best to look closely at an abnormality as soon as you see it and study it in all available views, before completing your search. This makes the rest of your search more meaningful and also prevents the common pitfall of thinking about the abnormality while you are viewing the remainder of the film, thus missing everything except the original abnormality.

PRINCIPLES OF VISIBILITY

The chest radiograph represents significant compromise in technique when compared with other plain film studies. In order to optimize the visualization of the vessels and airway walls in the lung, a high energy beam is used that prevents visibility of many tissue density differences. While abdominal and soft tissue films easily demonstrate the difference between fat and soft tissue, the compromise of the chest film precludes this, leaving only three fundamental densities: (1) air, (2) bone, and (3) everything in between these extremes including fat, water, other fluid, soft tissue such as muscle, and solid organs or masses.

Air on the chest film is present in only a few places: lungs, major airways, and abdominal viscera. Bones are, of course, only present in the periphery of the thorax. Since we cannot differentiate among structures more dense than air but less dense than bone, it follows that borders of all intermediate density structures are only seen clearly when they come up against an air-containing structure. Since most abnormalities are of soft tissue or fluid density, this means that an abnormality will not be clearly visible unless there is air on one or the other side of the lesion in the projection being viewed.

The only other way to see an abnormality is for there to be calcification (bone density) at or near its edge or for bone to be displaced or eroded. Often abnormal structures are only visible because they displace other structures of similar density. This is the case with many mediastinal masses, especially enlarged lymph nodes. One of the great values of the lateral chest view is that it permits us to see an abnormality which has air in front or behind it, but may not have air to its left or right, making it invisible on the frontal view.

The most obvious maxim derived from these principles is that structures are most visible on the chest film when they are surrounded by air in the lung fields. The small structures that are most visible are thus the vessels and those airway walls that are just large enough to be

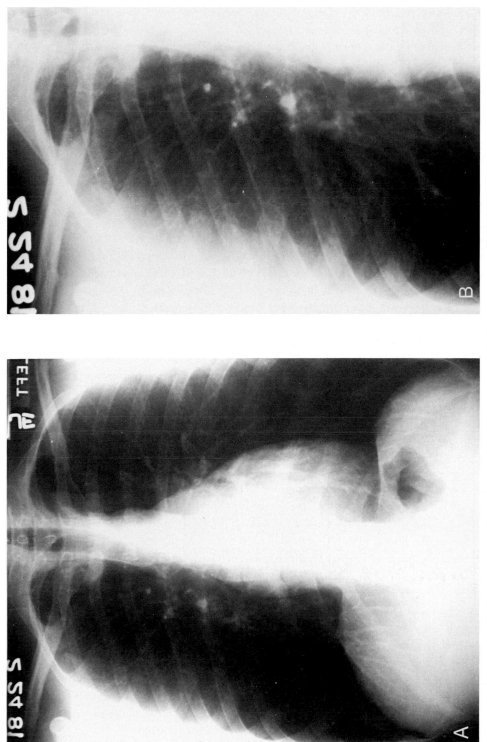

Figure 6-1.   Normal chest film **(A)** with close-up of right upper lung field **(B)** These are normal pulmonary markings; note that they all emanate from the pulmonary hilum and diverge from that point. The "nodular" densities, especially prominent in the hilum, are vessels seen on end. Note that vessels leading to and from them are similar to the "nodules" in diameter.

resolved. These constitute the "lung markings" and are the only normal structures that are *always* visible in the lung fields (Fig. 6-1).

In differentiating these normal markings from abnormal lines or nodular densities, one must remember that the vessels and bronchi all eminate from the hila and thus basically travel in a branching pattern, separating into the periphery of the lung fields. Abnormal lines in the lung generally run in directions other than towards the hilum. Nodules and masses are densities that are larger than the diameter of the vessels in that part of the lung or are clearly distinct from the vessels. Use of this rule permits differentiation of real abnormalities from vessels seen on end. Remember to look for an abnormality in *both* views in order to confirm its existence and to localize it specifically.

A Word About Definitions

The most ambiguous word in chest radiology is *alveolar*. To radiologists, it usually is used to refer to the lumen of the air space surrounded by the alveolar wall. To the pathologist, however, the term *alveolus* usually includes the wall as well as the lumen. The distinction is important because thickening of the alveolar walls appears as an *interstitial pattern* on radiographs. Because of this ambiguity, the term *consolidation* is increasingly replacing *alveolar pattern* in recent literature.

Another source of confusion is the word *airway*, which should always be used to refer to the trachea, bronchi, and bronchioles, as differentiated from *airspaces*, which are the lumens of the alveoli. This distinction is also important because airspace filling patterns *(consolidations)* are very different from airway patterns.[1,2]

BASIC APPROACH TO ABNORMAL LUNG FIELDS

If you study the chest film in the manner described above, you should be able to detect abnormal lucency or density within the lung fields whenever either exists. The regions in which one is most likely to miss lesions is behind the heart on the frontal film and almost anywhere on the lateral film. Be sure your search includes these areas.

Pulmonary abnormalities may be divided into five basic categories, the first five in Table 6-1. For completeness, the table includes four other types of abnormalities that are usually distinguishable from those involving the lung fields themselves. Each of these will be briefly discussed following a more complete analysis of the abnormal lungs.

Whenever an abnormal density or lucency is visible over the lung field, its location within the lungs may be confirmed on the lateral view and, occasionally, may require additional views such as oblique views or computed tomograms. Once location within the lung is confirmed or suspected, the most applicable of the five basic patterns should be chosen. In most cases, one pattern will be dominant and represent the starting point for differential diagnosis. If more than one pattern is evident, the differential diagnosis must include abnormalities typically represented by each of the patterns visible.

It is always best to view chest films with little or no information to bias our interpretation.

TABLE 6-1. ABNORMAL CHEST FILM
PATTERNS

Mass	Pleural Space
	Effusions
Consolidation	Thickening
	Masses
Interstitial	
Lines	Mediastinum
Nodules	Masses
Destructive	
	Heart and Pericardium
Airway	Shape
Obstruction	Size
Air Trapping	
	Periphery
Vascular	Bones
Overperfusion	Soft Tissues
Underperfusion	Abdomen

Abnormalities are often ignored if they appear contrary to our clinical expectations, and, conversely, normal areas may be interpreted as abnormal if we have already decided that there is a high probability of clinical abnormality in that region. Clinical information is vital and helpful primarily in determining whether a given differential diagnosis is logical and reasonable. For this reason, the more information available when the film is interpreted, the more information one can obtain from the film. It is best, however, to bring this information into use only after the film has been searched and the diagnostic possibilities are in mind for the pattern or patterns visible.

MASS

The term *mass* is probably the most "loaded" term used in the description of chest films. Most people immediately think of cancer when they see or hear the word mass. The term should be used whenever there is a localized pulmonary density which could conceivably be malignant. It is impossible to ignore a radiology report, either oral or written, that includes the term *mass* even if the patient has no symptoms referable to the chest. If a patient is radiographed without the clinical suspicion of chest disease, use of an alternative term such as *density* or even *infiltrate* may easily cause the lesion to be ignored. Substituting the word *mass* necessitates further investigation on both medical and probably legal grounds.

Thus, a mass may be defined as any localized density not completely surrounded by lung fissures or the pleura. In case of doubt, a density should always be called a mass rather than an infiltrate, as the latter term usually connotes reversible lung disease. Everyone knows that some infiltrative diseases, such as pneumonia, can appear as masses; more commonly forgotten is the equally vital fact that malignancies occasionally appear as localized infiltrates.

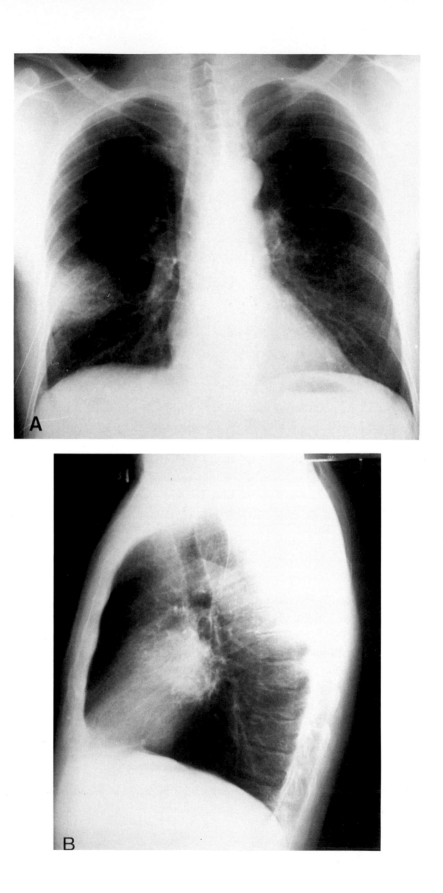

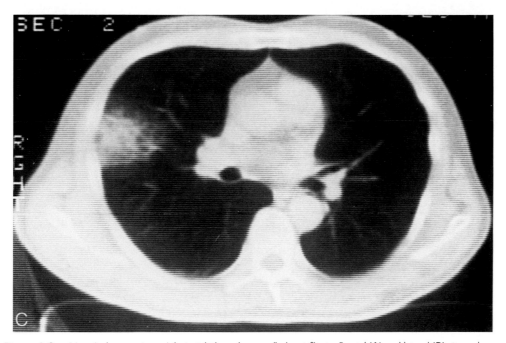

Figure 6-2. Mass (adenocarcinoma) that might have been called an infiltrate. Frontal (**A**) and lateral (**B**) views show localized density in the lateral segment of the right middle lobe. While the term *localized consolidation* would also have fit this appearance, this malignancy was further evaluated, in the absence of symptoms, because it was called a mass. A CT view through the lesion (**C**) similarly fails to distinguish between a mass and an infiltrate.

A typical mass that might have been called an infiltrate is illustrated in Figure 6-2. The patient was asymptomatic, and further investigation, which subsequently included bronchoscopy and biopsy, began with a chest CT that made the lesion appear even more mass-like than it did on plain film. Subsequent bronchoscopy did establish the diagnosis of adenocarcinoma, which fortunately was resectable. Had this abnormality been described as anything other than a *mass*, this cancer may have been ignored and left untreated.

The differential diagnosis of a pulmonary mass rests principally upon the clinical status of the patient. Such factors as age, history of smoking, sex, and the presence of other diseases are the most important determinants in the question of how to proceed following the detection of the mass on the plain film. In the case of most males over fifty years of age, the differential diagnosis of a pulmonary mass principally consists of malignancy and granuloma (which may be infectious like tuberculosis and histoplasmosis, or noninfectious like Wegener's granulomatosis). Other possibilities, as shown in Table 6-2, include benign neoplasms and congenital abnormalities, both of which are more common in younger individuals. Active inflammation, especially infection, is most important to consider when there are symptoms or findings referable to the region of the abnormality. Risk factors for malignancy all raise the likelihood of that diagnosis and may necessitate interventional evaluation as soon as a mass is suspected radiographically.

Specific radiographic features of masses are numerous, but they are usually less clinically

TABLE 6-2. PRINCIPAL CAUSES OF PULMONARY MASSES

Malignancy
Primary
Metastatic

Granulomatous Diseases
Infectious
Mycobacterial
Fungal
Bacterial
Noninfectious
eg. Sarcoid

Other Inflammation
eg. Pneumonia
Abscess

Benign Neoplasms
eg. Hamartomas

Congenital Abnormalities
eg. Sequestrations

important than the clinical parameters including age, sex, symptoms, concurrent diseases, and risk factors for cancer listed in Table 6-2. Characteristics include densities, edge sharpness, presence of lobulation, possible cavitation, and specific location. Only two appearance features of masses are considered crucial: (1) the presence of central and lamellar (ring-like) calcifications, and (2) stability or regression of the size of the lesion. If the lesion is calcified or is smaller or completely unchanged in comparison with previous films at least two years old, only the most flagrant of risk factors would warrant further evaluation. In most cases, calcification and stability indicate the need for follow up, but preclude the need for immediate investigation. Other appearance features do little if anything to alter the need for further evaluation of a suspected or confirmed pulmonary mass. Remember, it is far better to err on the side of overcaution with regard to masses, than to minimize or ignore their possible presence.

CONSOLIDATION

Consolidation is a synonym for the "alveolar" pattern originally described by Felson.[3] The term refers to the abnormality visible on chest films when the air spaces are filled with any substance of density greater than air, or are collapsed so that they are not filled at all. Air space filling is more common clinically than air space collapse, and the combination of both mechanisms is also relatively common. The appearance of consolidation is demonstrated in Figure 6-3. The abnormality consists of abnormal pulmonary density which obscures

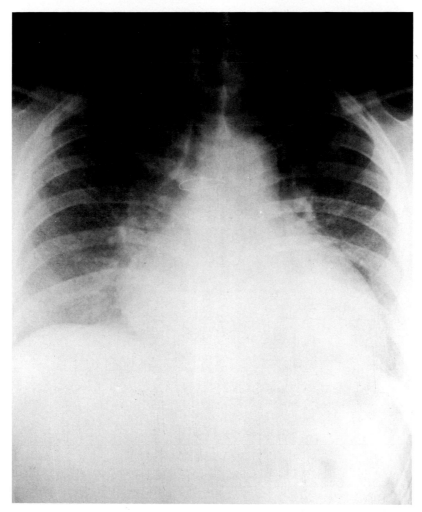

Figure 6-3. Consolidation of both lungs, caused by congestive heart failure. This patient, with a cardiomyopathy, shows typical findings of pulmonary edema producing diffuse consolidation. Notice the air-filled bronchi (bronchograms) most easily visible in the right upper lung field.

pulmonary vessels as it surrounds them with density similar to their own. Consolidations are coalescent in that they represent large cloud-like densities rather than small individual densities that may be called nodules (to be discussed later). Consolidation thus obscures all lung markings that it surrounds, with the exception of air in the lumen of any airway which remains patent. Remember, air will always be visible when surrounded by another basic density, and "air bronchograms" thus represent air within airways surrounded by consolidated air spaces.

Other characteristics of consolidations beside coalescence include soft, fluffy edges. Consolidations may have sharp borders if, and only if, they reach the edge of a lobe or segment and stop abruptly at the fissure or pleural surface. In this circumstance, the

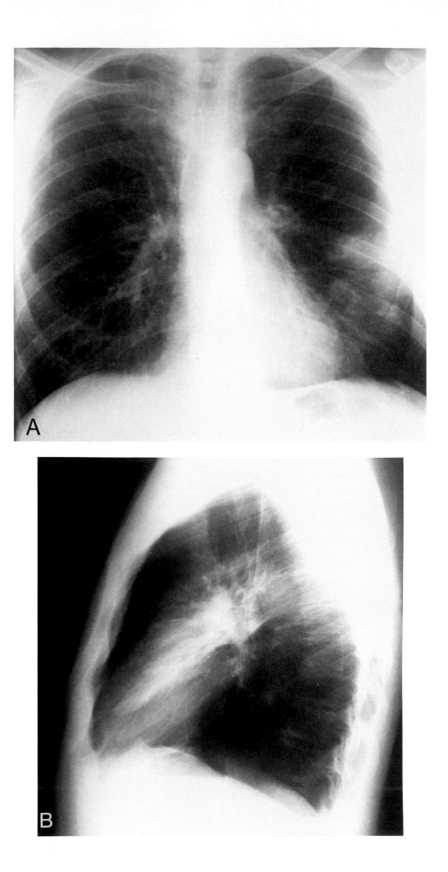

TABLE 6-3. PRINCIPAL CAUSES OF CONSOLIDATION

Blood
    Embolism
    Trauma

Pus
    Pneumonias

Water
    Congestion
    RDS

Protein
    Alveolar Proteinosis

Cells
    Alveolar Cell Carcinoma
    Lymphoma

consolidation will have sharp borders and usually resemble the shape and location of a specific lobe or segment of the lung (Fig. 6-4). Such "segmental" consolidations include many pneumonias and pulmonary infarcts. "Nonsegmental" and diffuse consolidations are not limited to specific nameable segments or lobes.

The differential diagnosis of a consolidation principally consists of the three substances denser than air that may fill air spaces: blood, pus, and water. Blood fills air spaces most commonly in embolic disease (in which case it is segmental) and as contusions or hematomata in trauma. Pus in the air spaces is usually the exudate of a pneumonia. Water fills air spaces by three distinct mechanisms: near drowning, excessive circulation ("congestion"), and excessive leakiness of capillaries (respiratory distress syndrome). While near drowning is usually clinically obvious, the differentiation of congestion from capillary leakage may be very difficult. When congestion causes consolidative patterns, vascular patterns (discussed below) of over-circulation may be evident if the vessels are distended; such vascular distention is usually absent in the respiratory distress syndromes. Unfortunately, there may be no radiographic difference between these two mechanisms, and clinical evaluation such as the use of Swan-Ganz catheter measurement of capillary wedge pressure may be required.

When the clinical evaluation of the possibilities of blood, pus, or water fail to reveal a clinical diagnosis, there are two less common possibilities as shown in Table 6-3. These are *protein* as in alveolar proteinosis[4] and *cells* as in alveolar cell carcinoma[5] and lymphoma.[6] These two malignant diseases tend to fill air spaces and are thus excellent examples of malignancies presenting as infiltrates rather than as masses.

←————————————————————————————————

Figure 6-4. Segmental consolidation, pneumonia, lingula. Frontal **(A)** and lateral **(B)** views show localized consolidation, with air bronchograms, best seen just above the major fissure that separates the lingula from the left lower lobe.

In summary, when you see a large coalescent density with or without sharp borders, and especially if you can see an air bronchogram, you should use the term *consolidation* and include a differential diagnosis of blood, pus, water, protein, or cells. Remember to consider the possibility that you are viewing a mass and that you should use the term *mass* whenever you are in doubt between that and a small consolidation.

INTERSTITIAL PATTERNS

Intersitital patterns all represent thickening of the interstices of the lung: septae, alveolar walls, connective tissue surrounding bronchi and vessels, and, usually, pleura. Such thickening may be caused by inflammation, malignancy, edema, or fibrosis and may involve reversible distention or irreversible destruction. Interstitial patterns are divided into three types: (1) lines or reticulations, (2) nodules, and (3) the pattern of destruction. Destroyed lung is often indistinguishable radiographically from lungs in which the interstitium is potentially reversibly distended. Late destruction is usually distinctive but is not sufficiently common or important to include in this discussion. Excellent discussions of the destructive interstitial pattern may be found elsewhere.[7,8,9]

INTERSTITIAL LINES

One of the most difficult problems in interpreting chest films is the differentiation of abnormal interstitial lines from the normal lines that represent pulmonary markings. The orientation of the pulmonary markings, as described above and shown in Figure 6-1, is that all vessels and airways branch from the hila. Interstitial lines are recognized whenever there are lines running in every possible direction *(reticulations)* or when there are nonvascular, nonbronchial lines in the periphery, usually representing thickened septae (Fig. 6-5).

The septal lines were originally described by Kerley and are thus often called *Kerley lines.* Most important are the "B" lines which are horizontal, short, and are usually best seen in the periphery of the lung bases. They extend laterally to the pleural surface and do not merge medially with the bronchi or vessels. Reticulations and septal lines are the hallmarks of the interstitial patterns.

The differential diagnosis of interstitial lines is best summarized by the term *life lines.* The pattern is *line* and the differential diagnosis is *life.* The specific causes are listed in Table 6-4. It is often exceedingly difficult to detect appearance differences among the four possible categories of diagnosis. Remember that the category *inflammation* includes a wide variety of specific diseases encompassing infections such as viral and mycoplasmal, as well as noninfectious inflammations which may be allergic, vasculitic, or ideopathic. A complete list of the possibilities is not usually clinically useful, as clinical parameters often suggest one or several specific diagnoses. When necessary, lists may be consulted in pulmonary radiology textbooks.[2,9]

Interstitial lines are often seen in combination with other pulmonary patterns. The combination often suggests the diagnosis, as in the case of congestive heart failure, in which both vascular and interstitial line patterns may be seen together. Further, a consolidation

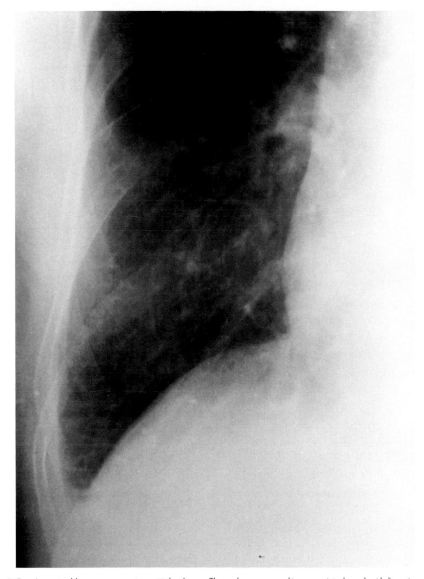

Figure 6-5. Interstitial linear pattern, interstitial edema. The pulmonary markings are interlaced with lines in every other direction (reticulations). The linear densities in the costophrenic angles are typical septal (Kerley B) lines.

may obscure interstitial lines because a lack of air within the air spaces prevents our visualizing the abnormal lines.

INTERSTITIAL NODULES

Many descriptions of abnormal pulmonary patterns include *nodules* as a distinct category among the patterns. Since nodules may be caused by a wide variety of different mechanisms

TABLE 6-4. PRINCIPAL CAUSES OF INTERSTITIAL LINES

"Life Lines"

"L"   Lymphangitic Metastases

"I"   Inflammation, "Interstitial Pneumonitis"
      Infections, such as viral
      Allergies to drugs, organic dusts
      Vasculitis, such as lupus, rheumatoid
      Ideopathic
      Others

"F"   Fibrosis

"E"   Edema

of pulmonary disease, it is preferable to distinguish between small, sharp, numerous nodules and large, hazy, ill-defined, less numerous, and unevenly distributed nodules.

The small, sharp nodules are most likely to have originated within the interstices of the lung. They differ in appearance from interstitial lines because the lines represent diffuse interstitial thickening, while the nodules are seen when the thickening is discrete, particulate, or focal. Such nodules are shown in Figure 6-6. Large, hazy nodules may also originate in the interstitium but become ill-defined and enlarged as they affect air spaces or airways more directly.

The differential diagnosis of interstitial nodules is relatively brief and is out lined in Table 6-5. The forms of pneumoconiosis that produce such nodules are usually dust exposures which were obvious to the patient and can be confirmed by obtaining the relevent history. Absence of such history leaves us with a differential diagnosis of metastases and granulomas. As a general rule, the smaller, sharper, and more numerous the nodules appear, the more likely they are to be granulomas rather than metastases. The smallest and most numerous nodules constitute the miliary pattern, which is usually caused by tiny granulomas spread by the blood stream. In most cases, the differentiation of granulomas from metastases requires clinical correlation, and often biopsy.

AIRWAY PATTERNS

Patterns of abnormal airways represent the most complicated of the abnormal pulmonary patterns.[10] They also represent the pattern most often ignored in descriptions of abnormal lungs. The reason for this exclusion is probably related to the multiplicity of features attributable to abnormal airways and to the differences among airway patterns seen in obstruction of airways of different sizes. The size and shape of the abnormality visible is dictated by the size and location of the obstructed airway.

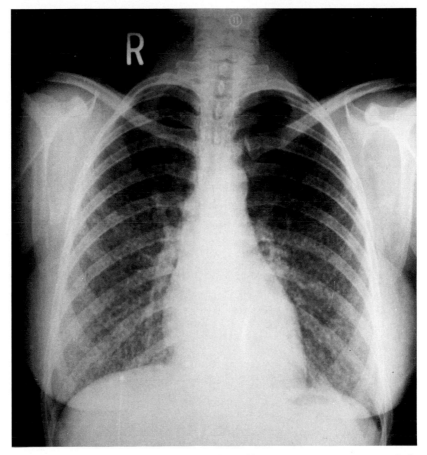

Figure 6-6.   Diffuse interstitial nodules of leiomyomatosis. The nodules are too numerous to count, small, sharply demarcated when they are not overlapping, and evenly distributed. They are typical of interstitial nodules that could be granulomatous or metastatic, if not pneumoconiosis.

TABLE 6-5. PRINCIPAL CAUSES OF INTERSTITIAL NODULES

Metastases
  Hematogenous Spread

Granulomas
  Infectious
  Noninfectious

Pneumoconiosis

If the airway is completely obstructed, the portion of the lung served by that airway tends to fill with secretions and thus increases in density. If the airway so obstructed is a large principal airway, such as a lobar bronchus, the entire portion of lung distal to the obstruction will either fill with secretions or collapse, since no air is entering or exiting from that portion of the lung. Thus, airway patterns include the typical appearance of collapse, as exemplified in Figure 6-7. Patterns of collapse superficially resemble consolidations but usually fail to demonstrate air bronchograms, since the airway is obstructed and does not usually fill with air. It is not always possible to distinguish the pattern of complete obstruction of a large airway from that of consolidation. This, for example, leads to the common problem of being unable to detect radiographically the difference between pneumonia and atelectasis.

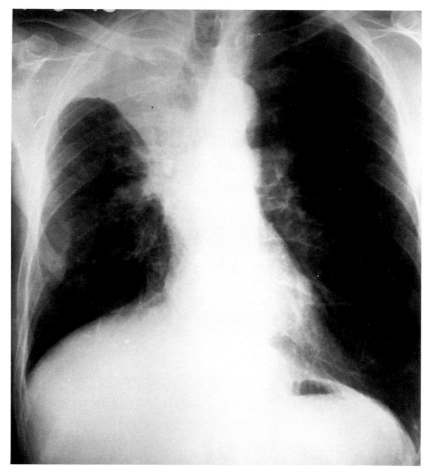

Figure 6-7.   Right upper lobe collapse. The density in the right upper lung field is produced by collapsed lung and thus resembles a consolidation without air bronchograms. Note that the mediastinum, especially the trachea, is deviated toward the density indicating volume loss in the adjacent lung, rather than a mass. The right hemidiaphragm is elevated and the overall volume of the right hemithorax is reduced. The secondary signs all aid in determining that this is a pattern of complete airway obstruction rather than alveolar consolidation.

TABLE 6-6. AIRWAY PATTERNS

Complete Obstruction — Densities
  Large Airways
    Collapse Patterns
  Small Airways
    Patchy Densities

Partial Obstruction — Lucencies
  Diffuse
    COPD
    Hyperexpansion
  Localized
    Cysts
    Bullae
    Pneumatoceles

Wall Thickening
  Bronchitis
  Bronchiectasis

If a bronchus is incompletely obstructed, the result is often air trapping (lucency) in the lung served by that airway. Bronchi are more narrow during expiration than inspiration, allowing air to enter distal air spaces but not to exit. Thus, airway patterns are often lucencies rather than densities and may be manifest as areas of localized air trapping or diffuse hyperexpansion of one or both lungs (Fig. 6-8). The most common disease producing hyperexpansion is chronic obstructive pulmonary disease (COPD). From a strictly pragmatic view, the radiographic finding most predictive of pulmonary function test obstructive findings is flattening of the hemidiaphragms, which is best visible on the lateral view. Other findings include increased height of lung fields, increased AP diameter, and relative increased spreading and decreased diameter of pulmonary vessels.[11]

The most complicated airway patterns result from partial or total obstruction of small airways, especially the bronchioles. When the bronchiole is completely obstructed the peripheral lung that is filled with secretions is relatively small and thus resembles a nodular density. Therefore, the appearance of small airway disease such as bronchiolitis is that of the large, hazy, ill-defined nodules mentioned above in distinction to interstitial nodules. The most common cause of such patchy, unsharp densities is small airway disease (Fig. 6-9). This pattern may also be produced by patchy consolidations. In general, the small airways are obstructed when such a pattern is visible, even though other abnormalities may also be present.

A useful generalization is that the inability to classify an abnormal pulmonary pattern as consolidative or interstitial often suggests that the abnormality is primarily that of small airway obstruction. The tendency of small airway disease to mimic and overlap with other patterns is one of the greatest sources of confusion in chest radiology.[10] It is the primary

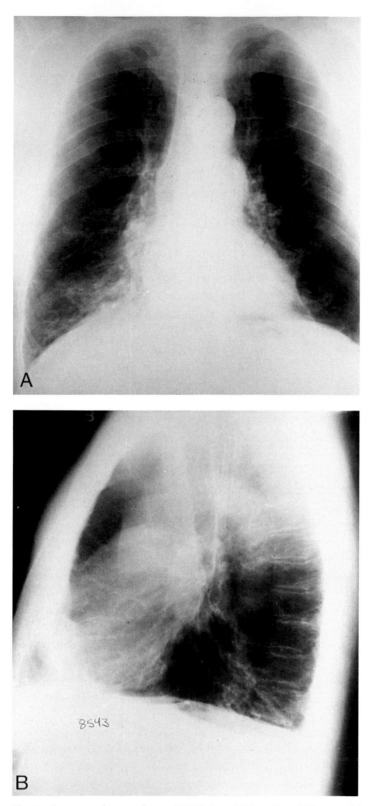

Figure 6-8. Chronic obstructive pulmonary disease (COPD). Frontal **(A)** and lateral **(B)** views of the chest show overexpansion of the lungs and, especially on the lateral views, flattening of the hemidiaphragms. The pulmonary arteries and heart are slightly enlarged, suggesting early pulmonary hypertension and cor pulmonale.

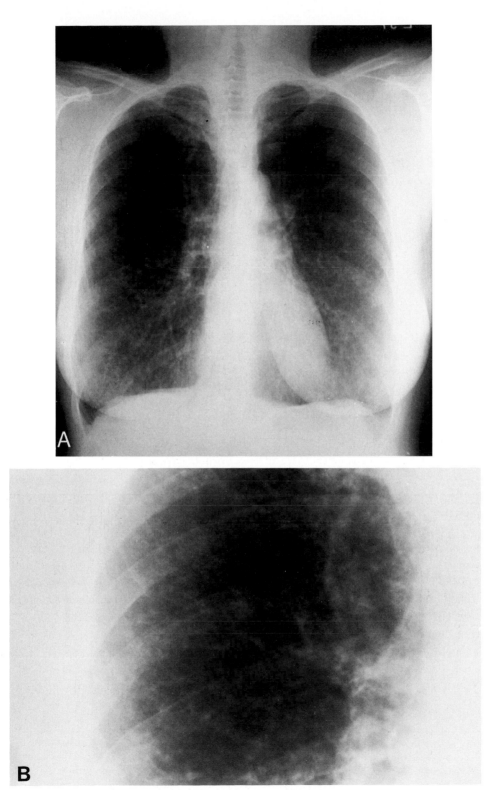

Figure 6-9. Small airway obstruction caused by bronchiolitis. Frontal **(A)** and close-up **(B)** views show small, irregular, and poorly defined nodules that usually represent obstruction of small airways. They are more likely to represent airway obstruction rather than focal interstitial abnormality.

TABLE 6-7. VASCULAR PATTERNS

Distention — Overcirculation, Increased Vascular Pressure
  Congestion
  Pulmonary Hypertension
    Arterial
    Venous
  Shunt Vascularity

Diminution — Undercirculation
  Thrombosis/Embolization
  Underdeveloped Circulation
  COPD

reason why, as noted above, many descriptions of abnormal films have ignored the vital role of abnormal airways in producing abnormal pulmonary patterns.

Airway wall thickening, as in chronic bronchitis or in bronchiectasis, may cause linear or circular densities in the lung fields. Such densities are oriented along bronchial pathways and may be double, parallel lines ("tram tracks").

VASCULAR PATTERNS

Pulmonary vessels are seen in direct proportion to the amount of blood they are carrying. Empty vessels are usually not visible at all because their walls are too thin to be resolved on a standard chest radiograph. Abnormal vascular pattern are thus attributable to distention of vessels (over-circulation) or diminution of vessels (under-circulation). The varieties are summarized in Table 6-7.

Over-circulation vascular patterns occur most commonly when the pulmonary vessels are congested by cardiac failure, renal failure, or simple over-hydration. The vessels in the upper lung fields distend more than those in the lower lung fields because they normally carry less blood, and because many upper lung field vessels are barely profused at all in the normal "resting state." As shown in Figure 6-10, the most common cause of accentuated vessels is congestion, but abnormal flow, such as that produced by the excess bloodflow of a left-to-right cardiac shunt, may cause the same basic pattern. Under-perfusion with diminution of vessels may be generalized as in severe COPD or localized when a specific vessel is obstructed, as by an embolus. Thus, vascular diminution may be quite similar in appearance to patterns of air trapping. In general, areas of diminished vessels have no discrete borders,

Figure 6-10. Vascular accentuation pattern of mild pulmonary congestion. Frontal **(A)** and lateral **(B)** views of a patient with cardiac disease show enlarged vessels in the upper lung fields on both views, as well as widening of the upper mediastinum on the frontal view ("widened vascular pedicle" of distended systemic veins). The increased blood flow in the upper lung field pulmonary veins is responsible for the large size and prominence of these structures in comparison with the normal appearance seen in Figure 6-1.

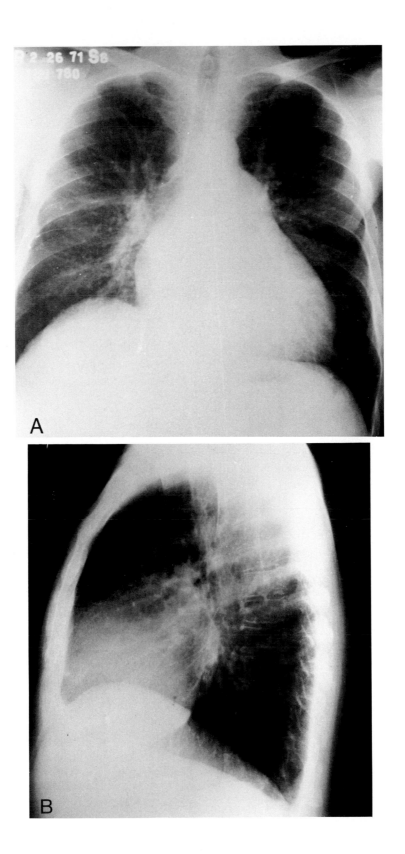

A

B

while bullous cavities and other areas of air trapping tend to have sharp, visible borders.

Patterns of abnormal vascular distribution include bronchial artery circulation in severe congenital heart disease. Far more commonly seen is pulmonary arterial hypertension with large central arteries and pruned peripheral arteries due to increased resistance in pulmonary arterioles.

Vascular patterns are thus relatively easy to recognize. Remember that abnormal vessel patterns are often seen in addition to other visible patterns, and they may aid the differential diagnosis by suggesting those specific causes, among the possibilities, in which abnormal blood flow is a part of the disease process.

APPEARANCE OF THE PLEURAL SPACE

Diseases of the pleural space are seen as pleural masses, nodularity, thickening, or fluid. Diffuse thickening and nodularity of the pleura, whether it involves the visceral pleura or the parietal pleura or both, is usually visible on any view of the chest, in the periphery just inside the ribs (Fig. 6-11). The lower portion of the lateral lung field is the area where diffuse pleural space thickening is most easily visible. Since the pleural space only has air on one side of it, all its abnormalities are less easily visible than abnormalities in the lung field that are completely surrounded by air in all projections.

It is often difficult, and sometimes impossible, to differentiate pleural abnormalities from those in the peripheral lung or in the chest wall. Secondary involvement of ribs and other bones in the chest wall, or of pulmonary markings in the lung fields, may be helpful but is not always definitive. Computed tomography presents the best imaging modality to define the specific location and extent of peripheral chest abnormalities, but it may also sometimes mislead. Generally, pleural lesions take the shape of the outer lung margin and are therefore elongated and often lenticulate; they are rarely spherical or cylindrical. Thus, pleural lesions tend to have a different shape in different views, including the standard frontal and lateral views of the chest. A lesion which appears of similar shape and diameter in all views is more likely to be located in the lung than the pleura. While violations of this rule occur, it is most useful in differentiating infections of lung, especially cavitary abscesses, from those of the pleural space, such as a fistula.

It is also not always possible to differentiate pleural fluid from solid pleural masses or thickening. Decubitus films are often helpful for seeing movement of fluid and verifying that the fluid may flow. Loculated fluid collections and those that are highly viscous may not flow at all. It is often useful to obtain a view with the affected side uppermost. This permits viewing the pleural space, adjacent chest wall, and adjacent lung field with the fluid that is mobile having moved to the dependent section of that hemithorax. This view is especially helpful for

---

Figure 6-11.   Left pleural effusion with loculation. Frontal **(A)** and right lateral decubitus **(B)** views of the chest show a large loculated fluid collection caused by highly viscous blood in the left pleural space. A previously unsuspected rib fracture is evident on the lateral view in the far periphery. A free-flowing effusion would have migrated toward the mediastinum on the decubitus view.

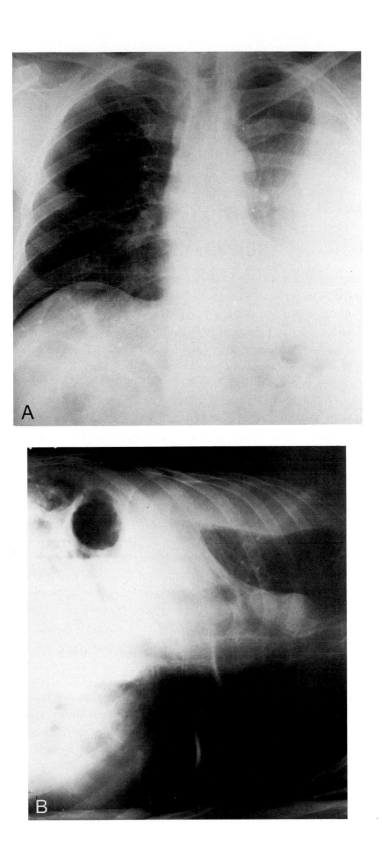

evaluating the possibility of a pulmonary consolidation, mass, or other abnormality that may be hidden by the fluid. It should not be attempted, however, if there is clinical evidence that exudate could spread to uninvolved areas of lung (see Fig. 6-11).

Truly solid pleural thickenings are usually inflammatory, traumatic, fibrotic (which may result from either of the other two), or malignant. The more nodular and irregular the pleural surface appears, the more likely the disease is to be malignant, but there are many exceptions to this rule. Always remember to look carefully for adjacent pulmonary abnormalities that may aid in choosing diagnostic possibilities.

APPEARANCE OF THE MEDIASTINUM

As explained above in the section on basic principles, mediastinal masses are only visible on plain films when they displace air-containing structures, namely the lungs or major airways. The presence of a mediastinal mass is often suspected on the basis of diffuse mediastinal widening or displacement of normal structures into abnormal positions. Thus, many mediastinal masses are difficult to detect or may cause no visible abnormality at all. Computed tomography of the mediastinum is far more sensitive than plain films for the detection of virtually all mediastinal abnormalities (Fig. 6-12).

Most mediastinal abnormalities are far less common than abnormalities of the lungs and pleural space. An exception is that lymph node enlargement in the mediastinum occurs frequently as a result of both malignant and inflammatory diseases, including infections. Hilar lymph node enlargement always suggests the possibility of mediastinal lymph node involvement, even if the mediastinum looks completely normal. Places where mediastinal lymph nodes are most easily visible include the small notch between the aortic and pulmonary artery protuberances on the left side of the mediastinum (a region sometimes called the aortico-pulmonary window), and the thin line that borders the right side of the trachea (the right paratracheal stripe). Nodularity of these two regions usually suggests diffuse lymph node enlargement; nodes in these two areas are most visible, as they are likely to displace lung as soon as they enlarge.

The most common mediastinal masses are listed in Table 6-8 by location and density as judged by computed tomography. More comprehensive lists are available elsewhere.[12]

APPEARANCE OF THE HEART AND PERICARDIUM

Abnormalities of the heart and pericardium consist principally of enlargement of all or part of their shadows. It is often impossible to differentiate abnormalities of these structures from those of other structures in the adjacent mediastinum or pleura. Diffuse cardiac enlargement is also indistinguishable from pericardial effusion. Ultrasound is far more specific than chest radiography for detection of pericardial effusions, and CT is excellent for depiction of all pericardial abnormalities.

The value of plain films in the diagnosis of cardiac abnormalities has decreased markedly in favor of other imaging modalities and laboratory procedures. In many cases, plain radiography in cardiac disease is useful primarily in showing calcification of coronary vessels, valves, and the myocardium, and in evaluating pulmonary blood flow. Since most diffuse cardiac abnormalities affect pulmonary venous or arterial pressures, or both, the presence of pulmonary vascular patterns is an essential part of the evaluation of any patient with known or suspected cardiac or pericardial disease.

APPEARANCE OF THE PERIPHERY

Chest films generally include suboptimal views of the soft tissues surrounding the chest and of the upper abdomen. The most important soft tissues to evaluate are those in the neck and upper chest, since abnormalities in this region are common, often associated with abnormalities elsewhere in the chest, and may be less clinically obvious than lesions in the soft tissues

TABLE 6-8. COMMON MEDIASTINAL MASSES — CT DENSITIES

	FAT	WATER/ FLUID	SOFT TISSUE	VASCULAR	MINERAL
ANTERIOR	Lipoma	Cystic masses	Thymic lesions	Anomalies	Benign lymph nodes
			Teratoid lesions		
			Lymphomas		
ANTERIOR DIAPHRAGM		Pericardial cysts			
DIAPHRAGM		Pancreatic pseudocyst	Hiatal hernia		
SUPERIOR			Thyroid masses	Anomalies	Thyroid masses
MIDDLE	Lipoma	Cysts	Esophageal masses		Benign lymph nodes
			Lymph nodes		Vessels
POSTERIOR			Neurogenic tumors	Dissection Aneurysm	Vessels
DIFFUSE	Lipomatosis		Sclerosing mediastinitis		

elsewhere or in the abdomen (Fig. 6-13). Particular attention should always be directed toward the airway in the neck, as compromise or deviation is a common cause of symptoms of pulmonary disease.

Subdiaphragmatic abnormalities suspected or clearly visible should be further evaluated for the possible presence of visceral obstruction, such as bowel dilatation, and for displacement that might suggest the presence of an enlarged organ or mass. Films specific to the abdomen should always be requested when the gas pattern at the bottom of the chest film appears abnormal. Abdomen films also provide increased penetration of the bases of the lungs, particularly the portion behind the diaphragms. With standard chest x-ray technique,

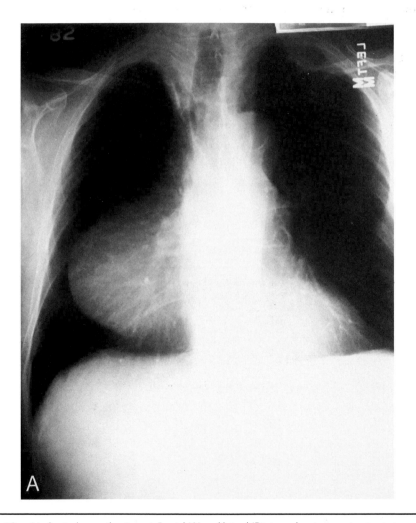

Figure 6-12.   Mediastinal mass; thymic cyst. Frontal **(A)** and lateral **(B)** views showing prominent anterior mediastinal mass, markedly displacing the right lung. A CT scan **(C)** through the lesion shows its density to be greater than that of the fat in the chest wall but less than that of the muscles and mediastinal blood vessels. This indicates that the lesion is filled with fluid, a finding that cannot be determined by the plain films.

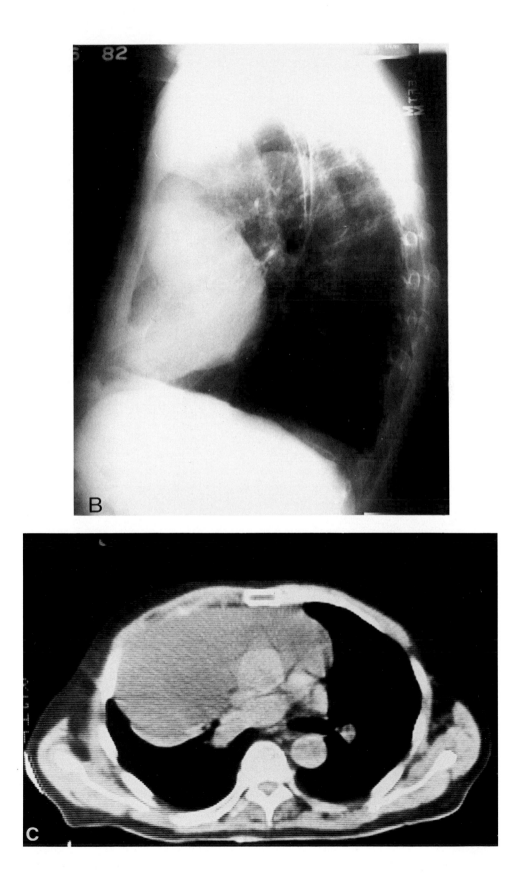

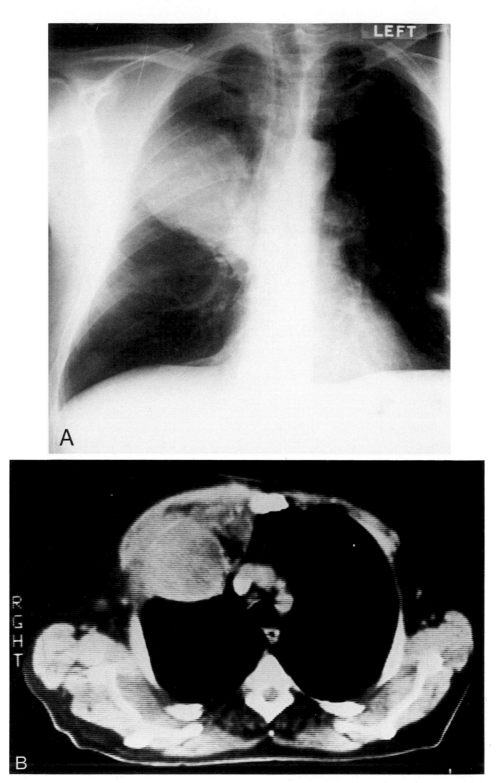

Figure 6-13. Mass in lung, a bronchogenic carcinoma, with direct spread to the anterior chest wall. The frontal view of the chest **(A)** does not clearly show chest wall invasion, although the anterior third rib is not visible (a very subtle finding). The chest wall invasion is obvious with use of CT **(B)**, confirming rib destruction as well as soft tissue invasion.

the filtering of the x-ray beam by the upper abdomen may conceal masses and infiltrates that would be visible elsewhere in the lungs. While lateral chest films usually show abnormalities in the lowest lung fields, a view of the lower chest on a standard abdominal film will usually demonstrate the frontal view of the lower lung markings and any possible abnormalities in this area. It is often impossible to differentiate abnormalities of these structures from those of other structures in the adjacent mediastinum or pleura.

COST EFFECTIVENESS

A source of considerable controversy is the question of when to obtain plain chest films of asymptomatic patients. There is never a question of the necessity for frontal and lateral views of the chest in any patient who has symptoms of pulmonary disease whose disease is not fully diagnosed and understood. Admission, preoperative, and "routine" chest films are probably unnecessary in young individuals who have no history of chest disease, are not immune-compromised, and have never smoked. "Routine" chest films are probably worth obtaining in any individual who is at significant risk of bronchogenic carcinoma by virtue of a history of smoking, concurrent disease, or exposure to substances, such as asbestos, that are known to increase the incidence of chest malignancy.

Care should be taken not to repeat the chest films more often than necessary; the interval for reexamination must be based on the individual case. Follow-up examinations in patients with pneumonia are most important when there is a risk of malignancy, but they are often performed with excessive frequency merely to demonstrate improvement.

Any imaging procedure in the chest, including CT as well as initial or additional plain film studies, should only be performed when the results will be useful in altering clinical outcome. If you cannot reasonably conceive of how the results of the examination will change your treatment or further evaluation of the patient, you probably should not request the study.

SOME "TIPS" TO REMEMBER

1. Never ignore the lateral film. It usually provides the best view of the hila and is invaluable for confirmation of abnormalities, especially masses, suspected on the frontal view.
2. Be sure to use the film markers as a guide rather than the shape of the heart in placing the frontal views on the view box; pneumothoraces and abnormal inflation of lungs (as well as heart disease) can cause embarrassing errors when you mount the film backwards.
3. Don't forget to evaluate the periphery of the chest, whether you do it first or last.
4. If you are totally confused by a pulmonary pattern, it is probably an airway pattern.

5. Pulmonary embolism usually produces no specific abnormalities. It should be considered whenever clinically reasonable, regardless of the chest film findings.

6. There is no chest film that is incompatible with tuberculosis.

REFERENCES

1. Fleischner Society: Glossary of terms for thoracic radiology. Recommendations of the nomenclature committee. *AJR* 143:509–517, 1984.

2. Forrest JV, Feigin DS: *Essentials of Chest Radiology.* Philadelphia, W.B. Saunders Company, 1982.

3. Felson B: A new look at pattern recognition of diffuse pulmonary disease. *AJR* 133:183–189, 1979.

4. Rubin E, Weisbrod GL, Sanders DE: Pulmonary alveolar proteinosis. *Diagnostic Radiology* 135:35–41, 1980.

5. Berkman YM: The many facets of alveolar cell carcinoma of the lung. *Radiology* 92:793–798, 1969.

6. Reed JC, Madewell JE: The air bronchogram in interstitial disease of the lungs. *Radiology* 116(1):1–9, 1975.

7. Gaensler EA, Carrington CP, Coutu RE: Chronic interstitial pneumonia. *Clin Notes Respir Dis* 10(4):316, 1972.

8. Genereux GP: Pattern recognition in diffuse lung disease. A review of theory and practice. *Medical Radiography and Photography* 61(1–2):1–53, 1985.

9. Reed JC: *Chest Radiology: Patterns and Differential Diagnosis.* 2d ed. Chicago, Year Book Medical Publishers, 1981.

10. Friedman PJ: Radiology of the airways with emphasis on the small airways. *J Thorac Imag* 1(2):7–22, 1986.

11. Fraser RG: The radiologist and obstructive airway disease. Caldwell Lecture 1973. *AJR* 120:737–775, 1974.

12. Feigin DS, Padua EM: Mediastinal masses. A system for diagnosis based on computed tomography. *CT: The Journal of Comp Tomo* 10:11–21, 1986.

GASTROINTESTINAL RADIOLOGY

David J. Curtis

Any radiologic examination of the gastrointestinal tract begins with a history taken by the radiologist. The first question which the history determines to answer is *where?* The gastrointestinal tract begins with the lips and ends with the dentate line of the anus. Where is the most likely anatomic site along this tract which may best explain the symptoms of which the patient complains or which their laboratory data may suggest? The site of the problem may be approximated by the location of symptoms. The temporal relationship of factors affecting the principle symptoms may further localize the problem.

The second question which must be answered by the history is *what?* What is the most likely cause of the symptoms? Is it more likely to be a gastrointestinal transit problem (too fast or too slow), an absorptive/secretory problem, a structural problem affecting the integrity of the mucosa, a structural problem affecting the integrity of the lumen, or a mass within the parenchyma of a solid organ?

The third question which must be answered by the history and an assessment of the condition of the patient is *how?* How can we examine the appropriate portion of the anatomy in this patient with these symptoms which suggest our preconceived diagnosis?

THE HOWS OF THE IMAGING EXAMINATION

Since we cannot begin to discuss the appearances of different disease processes until we have determined what imaging procedures we will perform, we must first consider the imaging modalities available to us. The most important question to consider first is whether it is appropriate to perform any radiologic examination. If a radiologic examination will retard

113

definitive therapy, especially in a life-threatening situation, the most appropriate radiologic-examination may be none at all. An appropriate examination is one which will significantly alter or direct the intended therapy, not hinder it. An example of this situation is a penetrating wound of the abdomen. Exploratory surgery with its immediate therapeutic options will be indicated on clinical grounds, and radiologic examinations should be considered only when they will direct or possibly obviate the exploration, not delay it.

ANATOMY AND PATIENT POSITIONING

Once imaging has been concluded to be potentially useful, the first "how" decision to be determined is which imaging procedure would optimize the diagnostic considerations. The plain film constitutes the most basic gastrointestinal examination. Intrinsic gastrointestinal feces or air, periluminal and peritoneal fat, organ soft tissues, pathologic calcifications, and ingested metallic substances provide differential contrast which help identify normal anatomic and pathologic conditions.

Plain film examination of the oropharynx includes posteroanterior (PA) and lateral high kilovoltage views to accentuate the airway. The oral cavity, oropharynx, and laryngopharynx constitute the proximal swallowing tube. If a foreign body containing calcium or other radiopaque substance has been swallowed, a lower kilovoltage examination should be used to accentuate the ingested contrast.

The plain film examination of the esophagus should include a lateral chest view which evaluates the course of the retrotracheal and retrocardiac esophagus in an unobscured manner. A posteroanterior chest view, on the other hand, may elucidate intrathoracic abnormalities but usually doesn't add significant information about the esophageal bed, since the esophagus overlies the spine in this view.

The plain supine film of the abdomen should extend from the superior pubic ramus to the upper abdomen. If rectal disease is suspected, imaging even lower may be required. The abdominal cavity is anatomically defined by the diaphragm, the properitoneal fat lying within the peritoneum, and the pelvic floor which extends from the pubis to the coccyx. The liver is a homogeneous right upper quadrant (RUQ) soft tissue wedge extending from the costal flank and the diaphragm to the spine. The stomach fundus lies in the left costovertebral region immediately beneath the diaphragm, and the body of the stomach crosses the spine roughly paralleling the liver edge. The antrum empties into the duodenal bulb in the right costovertebral region. Lateral to the gastric fundus is the reniform splenic soft tissue. The spleen is of variable size and normally positioned in the left subphrenic costal flank.

The small bowel normally lies uniformly contained within the colonic borders in most individuals. The small bowel is usually gasless in the adult, while the normal colon contains varied amounts of feces and gas, outlining the infrahepatic, infragastric, and infrasplenic abdomen. The first portion of the colon, the cecum, overlies the right iliac wing. The cecum opens superiorly into the retroperitoneal flank-hugging ascending colon. A mediosuperior bend along the liver edge which extends from the inferolateral liver tip to the region of the liver hilum constitutes the hepatic flexure of the colon. The colon becomes intraperitoneal as the transverse colon, which drapes inferiorly from its proximally fixed portion adjacent to the gallbladder to its distally fixed portion adjacent to the splenic hilum. The splenic flexure constitutes the anteroposteriorly directed return of the colon into the retroperitoneum. The descending colon hugs the left flank and ends near the left sacroiliac joint. Here the colon becomes the mesenteric sigmoid segment which varies considerably in length from patient to patient. The termination of the sigmoid colon lies medial to and near its origin. The rectum is the midline retroperitoneal pelvic colon segment originating near the lumbosacral spinal transition.

The most commonly obtained second plain view of the abdomen is the erect view. This view includes the superior aspect of the diaphragm. Its purpose is to detect abdominal contents which are not altered in position or configuration from that noted on the supine film. Fixed organs (unchanged in position and configuration when compared to plain film) are a near-certain indication of pathology. Infradiaphragmatic gas free of the anatomic constraints of the gastric and colonic boundaries is indicative of a hollow gastrointestinal organ perforation, if history excludes prior surgical intervention. The presence of air/fluid levels of similar or different height are evidence of gas and liquid within the same loop of bowel. Other interpretations rely on bowel diameter and clinical history.

An erect chest view completes most "acute" abdominal series. Performed at higher kilovoltage than the abdominal views, it assures a second look at the diaphragm and allows evaluation of the thoracic cavity for evidence of disease which may mimic abdominal processes. For example, pneumonia may present with abdominal pain. Sympathetic effusions within the pleura may be found with intraabdominal processes such as ascites and pancreatitis.

Additional plain film options for imaging the abdomen include decubitus views. The decubitus most commonly utilized is the left, placing the patient's left side on the table and his right side up; the x-ray beam is parallel to the floor (horizontal rather than vertical). The left decubitus view allows air and gas to rise against the right flank and be imaged between the liver and the peritoneal surface of the abdomen. A decubitus view may be used to replace the erect view in more debilitated patients. The left decubitus view is preferable to the right for visualizing free peritoneal air, as there is more soft tissue (the liver) to contrast with the free air. The right decubitus view places the gas-filled descending colon against the left flank fat. Occasionally the descending colonic gas is difficult to distinguish from free intraperitoneal gas. However, the right decubitus view, which places the left-sided descending colon up, may be useful in determining the patency of the colonic lumen into the rectum in differentiating cases of adynamic ileus from obstruction (dynamic ileus).

In the prone position, the patient's rectum is superior, allowing assessment of distal colon lumen patency in the same manner as the right decubitus view. Individuals with significant abdominal distension caused by ascites or gas may not be able to assume this position. Similarly, individuals who have had recent abdominal surgery and still have drains in place may be unable to assume this position.

A right or left lateral view of the abdomen (vertical x-ray beam) may be useful in evaluating the anteroposterior position of an intraperitoneal mass or calcification. Similarly, these views may be useful occasionally in evaluating obstructions.

The pelvis is additionally imaged with a right lateral view which places the colonic gas in the descending, sigmoid, and rectal colonic segments. An angled prone view with the x-ray beam centered at S2 and perpendicular to the sacral body fills the rectosigmoid with gas and may assist in evaluating a distal sigmoid or rectal process.

Oblique views have limited usefulness in plain film evaluations of the abdomen. They may assist in determining the anteroposterior position of fine calcifications which may be invisible in true lateral views. A posteriorly positioned object appears to move away from the spine if the supine patient is turned away from the object of interest and toward the spine if the patient is turned toward the object. An object midway from the front to the back appears to move little or not at all. An anteriorly positioned object appears to move away from the spine if the patient is rolled toward the object and toward the spine if he is turned away from the object.

USE OF CONTRAST MATERIAL

Contrast material may be negative (air), isodense (water), or positive (iodine or barium). The choice of contrast is the second "how" question to be answered. The appropriateness of contrast use must be considered as it may interfere with some more definitive examination or worsen the patient's condition. Whenever contrast is considered, a plain film should be obtained to determine whether the natural contrast contained within the patient needs to be enhanced. There is no additional risk to the patient if enhancement of natural contrast is not required.

Air or gas can be introduced without significant risk to the patient if the means of introduction does not carry a risk (intubation, swallowing). Carbonated beverages and gas-forming powders can be swallowed with minimal risk in most individuals, and the rectum is intubated with minimal risk as well. Before gas or air is used, however, it must be determined that this form of contrast will answer the clinical question with a high degree of specificity. If the answer will not be provided with gas alone, positive contrast is indicated.

Positive contrast is of two basic types: solutions and suspensions. Solutions are almost uniformly iodinated benzene ring derivatives which are usually hypertonic. The isosmolar solutions are extremely expensive. The hypertonicity becomes hazardous to the patient if aspirated (large quantities may cause severe pulmonary edema), if used in small bowel obstructions (they stimulate peristalsis and may further distend bowel by drawing fluid into the bowel lumen), or if used in infants (they may cause dehydration). Dilution of iodinated contrast solutions lessens their density and may diminish their usefulness. Palatable solutions are expensive, and nasogastric intubation for delivery of less expensive intravenous solutions should be considered.

Barium suspensions of finely emulsified powders derive their tonicity from the solution with which they are mixed. Hence, isotonic saline solutions can produce isotonic barium suspensions instead of the hypotonic suspension created when tapwater is used. Barium suspensions maintain two advantages over iodine solutions: (1) they are more radiopaque, hence provide better contrast, and (2) they coat mucosal surfaces, hence give more mucosal detail.

Either positive contrast medium can be utilized to fill the bowel lumen, demonstrate patency, demonstrate lumen integrity, and demonstrate large growths or defects in mucosa. Barium, since it is particulate, will not be absorbed if extravasated. It is mildly fibrogenic and removed slowly or not at all by phagocytic action. Hence, barium is contraindicated if a large perforation is suspected, moreso in colonic (contaminated) perforations. Evidence of free gas within the peritoneum or peritonitis is a preexamination contraindication to barium. Iodinated contrast should be the first positive contrast used. If no extravasation is demonstrated, barium should be used to determine if a small perforation is present. Small controlled quantities of barium should be followed by larger quantities when aspiration or small bowel obstruction is considered. Colonic obstructions, or indeterminate colon-distal small bowel obstruction, should be evaluated by enema to assure that barium impactions do not occur in the colon proximal to an obstructing lesion.

Barium comes in multiple preparations in order to serve many purposes. All barium mixtures can be used to fill the bowel lumen; however, coating bariums are intended to be used in conjunction with air or gas as the lumen-filling medium. This double contrast method requires a lower kilovoltage evaluation than when a liquid barium solution is used to fill the lumen. Occasionally, a pasty barium mixture is used to evaluate the pharyngoesophagus. A 13mm barium tablet may be used to evaluate solid bolus transport in the pharyngoesophagus and to evaluate lumen diameter.

THE CHOICE OF EXAMINATION

The examination which will provide the most information at least risk and cost to the patient is the preferred examination. Bowel is most completely evaluated by barium examinations. Barium examinations are usually two-thirds the cost of CT or endoscopic examinations. Solid organs, extraluminal intraperitoneal processes, and known masses are best evaluated by CT. Usually, masses in children should be evaluated first by ultrasound. All studies ordered should be complementary, i.e., they should provide information not available by any other examination. More than one examination may be needed prior to arriving at a specific diagnosis and instituting definitive therapy.

CASE EXAMPLES OF GASTROINTESTINAL IMAGING

The following examples demonstrate the various imaging choices used to evaluate gastrointestinal symptoms in a variety of patients. Comments accompanying these illustrations refer to the basic principles described in the text of this chapter.

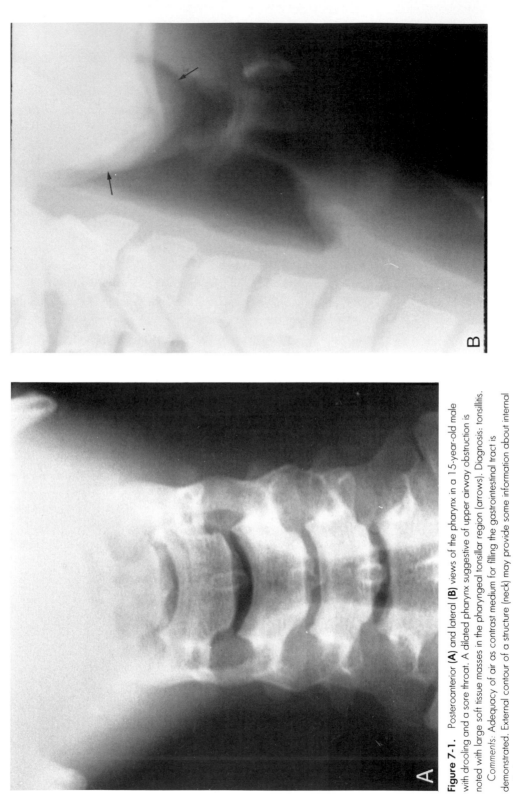

Figure 7-1. Posteroanterior (**A**) and lateral (**B**) views of the pharynx in a 15-year-old male with drooling and a sore throat. A dilated pharynx suggestive of upper airway obstruction is noted with large soft tissue masses in the pharyngeal tonsillar region (arrows). Diagnosis: tonsillitis.

Comments: Adequacy of air as contrast medium for filling the gastrointestinal tract is demonstrated. External contour of a structure (neck) may provide some information about internal pathology.

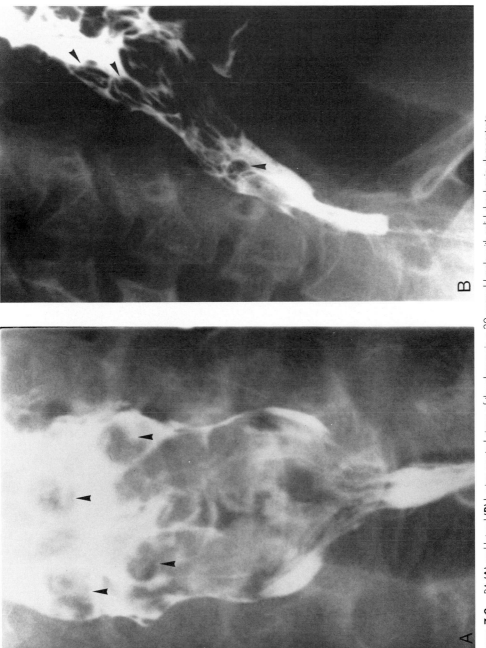

Figure 7-2. PA (**A**) and lateral (**B**) barium coated views of the pharynx in a 30-year-old male with solid dysphagia demonstrate haphazard mucosal pattern in much of the pharynx (arrowheads). A verrucous carcinoma of the pharynx was treated with total laryngectomy and jejunal interposition.

Comments: Pasty barium provides appropriate mucosal detail. This tumor would have been poorly detected radiologically without barium.

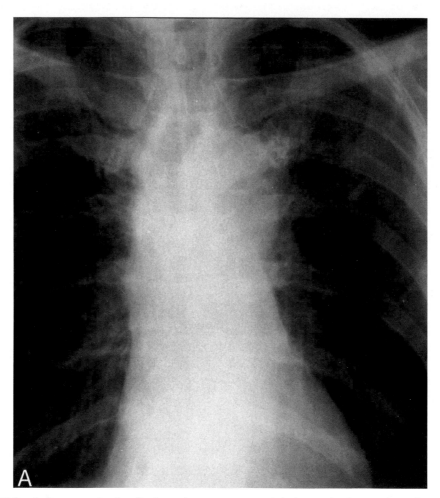

Figure 7-3.   A: Posteroanterior chest film shows changes consistent with the history of radiation to the mediastinum four months previously in a 68-year-old male with carcinoma of the esophagus. The changes include indistinct borders to the posterior mediastinum. The patient returns with dysphagia.

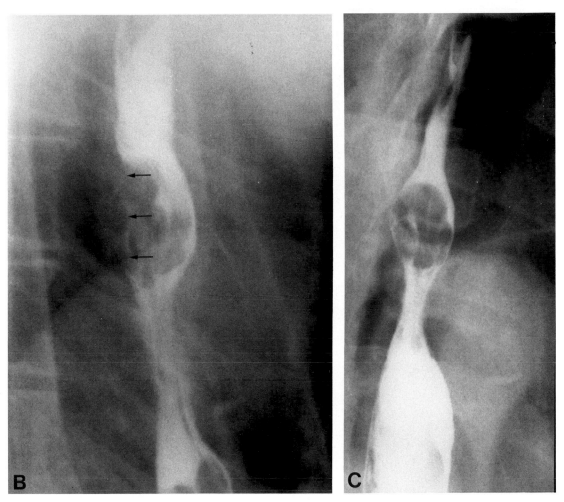

Figure 7-3.   B,C: Two views of a barium swallow obtained at 90° to each other show a nodular mass in the upper esophagus consistent with recurrent tumor mass.

Comments: Plain films provide the historic and anatomic context upon which basis the contrast films are interpreted. Two views 90° opposed are required to get information with three-dimensional characteristics. Since mural attachment is seen (B, arrows), this cannot be a swallowed object.

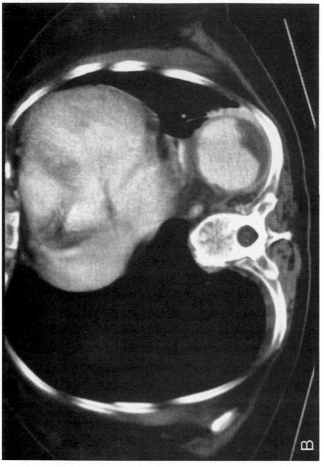

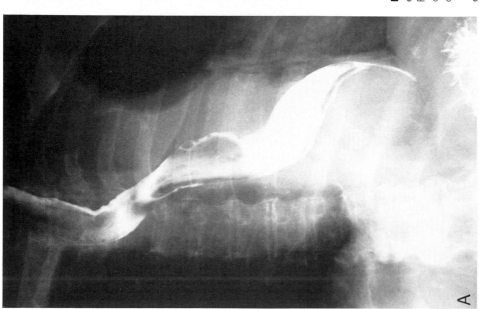

Figure 7-4. A: Barium swallow examination of an 83-year-old female experiencing dysphagia to solids. The esophagus is displaced laterally with narrowing of the distal lumen adjacent to an area of increased extraluminal density. Preliminary plain film examination of the chest showed left-sided mediastinal widening and cardiomegaly. **B,C,D:** A computed tomographic (CT) evaluation shows an aneurysmally dilated aorta with dissection of the lumen (arrowheads) displacing the esophagus (arrow). The acute onset of symptoms is probably due to the dissection.

Comment: The anatomic origin and physical nature of most masses affecting the gastrointestinal tract is usually best evaluated by CT if plain examination and routine barium examinations are not definitive.

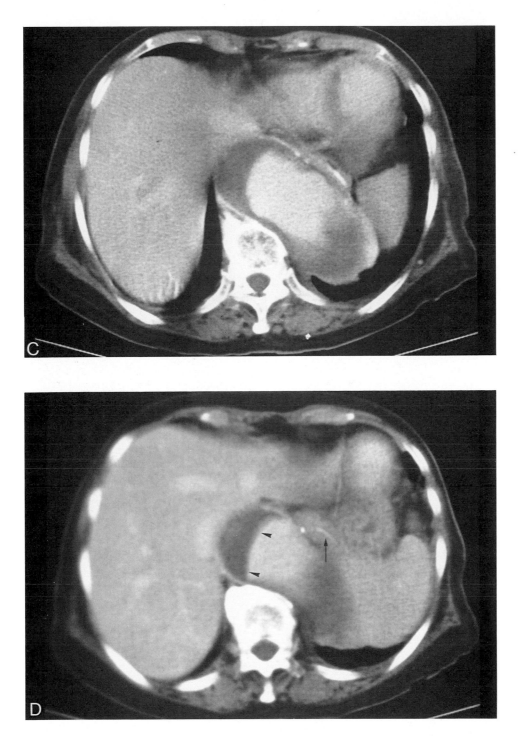

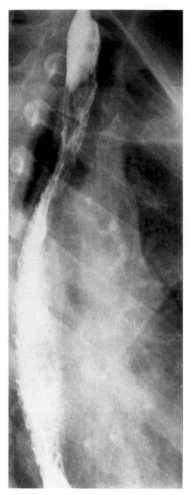

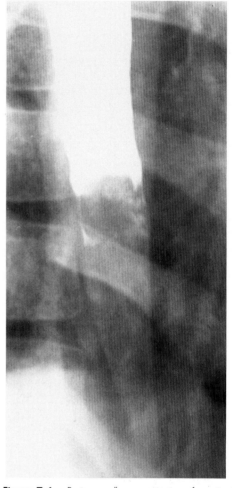

Figure 7-5. A 34-year-old male with AIDS complaining of dysphagia has a barium swallow which demonstrates narrowing of the esophagus and a nodular mucosal surface. Pain was experienced during the examination. Diagnosis: herpes esophagitis.

Comments: Gas-forming contrast media may create artifacts with similar appearances. Use of single contrast barium will exclude the possibility of such misinterpretation.

Figure 7-6. Barium swallow examination of a patient with sudden onset of chest discomfort following eating. An irregular obstructing mass is found. Diagnosis: meat impaction. A follow-up barium swallow exam or endoscopy will be required to rule out additional significant causative pathology such as tumor or stricture.

Comments: Carbonated beverages or gas-forming crystals will cure most distal impactions not associated with stricturing lesions, thus avoiding endoscopy. A foley catheter may be used in children or for more proximal obstructions in adults. The catheter is passed uninflated past the foreign object. The balloon is then inflated prior to pulling the catheter back out. Aspiration is to be avoided.

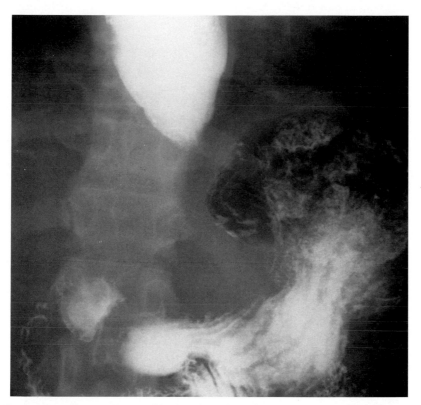

Figure 7-7. Barium swallow in a 22-year-old male with dysphagia shows a dilated debris-filled esophagus which empties incompletely and sporadically only in the erect position. No primary peristaltic wave was noted. The distal esophagus tapers symmetrically and smoothly in the region of the lower esophageal sphincter. These findings are consistent with achalasia.

   Comments: Motility is best evaluated by videotaping fluoroscopy. Much less fluoroscopic time is required to understand the nature of motility disturbances if several swallows are initially taped and independently reviewed. Dilatation of the esophagus is relative. The tracheal width accurately approximates the width of an average distended esophagus.

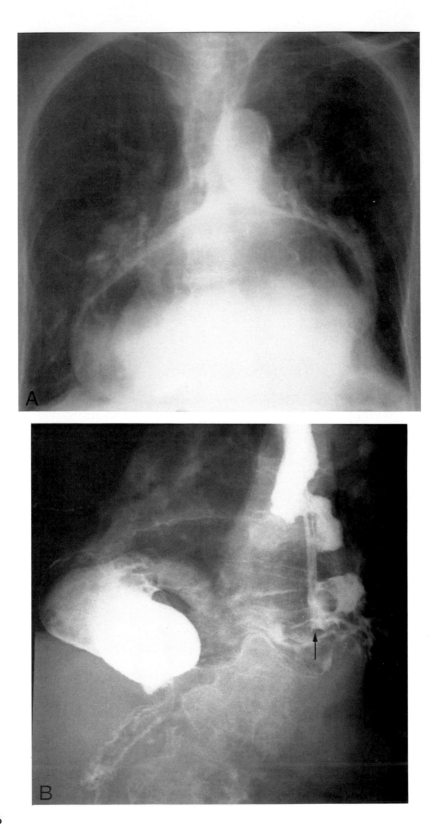

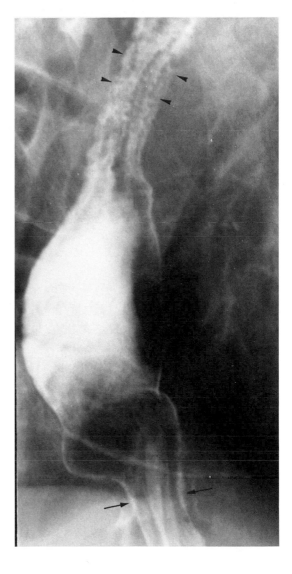

Figure 7-9. Barium swallow in a 72-year-old female with heartburn demonstrates gastric folds within a hiatal hernia above the diaphragm (arrows). Horizontal mucosal striations created by contractions of the longitudinally aligned muscularis mucosa are noted in the esophagus (arrowheads). This is called a "feline esophagus" since it resembles the structural ridges in the cat esophagus. This form of motility disturbance is suggestive of gastroesophageal reflux.

Comment: Gastroesophageal reflux is commonly observed during fluoroscopy. It is important to note its frequency, volume, and clearance.

Figure 7-8. **A:** A PA chest film in an 88-year-old female with chest pain. Air density is noted overlying the heart. A barium swallow followed an unsuccessful placement of a nasogastric tube. **B:** The barium demonstrates an intrathoracic stomach. The nasogastric tube is better positioned within the stomach (arrow). There was no obstruction to gastric emptying through the pylorus.

Comment: Occasionally, passage of tubes can be expedited by fluoroscopy; however, it is important to more fully elucidate bowel anatomy prior to any such attempt. Air may be sufficient contrast in these instances and should be considered prior to using positive contrast.

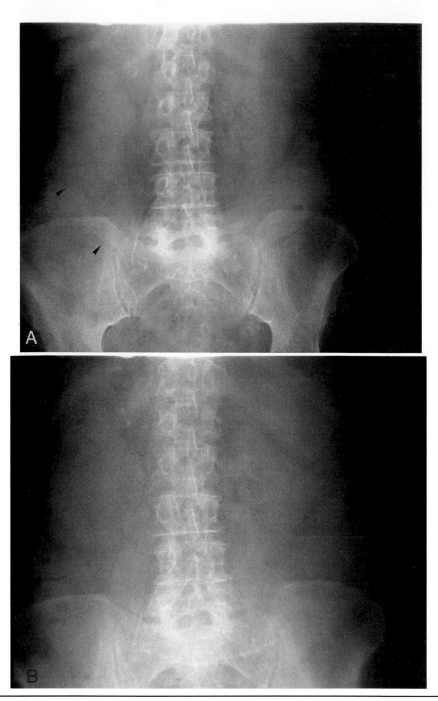

Figure 7-10. **A:** A plain film of the abdomen in a 73-year-old female with nausea and vomiting. This initial film is gasless except for minimal colon gas. An unusual arc-like border is noted over the right ilium (arrowheads). **B:** A film the following day shows still less gas within the abdomen, and the arc is seen lower on the ilium. **C:** Barium was given and outlines a stomach filling the abdomen. **D:** A right lateral view was obtained to allow the heavy barium to settle into the gastric antrum against the pylorus to determine its patency. A persistent collection of barium suggestive of an ulcer was noted on several spot films. A nasogastric tube was placed and 3000cc of greenish fluid was removed from the stomach in the fluoroscopy suite. No barium or air passed through the pylorus. Diagnosis: gastric outlet obstruction probably from ulcer disease.

A subsequent repeat barium examination was performed three days later, since endoscopy could not be scheduled sooner. Three antral and two duodenal ulcers were demonstrated.

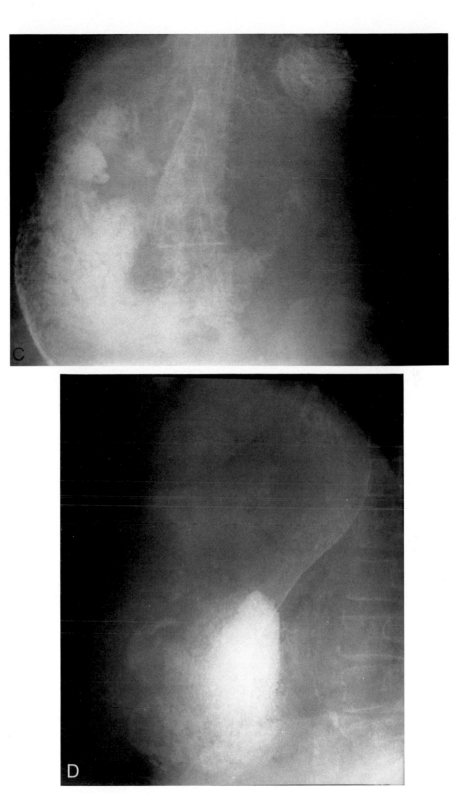

Figure 7-10. *Comments:* Barium is heavier than other fluids and can be directed by gravity even in adverse conditions like this. The information gained may be minimal but all that is required. Iodine solutions will be diluted and useless in situations such as this.

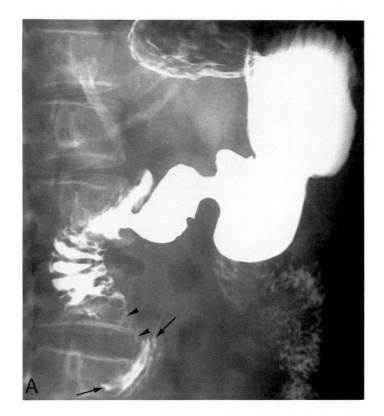

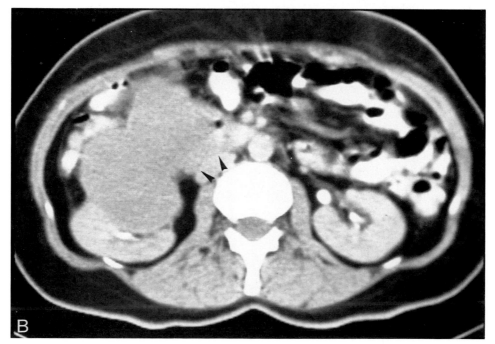

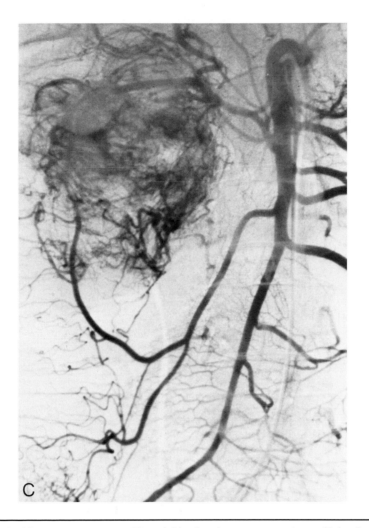

Figure 7-11.   A: A barium examination in a 50-year-old male with epigastric pain. A smoothly bordered eccentric narrowing of the descending duodenum (arrowheads) is seen with widening of the lumen distally (arrows). This is suggestive of a mural or extramural mass. **B:** CT examination shows compression of the right kidney by a mass which is discretely separate from the inferior vena cava (arrowheads). **C:** An angiogram showed no renal contribution to the tumor. Significant blood supply arises from the pancreaticoduodenal branch of the celiac axis, and a major contribution also comes from the right colic branch of the superior mesenteric artery. Diagnosis: a retroperitoneal leiomyosarcoma arising in the duodenum.

Comments: Angiography provides information useful in planning a surgical approach and may be most suggestive of the organ of origin. This work-up was entirely logical and appropriate in this mass affecting several organ systems and presenting with very nonspecific complaints.

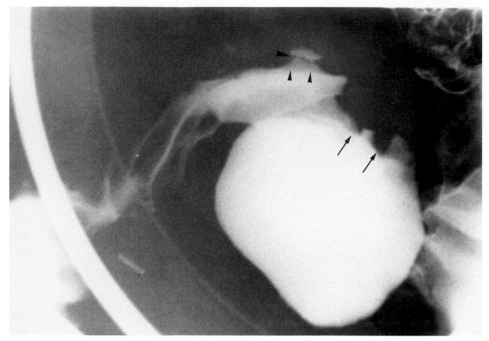

Figure 7-12. A barium examination of the duodenal bulb in a patient with epigastric pain. Two duodenal ulcers are seen with an ulcer collar (arrowheads), Hampton's mucosal line (large arrowhead), edema mound (arrows), and spasticity with adjacent fold thickening. Diagnosis: peptic ulcers.

Comments: Benign peptic ulcers are common and frequently found in the company of other ulcers, either within the prepyloric antrum or duodenal bulb (first portion of the duodenum).

Figure 7-13. **A:** Barium study in a 33-year-old Egyptian female seen for epigastric pain showing mild fold thickening within the stomach suggestive of gastritis. The proximal small bowel opacified as a part of the upper gastrointestinal examination was considered normal. **B:** A follow-up examination was performed because of vague persistent symptoms and demonstrated a normal stomach. Multiple smooth linear filling defects (arrows) were noted in the small bowel. The examination was continued to include the entire small bowel. Review of the previous study demonstrated the same findings (arrowheads). Diagnosis: unsuspected ascariasis.

Comments: All regions of the film may be pertinent to the patient's symptoms or of importance to the patient's welfare. Comparison with prior examinations may be the only way of confirming a diagnosis. Such review carries no risk. Barium will prevent adequate ova and parasite examinations for several weeks to months. However, two examinations showing the same problem should eliminate the need to further confirm the diagnosis and treatment can begin.

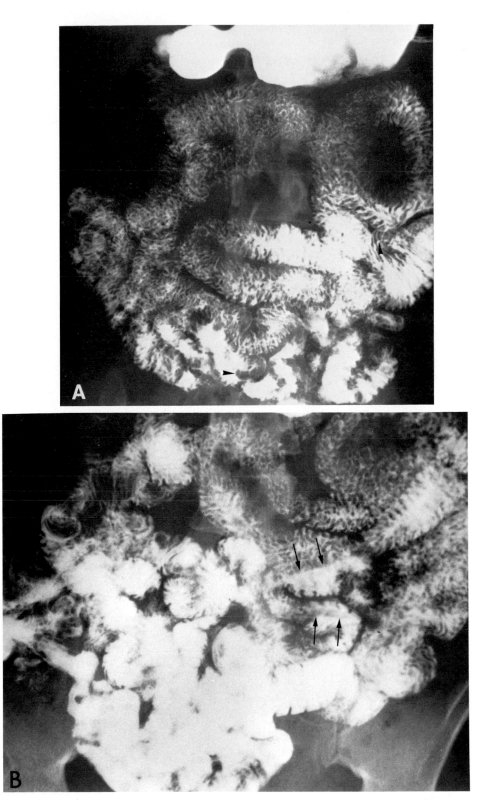

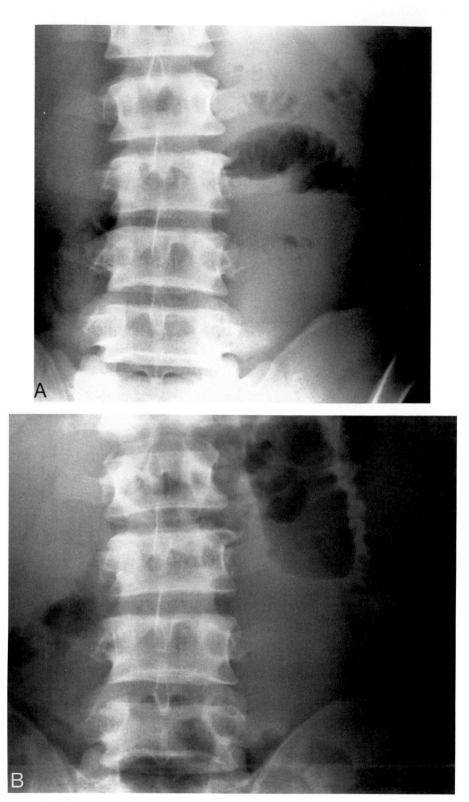

Figure 7-14. **A:** Plain film of the abdomen in a 17-year-old male with recent surgery for appendicitis, presently complaining of crampy abdominal pain. The initial film shows normal calibre left upper quadrant (LUQ) small bowel containing air and fluid which produce nonspecific fluid levels. **B:** One day later there is no significant change.

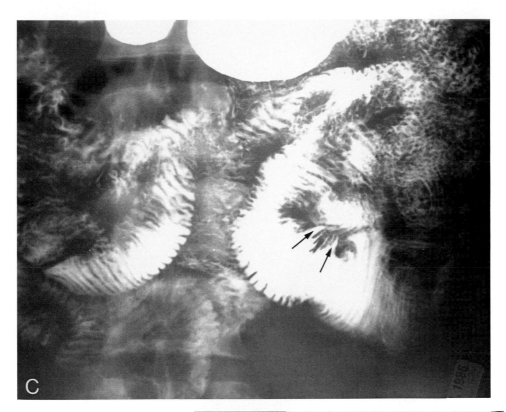

Figure 7-14 **C:** Two and three days from the initial examination the bowel lumen was unchanged in the same LUQ region despite a nasogastric tube being placed within the stomach. Feces and gas were still present in the rectal region. On the fourth day a barium study (C) demonstrates tethered loops of proximal jejunum (arrows). **D:** Dilated jejunal loops are found more distally, tapering to an eccentric point of obstruction which did not permit barium to pass overnight. Diagnosis: small bowel obstruction caused by adhesions.

Comments: Acceptable degrees of bowel distension may become unacceptable when compared and found to be unchanged from prior examinations. A small bowel enteroclysis (pumped in under pressure) would be hazardous in this situation.

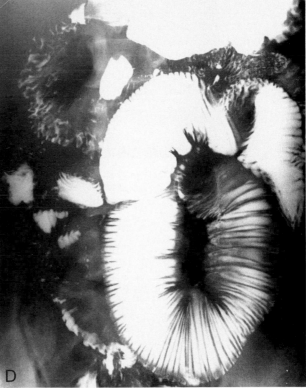

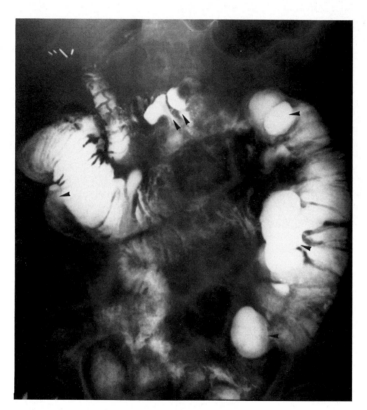

Figure 7-15.   A barium small bowel examination in an 82-year-old woman with diarrhea and macrocytic anemia. The small bowel is dilated. Large smooth outpouchings project from the bowel lumen filling with barium (arrowheads). The barium is diluted and forms clumps (flocculates). This is consistent with malabsorption caused by bacterial overgrowth in the large diverticula.

   Comment: Barium is the easiest means of evaluating the small bowel for malabsorption problems.

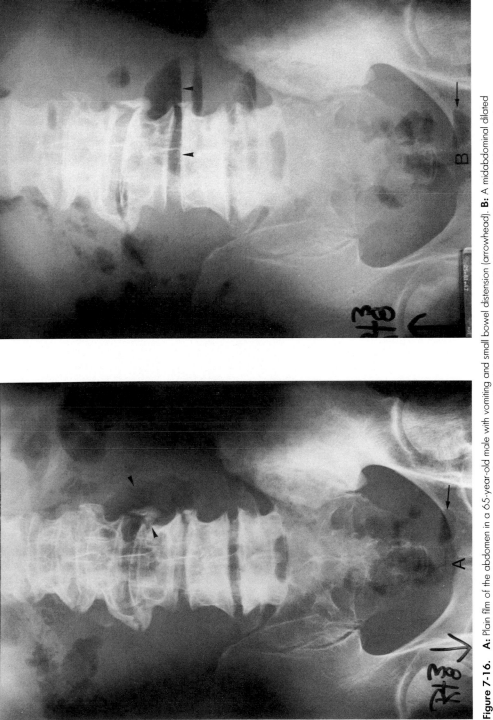

Figure 7-16. **A:** Plain film of the abdomen in a 65-year-old male with vomiting and small bowel distension (arrowhead). **B:** A midabdominal dilated fluid-filled loop appears smaller on the erect film since the fluid is one continuous level. Air is noted over the left pubic rami in the region of the inguinal canal on both films (arrows). Diagnosis: unsuspected strangulated left inguinal hernia.

Comment: Care in evaluating abdominal distension is mandatory. Searching the film for causes of the dilated bowel is the only way to detect the hernia.

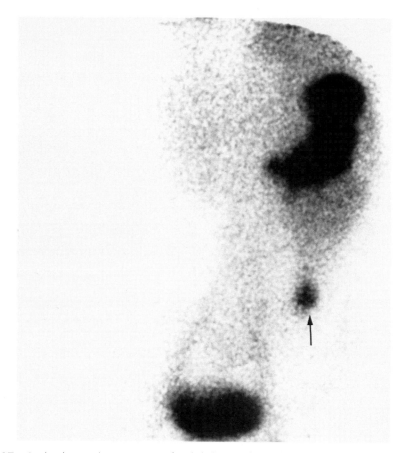

Figure 7-17.   Painless hematochezia in a young female led to a radionuclide scan with technetium (Tc^{99m}). The vascular phase of the scan was normal. Delayed imaging shows nuclide uptake in the left midabdomen below the region of gastric uptake (arrow). Diagnosis: Meckel's diverticulum with gastric mucosa.

   Comments: This scan is useful only if gastric mucosa is present. Gastric uptake must *not* be blocked with potassium perchlerate as it is for most technetium scans. The anatomic location of this Meckel's diverticulum is unusual. The scan is specific, however.

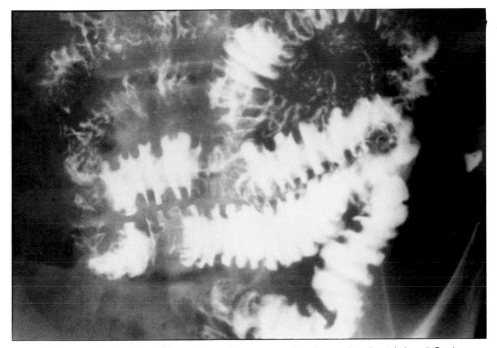

Figure 7-18. Barium examination of the small bowel in a young male with unexplained weight loss. Diffusely thickened and minimally nodular folds are demonstrated with no dilution of the intraluminal barium. Diagnosis: small bowel lymphoma.

Comment: Dilution of barium suggests secretory bowel problems. Its absence in this instance helps significantly in narrowing the differential diagnosis. A CT scan would be helpful to rule out adenopathy in the mesentery and retroperitoneum if palpable accessible disease were not present for biopsy.

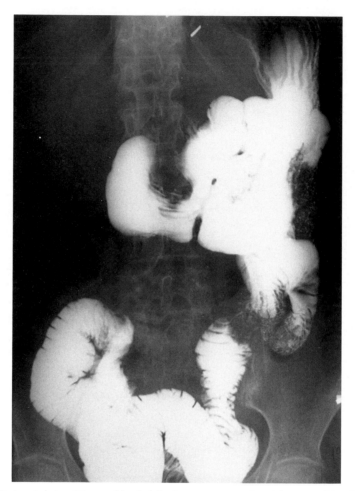

Figure 7-19.   Barium study in a 63-year-old male following gastrostomy with malabsorption. Dilated small bowel is plastered over the stomach consistent with the gastrostomy. Vagotomy clips are noted in the gastroesophageal region. The bowel dilatation extends further distally than might be expected from the vagotomy. No fold thickening is noted. The barium is not excessively diluted. Diagnosis: biopsy confirmed gluten enteropathy (nontropical sprue).

    Comments: Vagotomy generally does not produce secretory problems. It will cause bowel dilatation, however. The inconsistency of the extent of bowel dilatation with the prior vagotomy requires explanation; biopsy is the most efficient and direct approach to a definitive diagnosis.

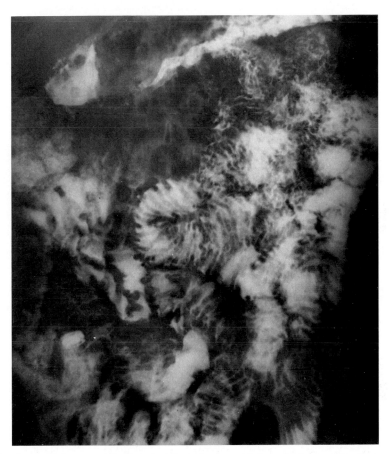

Figure 7-20.   Barium study in an adult male with abdominal pain, weight loss, diarrhea, and lymphadenopathy. The stomach and small bowel show diffuse fold thickening and nodularity with hyperactivity, evidenced by separation of barium into small aliquots. The barium is diluted consistent with hypersecretion. Diagnosis: biopsy showed PAS-positive, Sudan-negative macrophages consistent with Whipple's disease.

Comments: Fold thickening with nodularity and hypersecretion are important differential observations. Biopsy, again, is the most cost-effective next step.

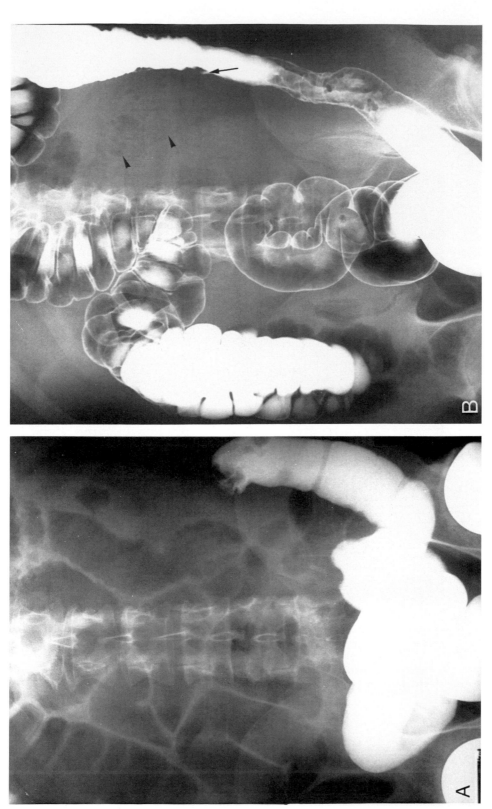

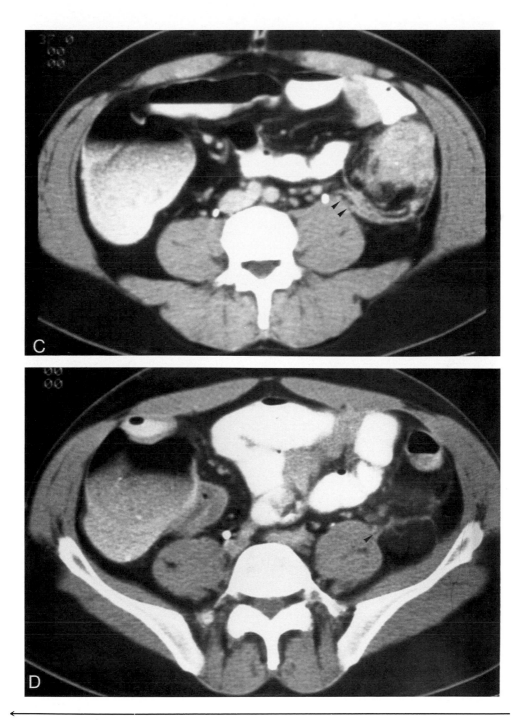

Figure 7-21. **A:** A single contrast barium examination in a 38-year-old male with distention and a history of Crohn's disease shows a complete obstruction to proximal flow of barium and dilatation of the gas-filled more proximal colon. The area of obstruction is finely irregular. Bilateral total hip replacements are seen. **B:** Films taken seven years previously show narrowing of the descending colon with linear ulcerations and an extraluminal sinus medial to the proximal descending colon in the region of the present obstruction (arrow). A mottled gas/soft tissue mass is noted medially as well (arrowheads). **C,D,E:** CT examination shows a retroperitoneal and mesenteric edematous change consistent with inflammatory disease (arrowheads). Diagnosis: total obstruction secondary to recurrent Crohn's disease.

143

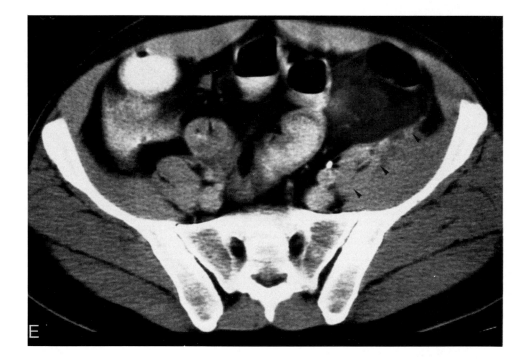

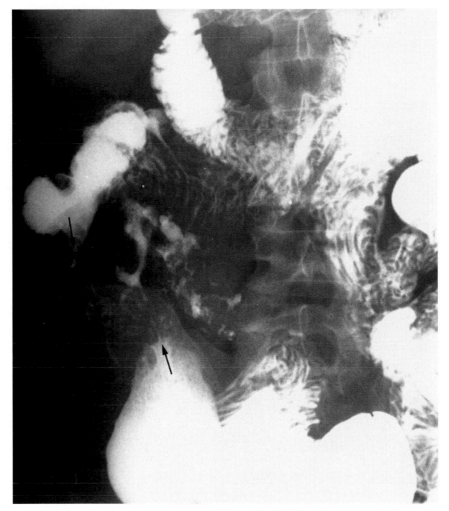

Figure 7-22.   Single contrast barium examination in a 47-year-old with Crohn's disease presenting with increasing crampy pain. A hemicolectomy 15 years previously had been asymptomatic. Diffuse fistulization and obstruction are present in the region of the ileocolostomy (arrows).

   Comment: Fistulae are poorly demonstrated with water-soluble contrast. Barium is required.

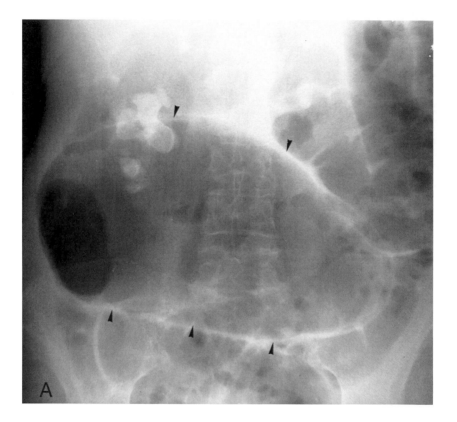

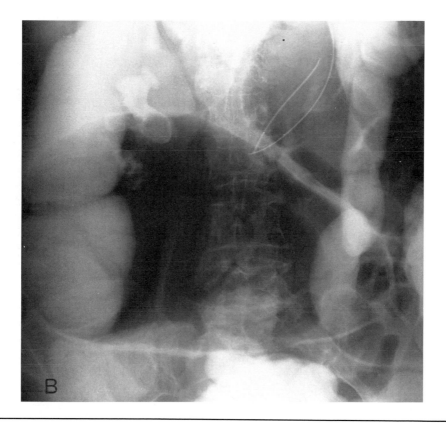

Figure 7-23. **A:** Plain abdominal examination in a 68-year-old female with known renal disease presenting with pain and increasing abdominal girth shows a 12cm midabdominal loop of bowel (arrowheads). Rectal and distal colonic gas are noted. **B:** A single contrast barium examination shows normal colon distal to the dilated gas-filled loop noted on plain film. Surgery was performed to decompress the dilated cecum. No obstruction was found. Diagnosis: Ogilvie's syndrome, or bascule, an ileus-like dilatation of the cecum in debilitated patients.

Comments: No contrast is needed in most patients. A left lateral decubitus positioning will frequently decompress these ceca. If there is no decompression in several hours, surgery may be necessary to avoid cecal rupture. Distension of the cecum is probably caused by the anterior position of the cecum relative to the ascending colon. This normal anatomic relationship and the inability of dilated bowel to push gas against gravity is accentuated by the patient's inability to change position because of pain or debility. The same inability to obtain patient position change is the only reason the cecum was not filled with barium. The left lateral position or semi-erect positioning during fluoroscopy should have been attempted.

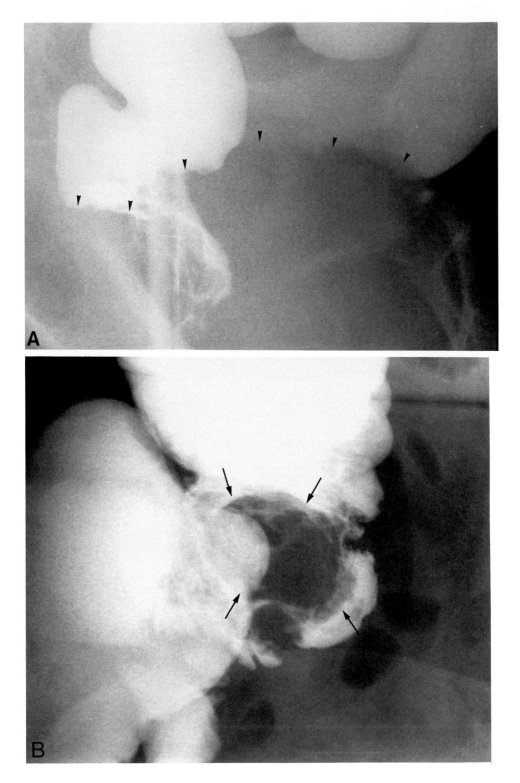

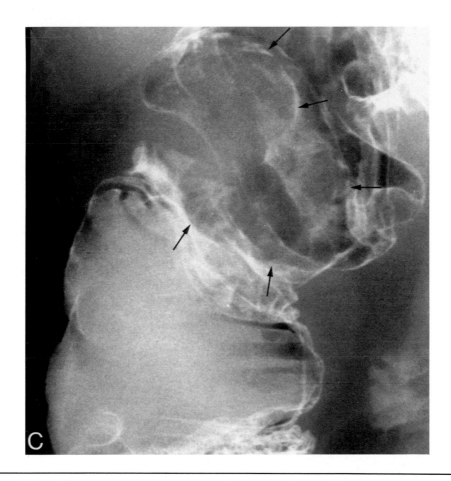

Figure 7-24. **A:** Barium and air contrast examination of the colon in a 66-year-old male with guaiac-positive stools shows a large rectal mass impinging on the bladder but obscured by the rectal tube (arrowheads). **B:** An ascending colon mass is well seen within the barium column (arrows). **C:** When outlined by air and coated with barium, the mass is somewhat more difficult to appreciate (arrows). Diagnosis: intraperitoneal spread of tumor to the pelvis from a colon mass.

Comments: The rectal tube may obscure rectal masses. Double contrast examinations must be examined closely to avoid missing large as well as small tumors. Tumors in the abdomen may spread transperitoneally as well as by direct, blood-borne, or lymphatic spread.

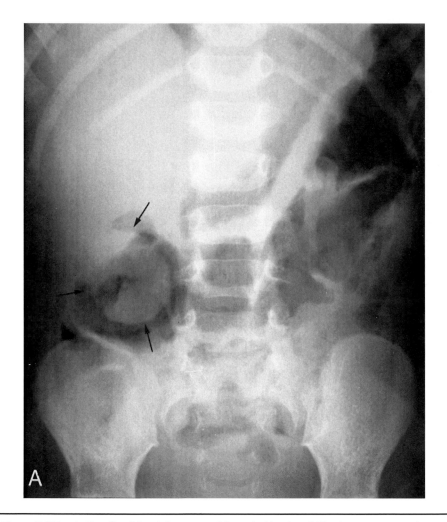

Figure 7-25.   A: Plain film of the abdomen in an 18-month-old male with bleeding per rectum and crampy abdominal pain shows an infrahepatic soft tissue density (arrows). **B:** Barium examination of the colon confirms the intraluminal nature of the density which could not be altered with time (arrows). Diagnosis: nonreducible intussusception.

Comments: The age of the patient frequently aids in determining the most likely diagnosis for a clinical presentation. Obstruction in a child between 6 months and 2 years of age is most likely caused by an idiopathic intussusception. A radiologic procedure is frequently therapeutic. If the intussusception had been reduced, it may not have recurred and surgery would have been avoided. Too vigorous an attempt at reduction, when symptoms have been present for over 12 hours may lead to perforation, however.

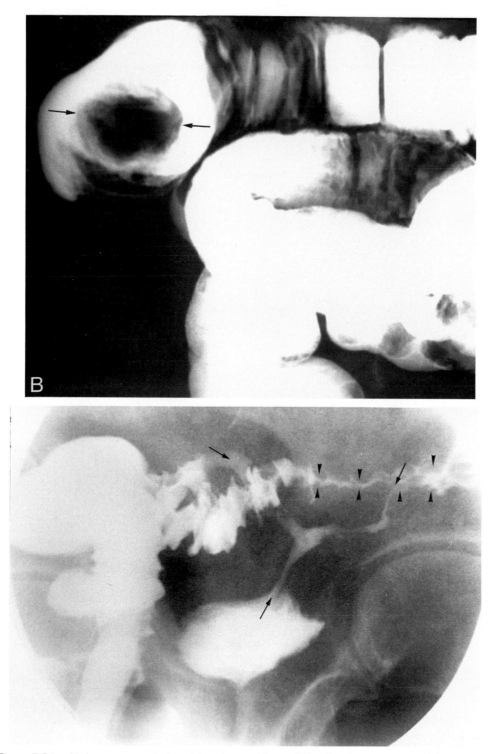

Figure 7-26. Single contrast examination of the colon in a 65-year-old female with pneumaturia and left lower quadrant pain demonstrates a fistulous tract from the sigmoid colon into the bladder (arrows). The adjacent sigmoid colon is narrowed as well (arrowheads). Diagnosis: diverticulitis with coloverical fistula.

Comments: Gas should be sought within the bladder. This study was performed as a surgical roadmap and to exclude tumor as the cause of the clinically apparent fistula. Occasionally the fistula will not fill. A retrograde cystogram would then be an appropriate examination.

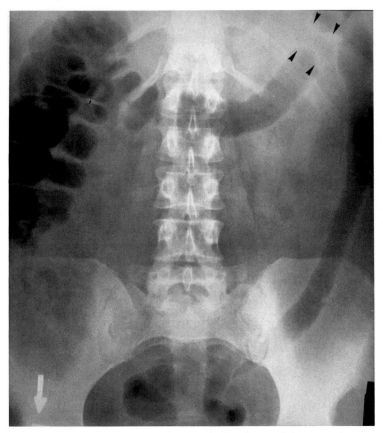

Figure 7-27.   Plain film of the abdomen in a young female with a long history of ulcerative colitis presenting with diarrhea shows narrowing and loss of normal colonic haustration from the mid-transverse colon distally. A soft tissue constriction of the colon in the splenic flexure region is consistent with carcinoma (arrowheads). (Courtesy of Anne Brower.)

    Comments: This is a plain film diagnostic examination. Barium examination will contribute nothing more. Biopsy is the next step.

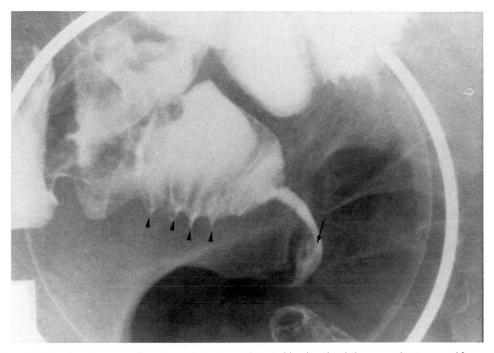

Figure 7-28.   A single contrast barium examination in a 43-year-old male with right lower quadrant pain and fever shows tethering of the base of the cecum (arrowheads) and incomplete filling of the appendix (arrow). These findings are consistent with acute appendicitis. Adenocarcinoma of the appendix with superimposed periappendiceal abscess was found at surgery.

Comments: The indication for surgery is clinical. The radiography is supportive. The clinical outcome is prospectively untenable because of the rarity of this tumor.

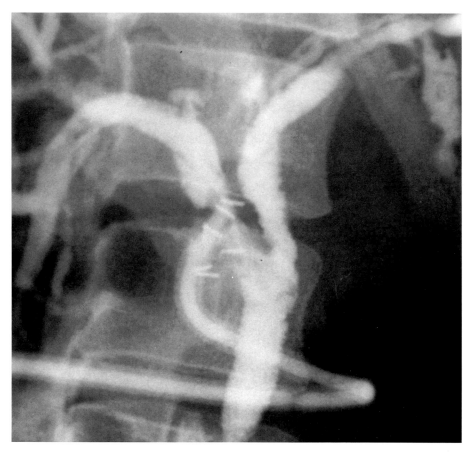

Figure 7-29.   T-tube cholangiogram using water soluble contrast demonstrates an irregularly narrowed biliary tree in a patient with AIDS and elevated bilirubin. Diagnosis: nocardia cholangitis.

Comments: Unusual diseases occur in AIDS. Infectious cholangitis cannot be radiologically separated from sclerosing cholangitis. In the context of AIDS, it should be suspected, however. The organism must be obtained by culture or biopsy.

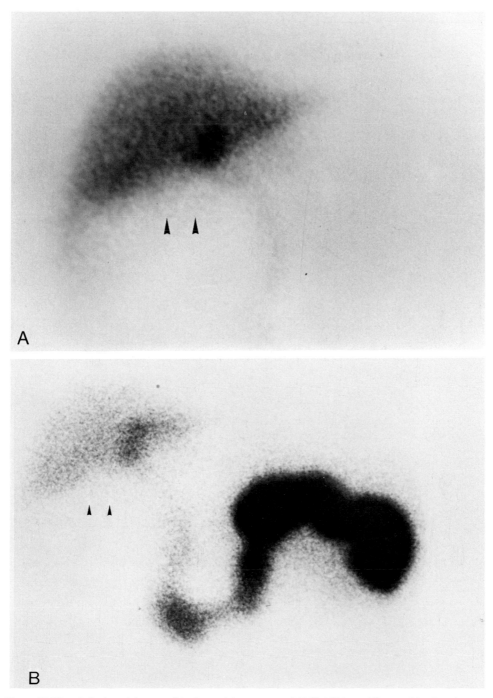

Figure 7-30.   **A:** Radionuclide scan of the hepatobiliary system with Tc^{99m} HIDA in a 72-year-old male with acute right upper quadrant pain and mild elevation of bilirubin. There is no activity in the gallbladder fossa through a 4-hour period (arrowheads). **B:** Hepatic activity steadily diminishes as small bowel activity increases. This is consistent with acute cholecystitis. (Arrowheads point to gallbladder fossa.)

   Comment: This is a classic presentation. However, on occasion, it may not represent acute cholecystitis.

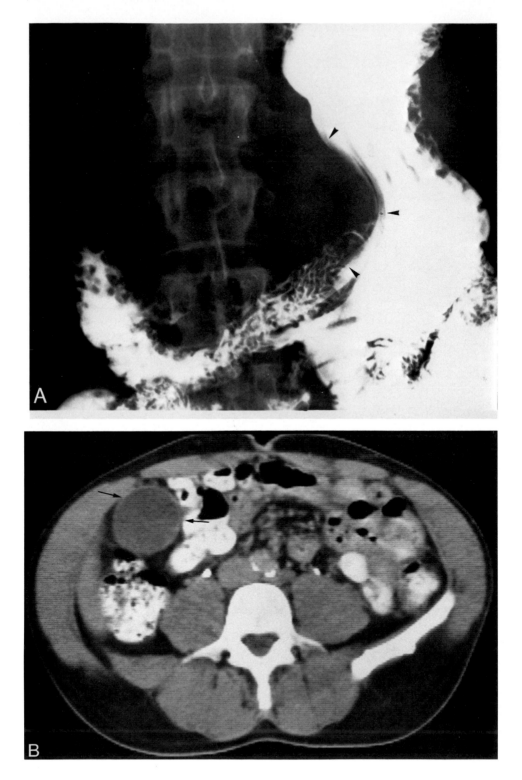

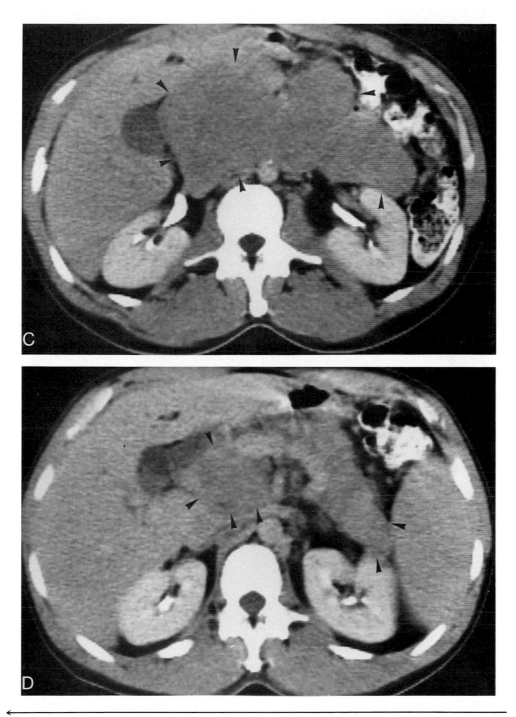

Figure 7-31. **A:** Barium study of the upper gastrointestinal system in a 47-year-old alcoholic with vague abdominal discomfort and weight loss suggests hepatic enlargement (arrowheads) and splenomegaly. **B:** CT scan of the pancreas to evaluate the cause of a mildly elevated bilirubin demonstrates an enlarged Courvoisier gallbladder (arrows) which is usually associated with carcinoma of the pancreas. **C,D:** Massive enlargement of the entire pancreas is noted (arrowheads).

Comments: The indiscernibility of a definite mass in the head of the pancreas is not unusual in carcinoma of the pancreas. Biopsy of the pancreas may also not confirm the diagnosis of carcinoma even when it is present.

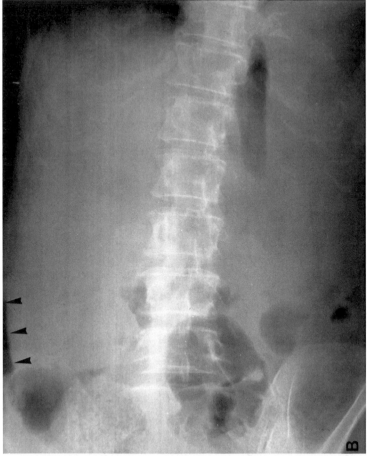

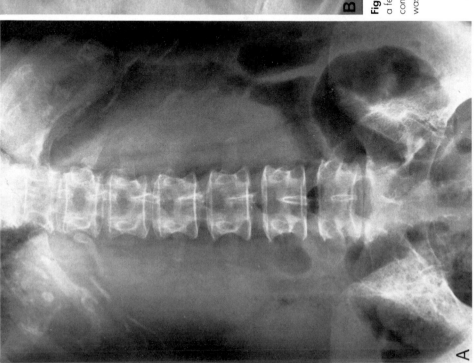

Figure 7-32. **A:** Plain abdominal film was unremarkable in a 62-year-old female on steroids who spiked a fever and developed abdominal distension. **B:** A left decubitus film was obtained because of the patient's condition. Not all of the right flank was imaged. A nonanatomic collection of gas overlying the right ilium was overlooked (arrowheads).

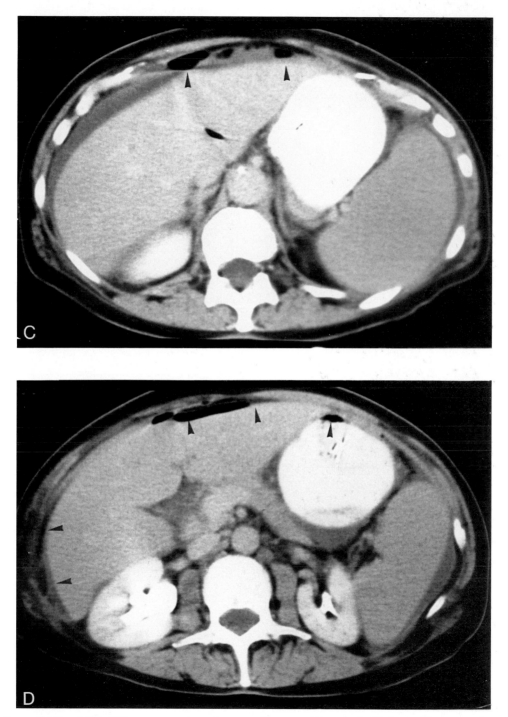

Figure 7-32. **C,D,E:** A CT scan was performed to pursue the cause of the patient's difficulties and demonstrated diffusely scattered pockets of free gas (arrowheads) within the abdomen responsible for the subtle mottling of the mid abdominal density just medial to the stomach on the plain film (see Fig. 7-32A).

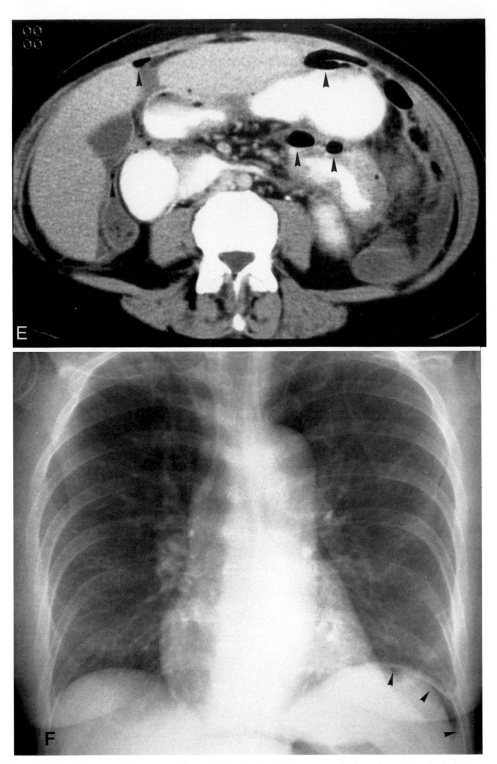

Figure 7-32. **F:** An erect chest x-ray performed following the CT demonstrated a laterally positioned subphrenic gas collection. Diagnosis: perforated steroid ulcer of the stomach.

Comment: Technical problems such as positioning may compromise a diagnosis. Each examination must be interpreted on its own merits. In this patient, prior abdominal disease has altered the usual localization of abdominal free air under the highest portion of the diaphragm.

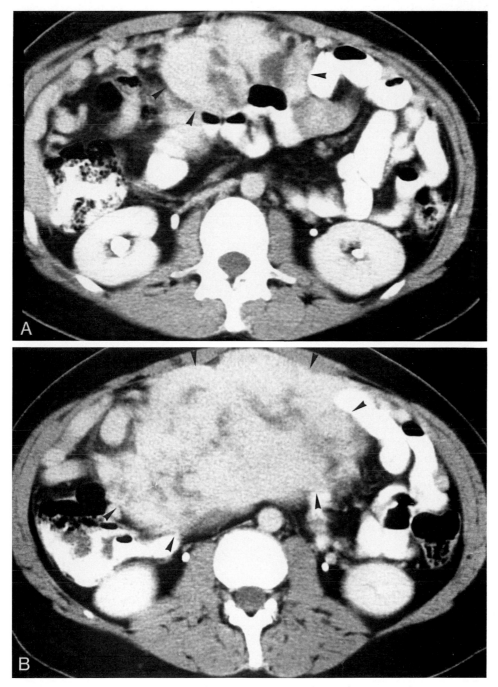

Figure 7-33. A,B,C,D: CT images of the abdomen in a woman with a history of increasing girth demonstrate a large abdominal mass (arrowheads).

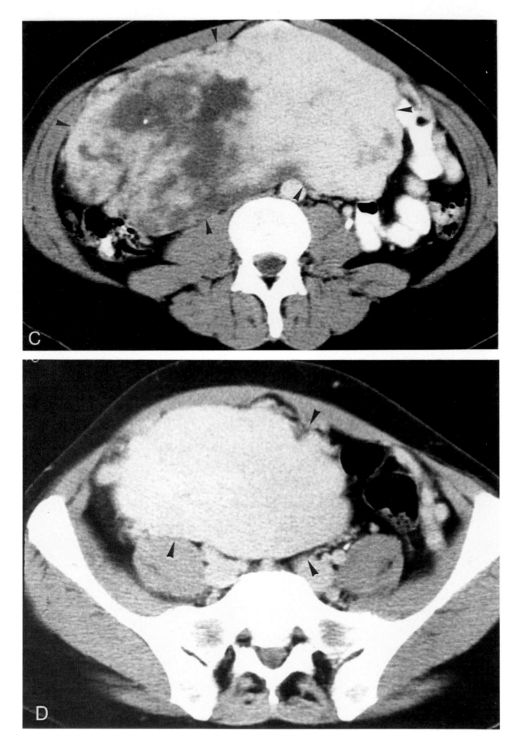

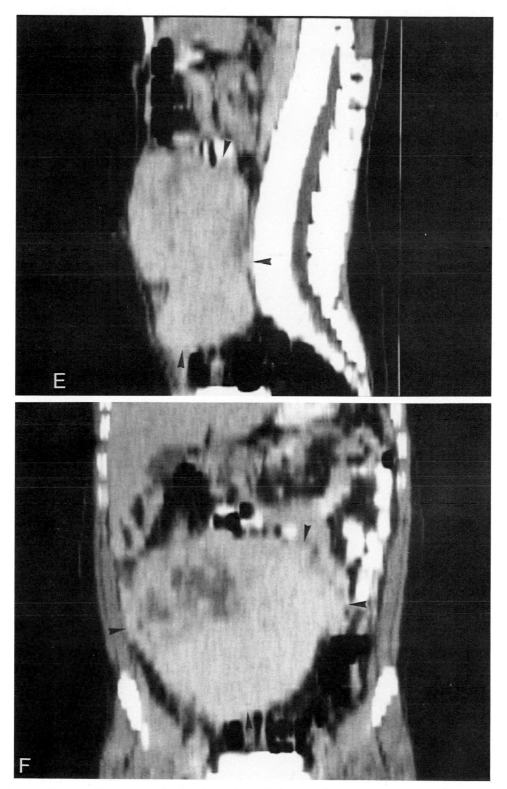

Figure 7-33.   E,F: The mass (arrowheads) is best understood when sagittal and coronal reconstructions are utilized. Diagnosis: omental cake metastasis of ovarian carcinoma.

Comment: CT provides the ability to reconstruct images into multiple planes of tomographic evaluation. This process makes the extent of disease, as seen here, more readily understandable.

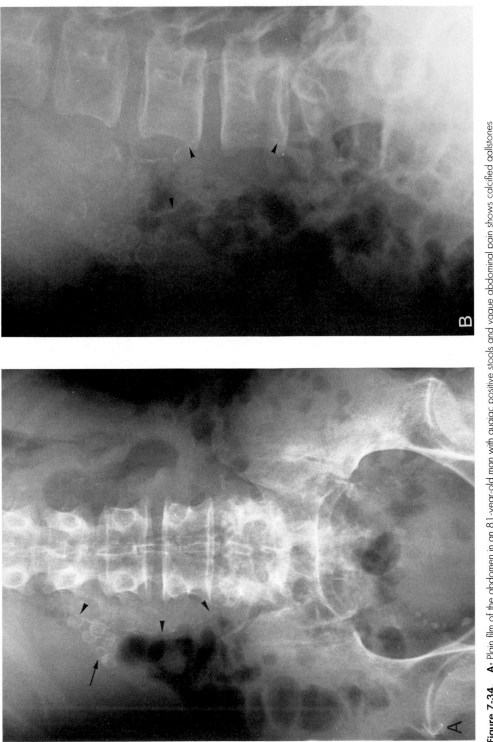

Figure 7-34. **A:** Plain film of the abdomen in an 81-year-old man with guaiac positive stools and vague abdominal pain shows calcified gallstones (arrow). Aortic calcifications are suggestive of an aneurysm (arrowheads). **B:** A lateral view was obtained to attempt to determine the aortic diameter and length of involvement. No calcification was present in this view, but a slight oblique off-lateral view demonstrated the 8×12cm aneurysm (arrowheads).

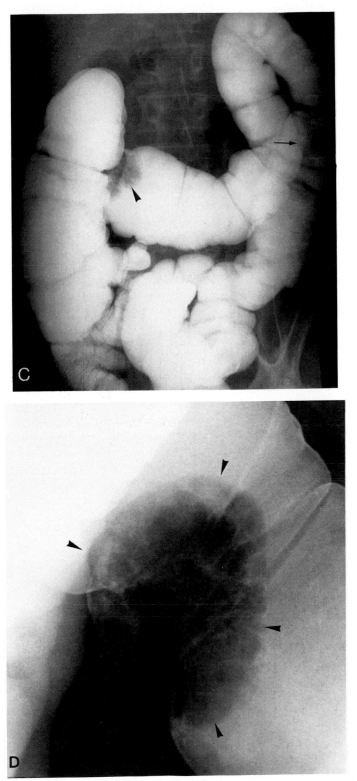

Figure 7-34. **C:** A single contrast barium enema to evaluate the patient for the guaiac positive stool found an 8cm villous tumor in the transverse colon (arrowhead) and a 2cm polyp on a stalk in the descending colon (arrow). **D:** Spot film of the villous adenoma (arrowheads) shows the barium extending deep into crevices, characteristic of this tumor.

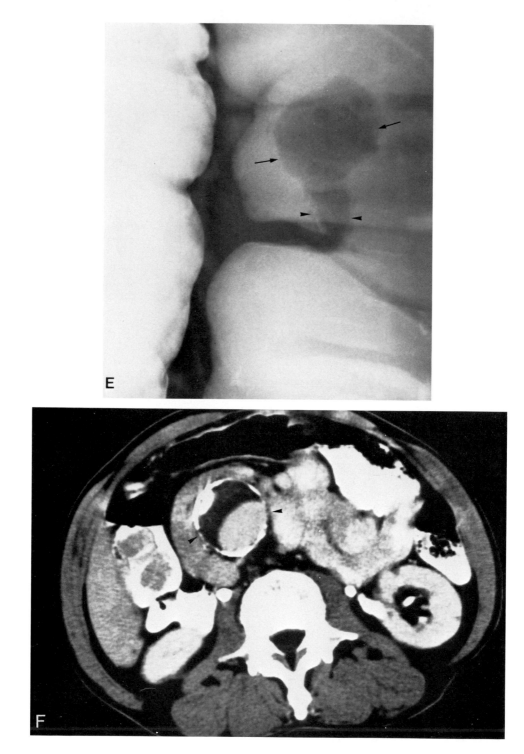

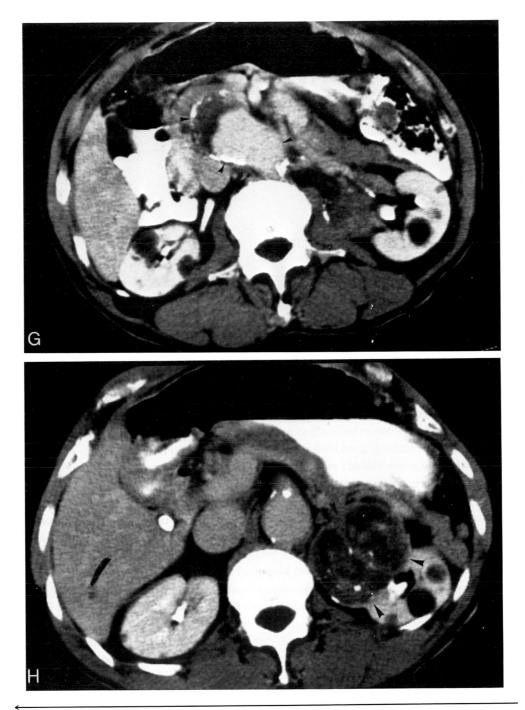

Figure 7-34. **E:** Spot film of the polyp (arrows) shows its stalk (arrowheads). **F,G,H:** CT of the abdomen to evaluate for liver metastases demonstrated the aortic aneurysm (arrowheads) and unsuspected carcinoma of the left kidney (arrowheads).

Comments: One diagnosis occasionally falls far short of the total clinical problem in a given patient. The most immediately lethal problem identified in this patient is the aneurysm. The aneurysm could be the cause of gastrointestinal bleeding; however, gastrointestinal evaluation is necessary to confirm this supposition.

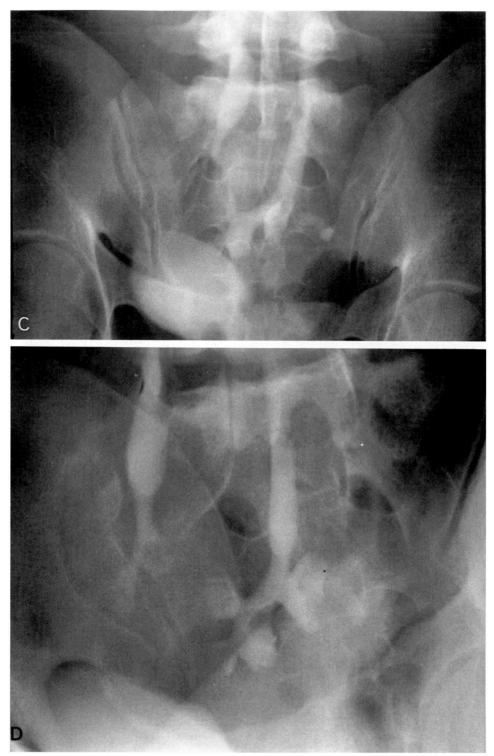

C

D

174

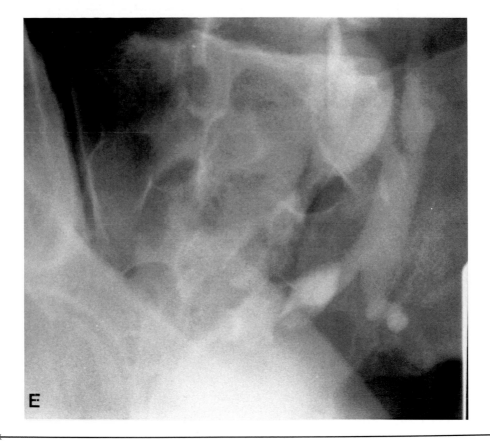

Figure 8-1. **C:** An angled view of the pelvis with the x-ray beam perpendicular to the sacrum and oblique views of the pelvis (see Figs. 8-1 D,E) demonstrate a pelvic fused kidney which is more susceptible to trauma because of its position across the spine. **D:** Inverted pyelocalyceal systems appear otherwise normal in the right posterior oblique (RPO) position. **E:** Both collecting systems are distorted by the left posterior oblique (LPO) positioning. Diagnosis: "pancake" kidney.

Comments: Fused kidneys usually are inferiorly positioned and malrotated. Multiple projections may be required to determine if other problems exist in such malformed kidneys.

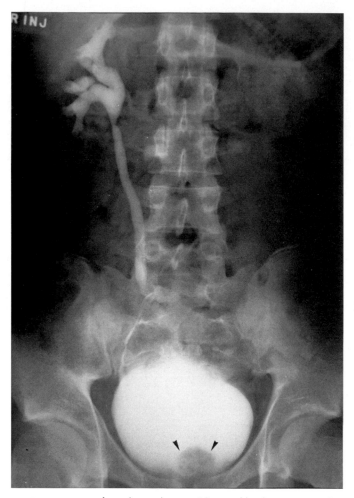

Figure 8-2.   An excretory urogram performed to evaluate an 18-year-old male presenting with urinary tract infection demonstrates only a right kidney. A filling defect of 1 cm size is observed in the left floor of the bladder (arrowheads). Agenesis of the left kidney is associated with seminal vesicle cyst in males and is frequently associated with unicornuate uterus in females.

   Comment: Ultrasound would further elucidate the nature of this filling defect.

Figure 8-3.   **A:** An excretory urogram in a 6-month-old child with a right upper quadrant mass, chronic urinary tract infections, and Klebsiella septicemia shows distortion, moderate obstruction, and anterolateral and inferior displacement of the right renal collecting systems (arrows). The bladder fills poorly (arrowheads). **B:** A lateral view shows a smooth mass within the bladder (arrowheads). Anteroinferior displacement of the right kidney is seen (arrows).

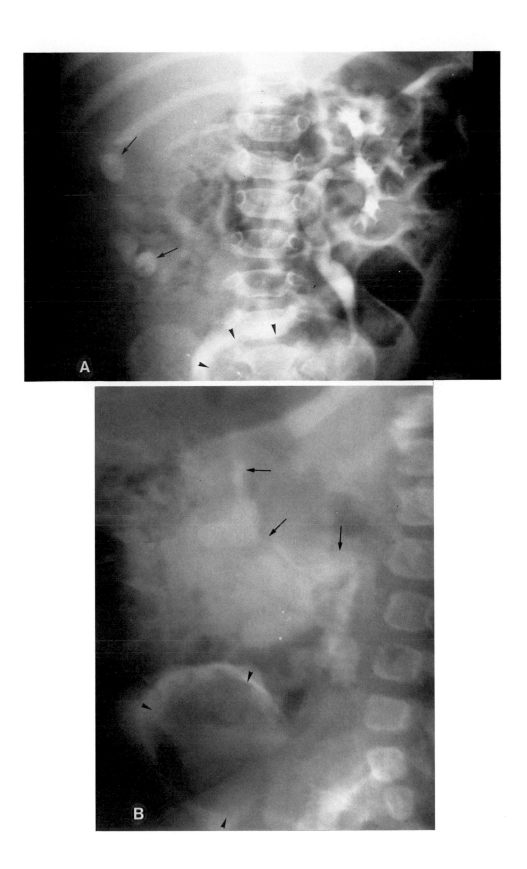

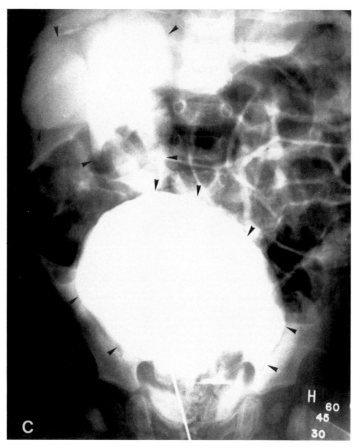

Figure 8-3.   C: A percutaneous cystostomy was performed with injection of a nonfunctioning dilated right upper pole infected ectopic ureterocele (arrowheads). Diagnosis: ectopic ureterocele with superinfection.

Comments: Normally an ultrasound study would be performed first to evaluate a pediatric abdominal mass. The lateral view helps determine mass effect on the right kidney and further elucidate the bladder mass.

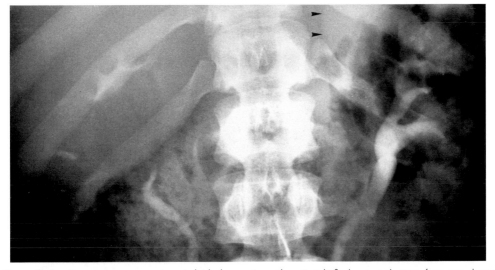

Figure 8-4.   An excretory urogram in an individual presenting with acute right flank pain and urinary frequency shows asymmetric distortion of the right collecting system compared with the normal distension on the left. An ill-defined renal margin on the right compared to the distinct left margin (arrowheads) and mild enlargement of the right kidney also suggest the diagnosis of acute pyelonephritis on the right.

Comments: The effacement of infundibula suggests mass (swollen renal parenchyma in this instance) within the kidney. Medullary fat will produce a similar effect, but its lesser density should be identifiable.

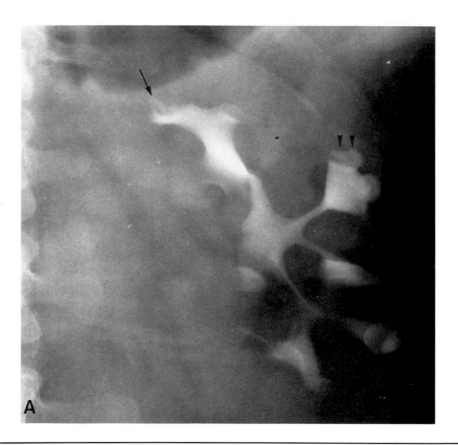

Figure 8-5.   A: An excretory urogram in an individual presenting with a history of recurrent urinary tract infections shows central (arrowheads) and forniceal (arrow) contrast within the papillae on the left. **B:** Nephrotomography improves renal outline definition (arrowheads) obscured by overlying colon gas. Its wavy appearance becomes apparent. **C:** The dense nephrogram phase of an arteriogram allows identification of renal corticomedullary junction (arrowheads). Loss of densely opacifying renal parenchyma is excessive enough that the undistorted lower pole calyx actually extends peripheral to the apparent renal border (arrow).

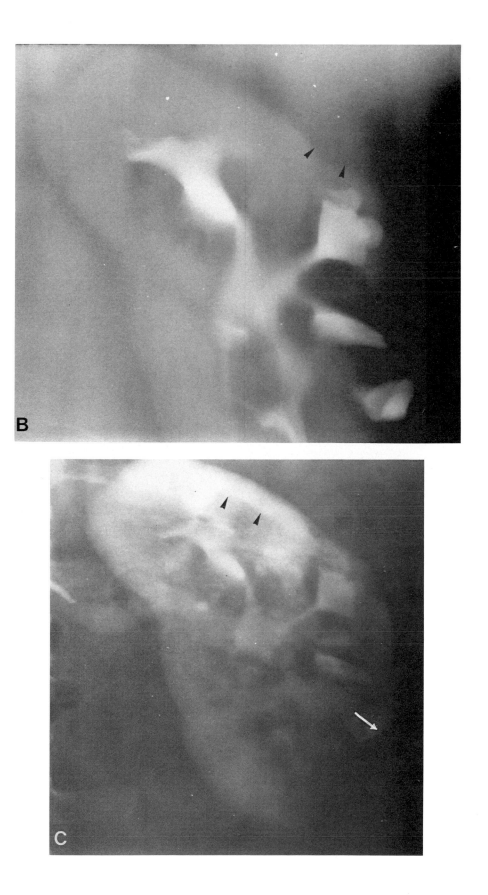

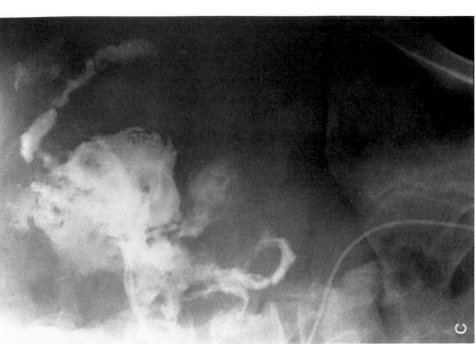

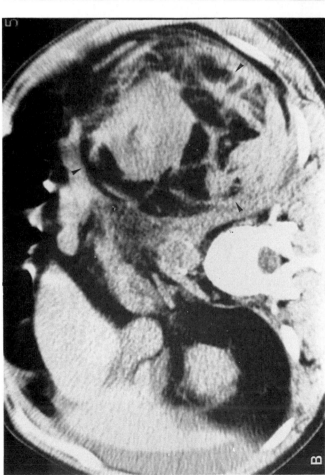

Figure 8-6. **B:** A CT scan shows a phlegmon with the renal structure centered within a spiderweb-like Gerota's fascia (arrowheads). **C:** A retrograde urogram shows extravasation of contrast into distorted renal tissue. Diagnosis: renal abscess.

Comments: The mass should have led to an initial CT study rather than a urogram. Renal function can be confirmed on contrast-enhanced CT. Retrograde examination was probably not necessary, since no obstructive changes were seen in the left kidney on CT.

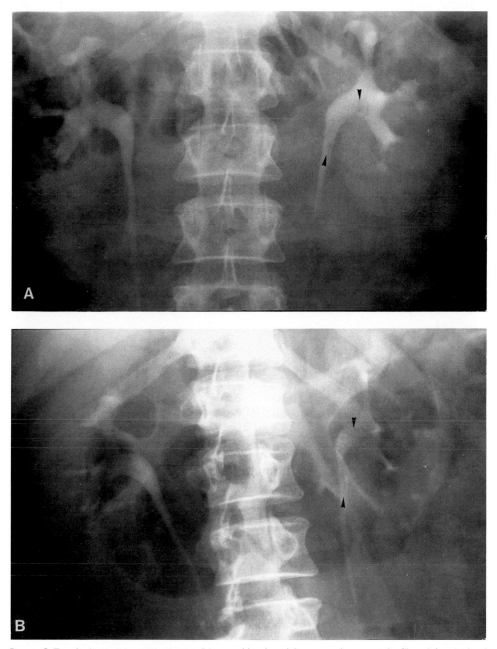

Figure 8-7. **A:** An excretory urogram in a 56-year-old male with hematuria shows irregular filling defects within the left renal pelvis and proximal ureter (arrowheads). **B:** An oblique view confirms the intrapelvic location of the filling defects (arrowheads). Diagnosis: papillary form of transitional cell carcinoma.

Comments: The intrarenal nature of the tumor must be confirmed by a second view in a different projection to exclude overlying bowel gas. A film taken at a different time also helps confirm its urinary tract location.

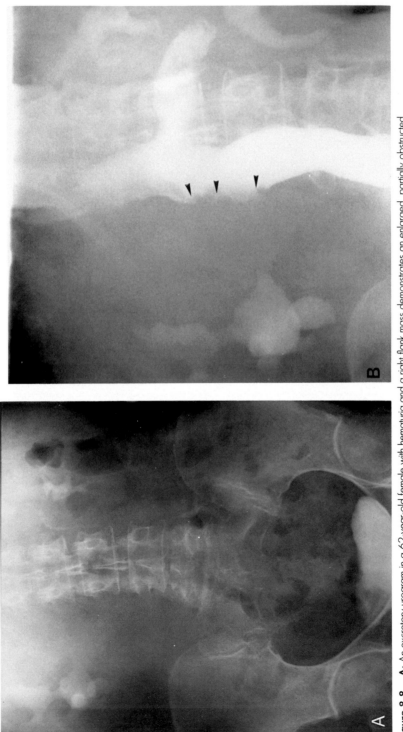

Figure 8-8. **A:** An excretory urogram in a 62-year-old female with hematuria and a right flank mass demonstrates an enlarged, partially obstructed, and laterally displaced right kidney. Bowel gas is displaced inferomedially away from the kidney as well. Angiography demonstrated vascular supply to the mass from the superior mesenteric artery and hepatic artery as well as from the renal artery. **B:** An inferior venocavagram demonstrates occlusion of the right renal vein (arrowheads). Diagnosis: renal cell carcinoma with renal vein obstruction.

Comments: Masses should usually be evaluated with CT first in adults. The inferior venocavagram might then be eliminated as unnecessary. The angiographic evaluations may show extensive parasitization that these tumors may undergo from adjacent structures.

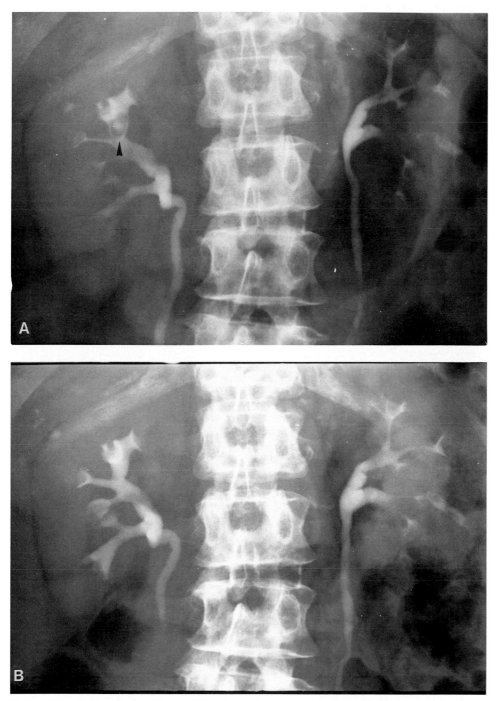

Figure 8-9. **A:** The patient, a 73-year-old female who is on coumadin, presented with gross hematuria. The excretory urogram shows filling defects within the right renal collecting system (arrowhead). **B:** A repeat urogram 2 weeks later shows no residual abnormality. Diagnosis: blood clot in collecting systems. No etiology other than medication.

Comment: Repeat examinations as well as delayed films can be used to differentiate between inconstant filling defects such as clot and constant problems such as tumor.

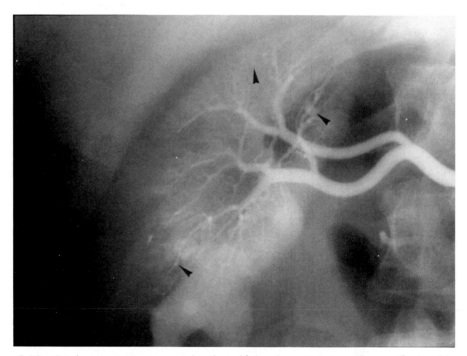

Figure 8-10.   Renal arteriogram in a young male with renal failure demonstrates incomplete opacification of the entire kidney. The selective angiogram injected only one of many renal arteries. Fine peripheral aneurysms (arrowheads) are noted. They are consistent with the diagnosis of polyarteritis nodosa. Additional aneurysms were also noted in the superior mesenteric artery and hepatic artery distributions as well. Diagnosis: polyarteritis nodosa.

Comment: This is one disease which may require arteriography for diagnosis, although biopsy may be sufficient.

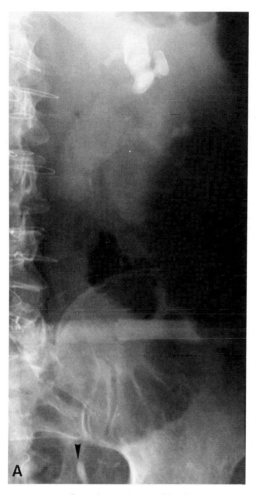

Figure 8-11. **A:** An excretory urogram performed in a 63-year-old male with a history of renal stones and acute onset of left flank pain demonstrates a delayed, but enhancing nephrogram with poor visualization of the pyelocalyceal systems at five hours.

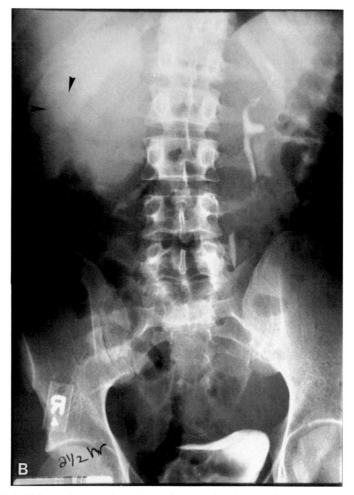

Figure 8-12. **B:** At $2\frac{1}{2}$ hours, the area of previous mottling (arrowheads) shows filling with contrast suggestive of massive pyelocaliectasis. A right bladder mass is suggested. Diagnosis: Obstructive uropathy with subacute hydronephrosis.

Comments: This demonstrates the total body opacification with initial injection and its ability to enhance vascular tissue (kidney) and not enhance avascular areas (dilated right renal collecting system). Later opacification of the nonopacified area confirms its connection with opacified urine.

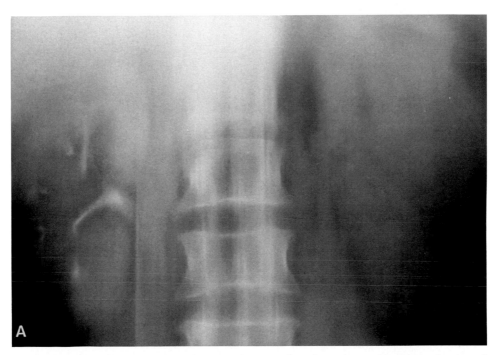

Figure 8-13. **A:** An excretory urogram with tomography was performed in a 52-year-old postsurgical patient with sudden onset of left flank pain and minimal hematuria. Nephrolithiasis was suspected. A poor nephrogram on the left which did not improve over 2 hours was seen. This is inconsistent with obstruction. An ultrasound study was requested to rule out obstruction. It was not needed in the work-up of this patient, since the nephrogram should increase in intensity if acute obstruction is the cause of the delayed pyelogram.

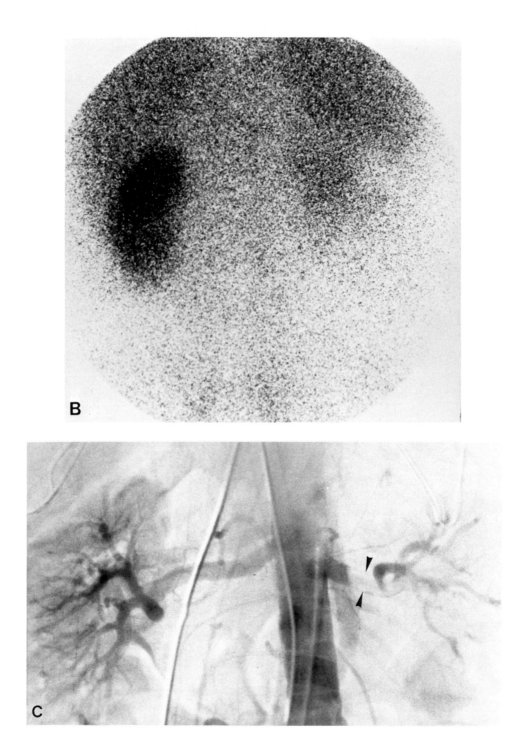

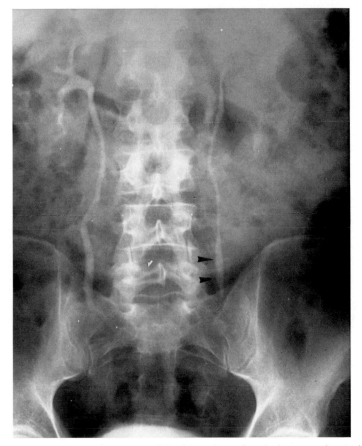

Figure 8-14.   An excretory urogram in a patient with back pain shows diminished ureteric volume with a prolonged poor nephrogram, slightly enlarged kidneys, poor pyelogram, and notched left ureter (arrowheads). Diagnosis: chronic renal vein thrombosis with venous collaterals indenting the ureter.

Comments: The renal sponge expands with venous occlusion. Contrast is present but urinary volume is diminished.

Figure 8-13.   B: A renal scan was done with a flow study which showed minimal radionuclide in the left kidney. A delayed film was obtained overnight at 12 hours with no change in the left renal uptake. This study was superfluous. **C:** A renal arteriogram, which was suggested at 2 hours, was finally performed and showed poor perfusion of the left kidney, with clot filling the main renal artery (arrowheads) in the subtraction-enhanced film. Diagnosis: acute renal artery thrombosis.

Comments: A poor nephrogram requires angiographic evaluation. The nuclide study is a "poor man's angiogram" without the risk of angiography. Evidence of poor perfusion on a nuclide examination needs further angiographic workup. If the clinical context suggests an acute episode, the vascular evaluation is urgent. Intervention can be undertaken immediately.

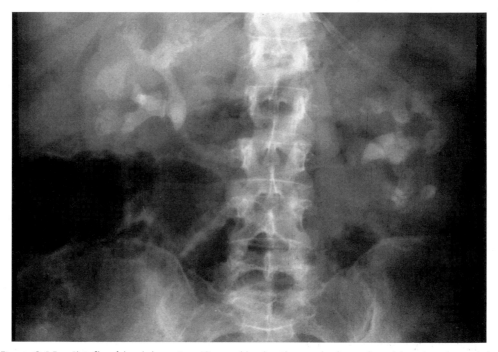

Figure 8-15. Plain film of the abdomen in a 49-year-old male with vague back pain shows bilateral staghorn calculi filling the pyelocalyceal collecting systems of the kidneys.
   Comment: Staghorn calculi mimic contrast.

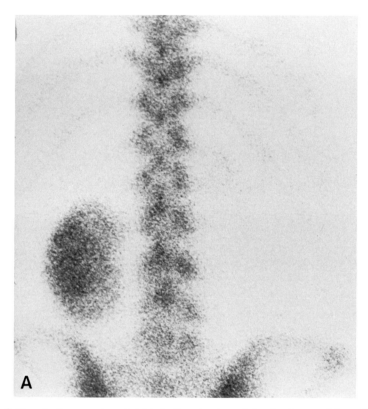

Figure 8-16. **A:** Bone scan in an individual with a chronic renal disorder shows no left renal function.

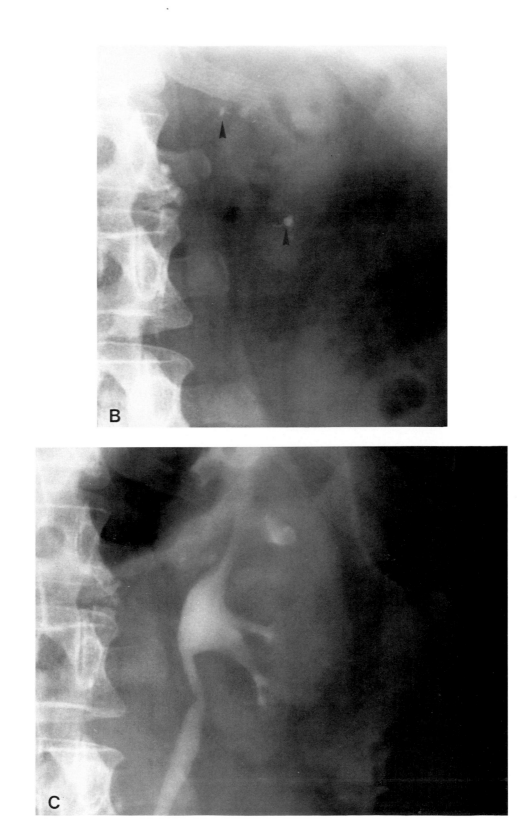

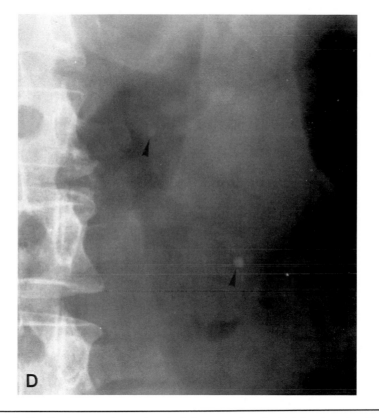

Figure 8-16.   B: Plain film shows renal parenchymal calcification overlying the left kidney (arrowheads).
C: Examination 2 years previously shows a larger kidney with function. **D:** Comparison of the positions of the calcifications suggests the degree of shrinkage. Diagnosis: renal infarction with shrinkage of renal parenchyma.

Comments: Bone scans frequently show incidental renal abnormalities. Renal calculi can be used to determine renal size as well as the renal outline. Renal size is diminished by atrophy because of arterial occlusion. More subtle loss of size may be seen in acute renal artery occlusion (compare to Figure 8-13).

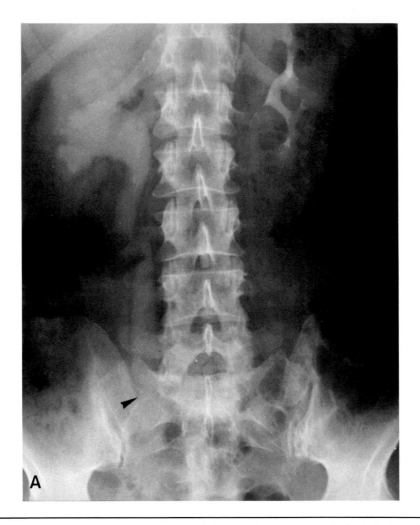

Figure 8-17.   A: An excretory urogram in a 49-year-old female with sterile pyuria and dull right flank pain shows marked ureteropyelocaliectasis extending into the true pelvis (arrowhead). **B:** A retrograde examination demonstrates a long irregular stricture in the distal right ureter with normal left collecting systems. Diagnosis: tuberculous ureteritis diagnosed on culture.

Comment: Retrograde examination may be the only adequate means of evaluating poorly visualized ureters.

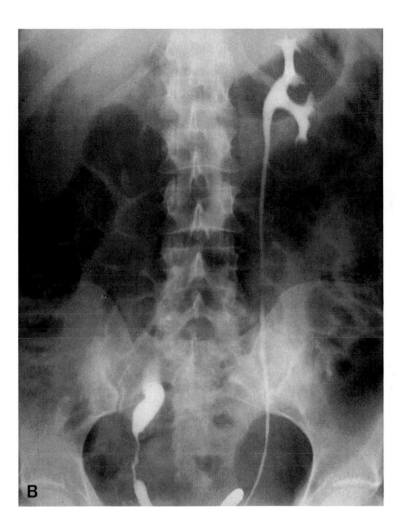

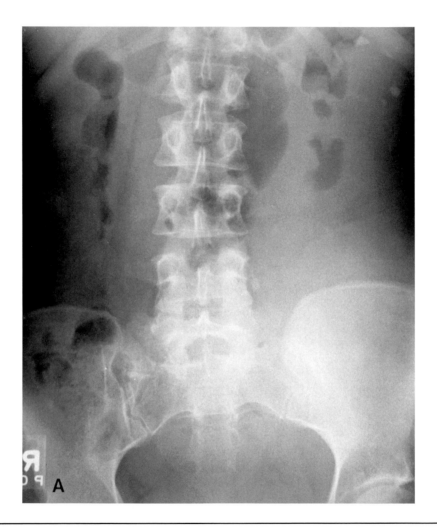

Figure 8-18. **A:** An excretory urogram was performed in this 32-year-old female with hematuria and a growing left flank discomfort following a left ureter stone removal attempt using a cystoscopically introduced basket. The plain film demonstrates left renal calculi and an infrarenal area of soft tissue density devoid of bowel gas. **B:** The area of density increases in density over 2 hours of the urographic examination, while a distorted left renal collecting system demonstrates pyelocaliectasis. Diagnosis: traumatic urinoma from ureteric perforation at the time of stone removal.

Comment: Density increasing with time indicates filling of an area with concentrated urine.

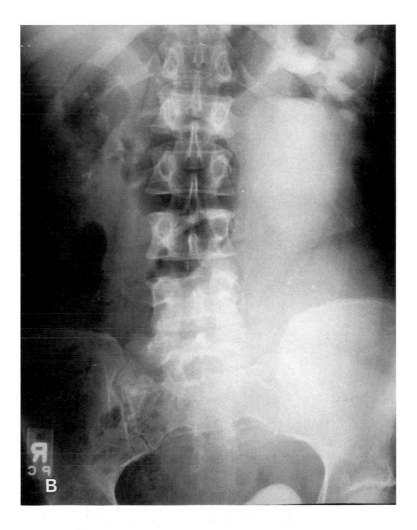

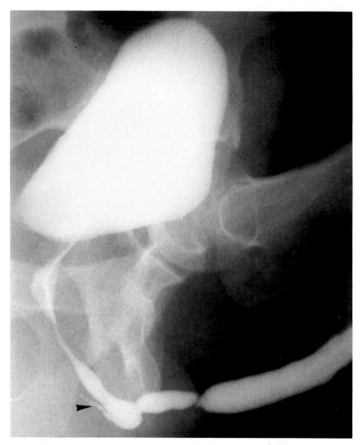

Figure 8-19.   Retrograde urethrogram in a 25-year-old male with a history of urethral discharge and diminishing urinary stream demonstrates (1) a stricture of the bulbopenile urethral junction, (2) a midbulbar urethral stricture, and (3) a premembranous extraurethral sinus (arrowhead). The prostatic urethra does not fill. Diagnosis: gonorrheal strictures and sinus.

   Comment: A voiding urethrogram is needed to evaluate the proximal urethra and further delineate the strictures and extraurethral sinus.

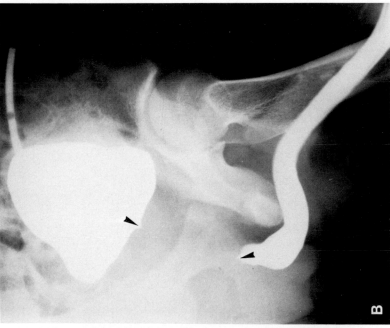

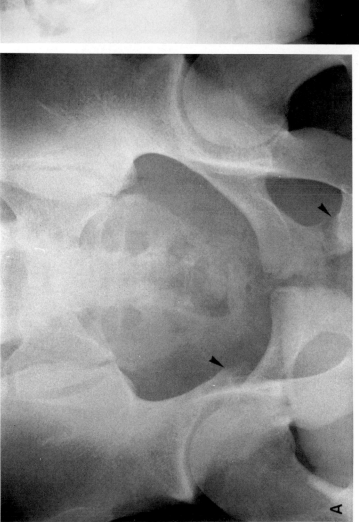

Figure 8-20. **A:** Anteroposterior view of the pelvis in a 21-year-old male who straddled a log bridge while attempting to cross it during a hike. Bilateral pubic fractures (arrowheads) with diastasis of the symphysis pubis are seen. **B:** A cystostomy was performed and a prograde and simultaneous retrograde urethrogram were performed, demonstrating a discontinuity of the urethral lumen without extravasation (arrowheads). Diagnosis: hematoma obstructing the membranous urethra. No definite rupture.

Comments: Full evaluation of the urethra may require prograde and retrograde examinations. Occasionally these can be carried out simultaneously.

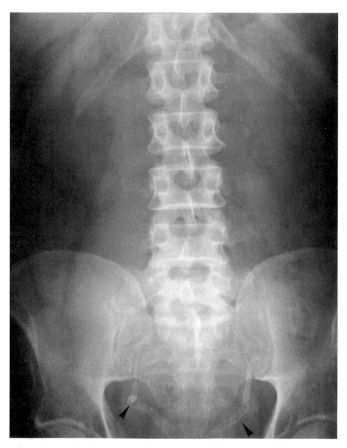

Figure 8-21. Plain film scout prior to the performance of a scheduled excretory urogram in a 44-year-old male demonstrates calcification of the vas deferens (arrowheads). This finding strongly suggests diabetes mellitus and the need to avoid dehydration and the subsequent risk of renal shut-down if contrast is injected.

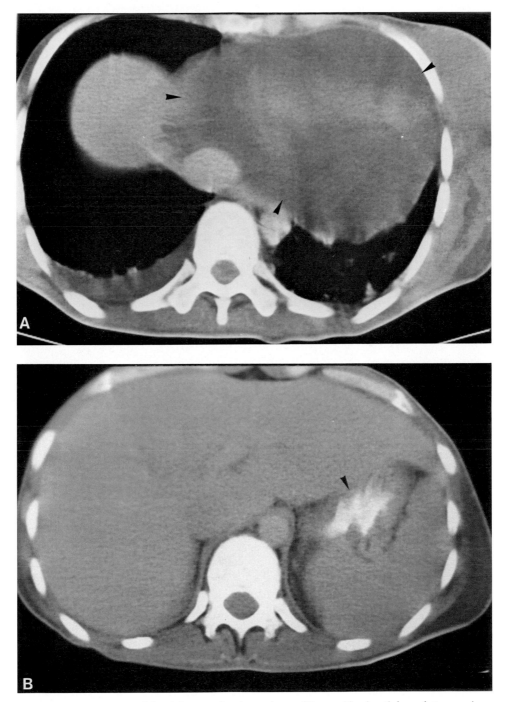

Figure 8-22. **A:** A CT scan of the abdomen ordered to evaluate a 31-year-old male with fever, fatigue, and a palpably enlarged liver demonstrates a pericardial effusion (arrowheads) and right pleural effusion. **B:** Hepatomegaly which displaces the stomach (arrowhead) posterolaterally is noted.

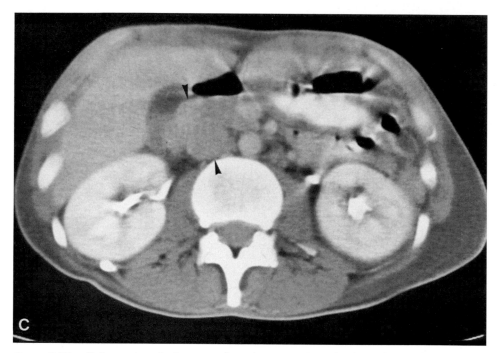

Figure 8-22.   C: Retroperitoneal indistinctness of vascular structures (arrowheads) is indicative of tumor and adenopathy. Diagnosis: lymphoma.

Comment: CT is the most useful modality for evaluating retroperitoneum and solid organs of the abdomen.

SONOGRAPHY IN DIAGNOSTIC MEDICAL IMAGING

Michael C. Hill

SONOGRAPHIC INSTRUMENTATION

Sonography uses a transducer (piezoelectric crystal) to emit and receive sound waves.[1,2] Each transducer is focused according to its use. It is focused in the near-field (high frequency, 7 to 10MHz) for imaging superficial organs like the thyroid, in the mid-field (5MHz) for structures like the gallbladder, and in the far-field (low frequency, 3MHz) for full evaluation of organs such as the liver or obstetrical patients who are near term.

The transducer is coupled to the patient's skin using an acoustic gel. Images are produced by directing the ultrasound beam through the area of interest. This can be done by (1) mechanically moving the transducer (mechanical sector scanner), (2) electronically guiding the beam without moving the transducer (phased array), or (3) using multiple fixed transducers (linear array). The image produced can be pie-shaped (sector scanner, phased array) or rectangular (linear array), with the latter providing the larger field of view which is optimal for obstetrical sonography (Fig. 9-1). The scanning rate of these instruments is fast enough to give us a "moving picture" of the anatomy being examined, and this is called real-time ultrasound.

Sound waves are reflected at interfaces of different density.[1,2,3] The greater the density difference, the greater the amount of reflection. The image produced by the transducer is displayed on a TV monitor in varying shades of gray, depending on the strength of the returning echo from each point of information in the image. This gives a gray-scale texture to the tissues. A *cystic* fluid-filled structure is echo-free and transmits sound through it very well (see Figs. 9-4, 9-21). A *solid* mass, however, has a varying number of internal echoes and attenuates the sound beam so that the through-transmission is poor (see Figs. 9-22, 9-24).

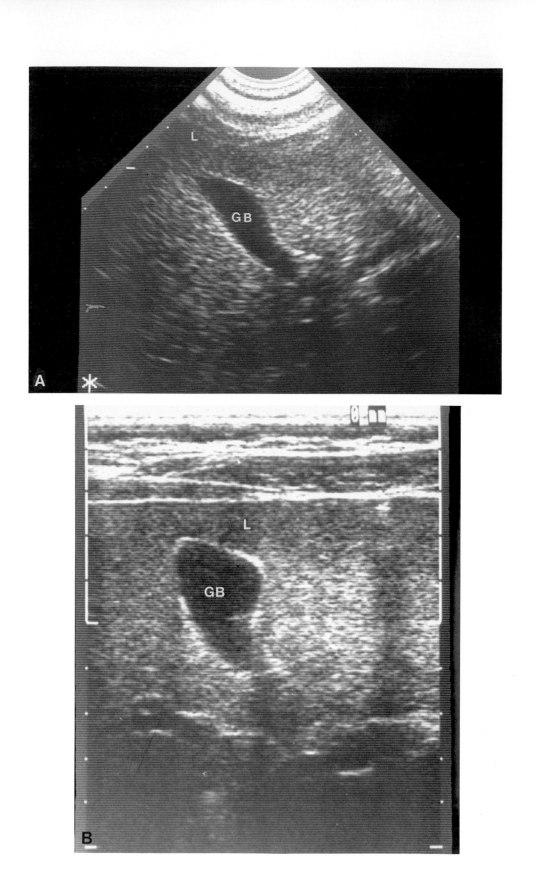

The amount of internal echoes (echogenicity) can be the same (isoechoic), less (hypoechoic), or more (hyperechoic) than the surrounding tissues. A *complex* mass has a combination of both cystic and solid elements (see Fig. 9-32). In the human body, bowel gas, barium, and bone prevent sonographic access to the underlying organs and tissues; the density difference between these and the soft tissues is so great that all of the sound is reflected (see Fig. 9-2A).

Doppler ultrasound allows one to determine the presence, direction, and rate of flow in a blood vessel (see Fig. 9-37). With duplex Doppler sonography, the vessels being evaluated can be visualized at the same time.

PATIENT PREPARATION

Examination of the liver, gallbladder, biliary tree, pancreas, and retroperitoneum optimally requires that the patient should be fasting for four hours prior to the sonographic examination (Figs. 9-2A – E).[1,2,3] To prevent dehydration, small amounts of clear liquid can be given up to one to two hours prior to the study. In an emergency situation (e.g., acute cholecystitis) these guidelines can be disregarded. In most instances (75 to 80 per cent), even if the patient has eaten, a diagnostic study can be performed. If the area of interest cannot be visualized, the study should be repeated with patient fasting. No patient preparation is necessary for a renal sonogram unless the urinary bladder is to be evaluated at the same time, for example, in renal colic. In such cases, the patient should be evaluated with a full bladder.

A pelvic sonogram requires that the patient's urinary bladder be filled by drinking three to four cups of water 20 to 30 minutes prior to the examination. This displaces gas-filled loops of bowel out of the pelvis and allows visualization of the uterus, ovaries, adnexa, and cul-de-sac (see Fig. 9-27). In an emergency situation (e.g., suspected ectopic pregnancy), where oral fluids should not be given because of possible surgery, intravenous fluids should be administered. Catheterization with retrograde filling of the bladder with a sterile isotonic saline solution should be reserved for those uncommon occurrences where an immediate emergency pelvic sonogram is requested.

Figure 9-1. Sector (A) versus linear (B) scans of the gallbladder (GB) and liver (L).

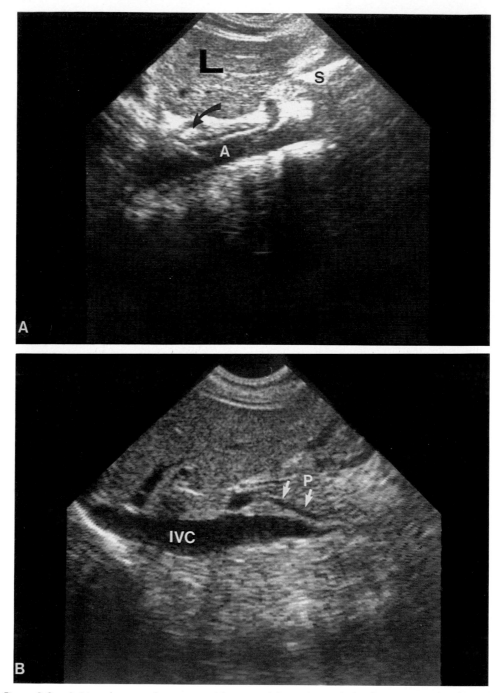

Figure 9-2.   A: Normal sonographic anatomy of the upper abdomen. Longitudinal midline sonogram showing the aorta (A), the esophagogastric junction (black arrow), and the liver (L). Note how the gas-filled stomach (S) prevents visualization of deeper anatomic structures. **B:** Longitudinal sonogram to the right of midline showing the inferior vena cava (IVC) and head of the pancreas (P) containing the distal end of the common bile duct (arrows).

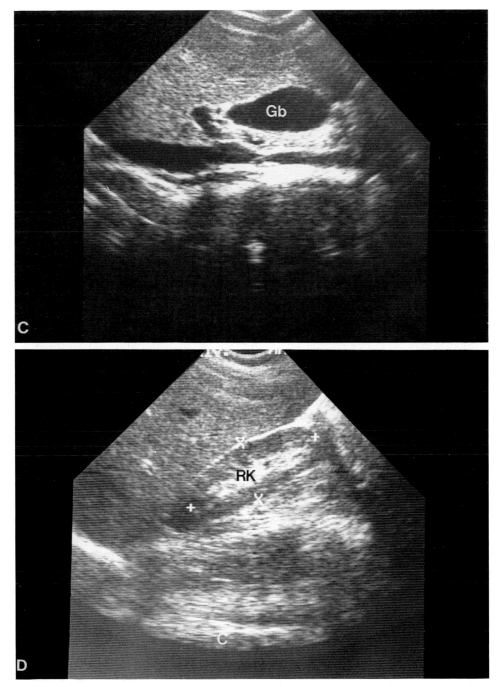

Figure 9-2. **C:** Longitudinal sonogram to the right of the area in Figure 9-2B showing the normal gallbladder (Gb). **D:** Longitudinal sonogram of the right kidney (RK), showing the echogenic renal sinus in the center of the kidney surrounded by the relatively hypoechoic renal parenchyma.

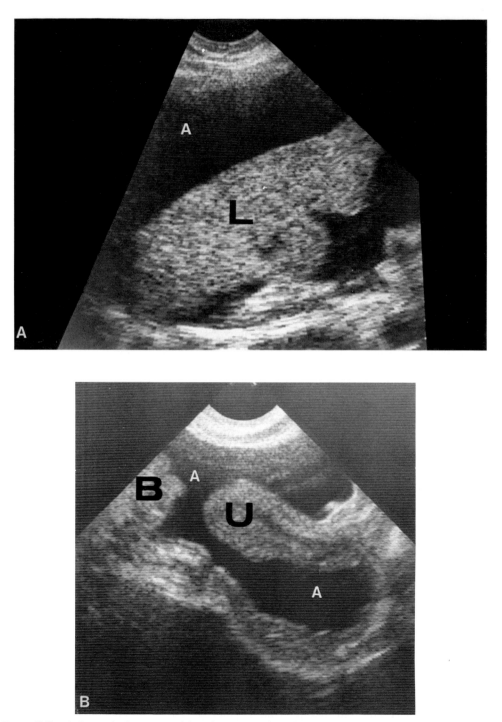

Figure 9-3.   A: Longitudinal sonogram of the right upper quadrant shows the liver (L) to have an abnormal echo texture compatible with cirrhosis, associated with ascites (A). **B:** Longitudinal sonogram of the pelvis reveals the uterus (U) surrounded by ascites (A). Loops of bowel (B).

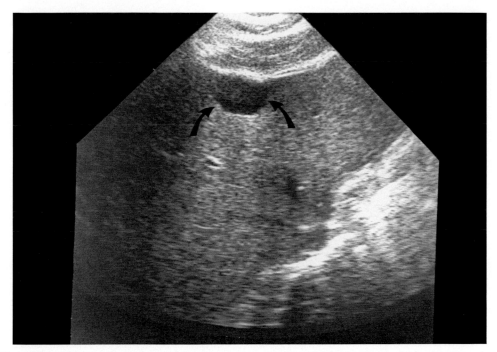

Figure 9-4.   Liver cyst. Sonogram reveals a cystic mass (arrows) with well-defined walls, an echo-free interior, and good through-transmission.

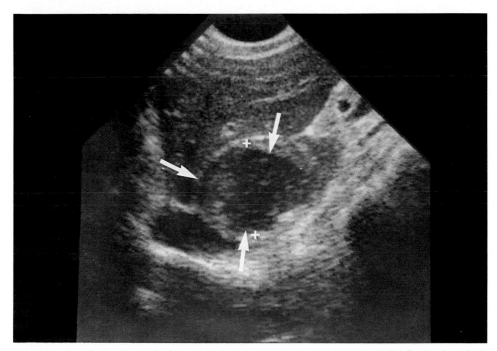

Figure 9-5.   Liver abscess. Longitudinal sonogram demonstrates a cystic mass (arrows) with ill-defined walls and a lot of internal echoes.

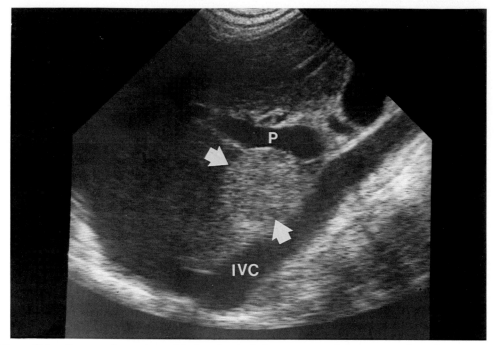

Figure 9-6. Cavernous hemangioma of the liver. Longitudinal sonogram reveals the presence of an echogenic mass (arrows) in the caudate lobe of the liver between the main portal vein (P) and the inferior vena cava (IVC).

abscesses such as coccidioidomycosis may occur in the liver. These abscesses are very small, usually less than 1cm, and have an echogenic center and a hypoechoic periphery.

A complex fluid collection in or around the liver will be found with a *hematoma*. With time, the hematoma becomes better defined and the echoes will disappear as the clot lyses. The diagnosis of a hematoma can be made when there is a history of trauma.

The sonographic appearance of a solid mass in the liver is nonspecific. It may be echogenic, hypoechoic, or isoechoic with the liver. It may also be complex in nature or have an echogenic center with a hypoechoic rim (bull's eye lesion). The most common solid benign lesion in the liver is a *cavernous hemangioma*. This is present in about 5 per cent of normal people and is usually single, but may be multiple (15 per cent). They usually measure less than 4 to 5cm, are echogenic, and have well-defined, sometimes lobulated margins (Fig. 9-6).[1,2,3] On close examination, small vascular channels can be identified within the mass. The sonographic diagnosis can be confirmed with a dynamic CT scan or a technetium-labeled red blood cell study.

Hepatic adenomas are found in glycogen storage disease and in women on birth control pills. These well-defined masses are difficult to identify sonographically and are hypoechoic or isoechoic with the liver. They can present with acute life-threatening hemorrhage, giving them a complex appearance which becomes more cystic with time as the clot involutes.[1,2,3]

Liver metastases are usually evident as such because they are most often multiple (Fig. 9-7). When solitary, they can be indistinguishable from other solid mass lesions of the

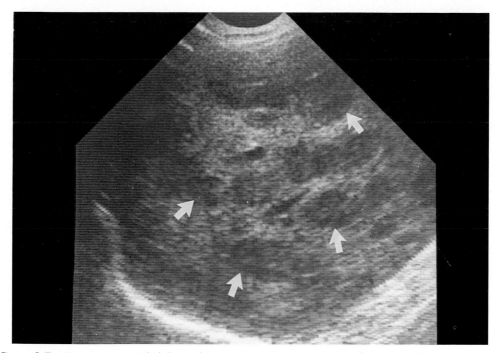

Figure 9-7.   Liver metastasis. Multiple hypoechoic areas (arrows) are present within the liver parenchyma.

liver.[1,2,3] Ultrasound is not as good overall as CT or a technetium sulfur colloid scan in screening the liver for metastatic disease.

Hepatoma can also present as a single solid or as multiple focal masses in the liver. There is often underlying chronic liver disease (cirrhosis or hepatitis), and the alpha fetoprotein will be elevated in the majority (85 per cent) of cases. Malignant hepatic masses may invade the portal vein or the hepatic veins (Budd-Chiari syndrome), and this can be recognized sonographically.

If the cause of a mass lesion in the liver cannot be determined by clinical history or other imaging modalities, an ultrasound/CT-guided biopsy will yield a pathological diagnosis in 90 per cent of patients.

SPLEEN

TECHNIQUE

Upper abdominal sonography.

INDICATIONS FOR EXAMINATION

(1) Suspected splenic mass; abscess; hematoma.

(2) Splenomegaly; left upper quadrant mass.

Sonography can be used to confirm that a left upper quadrant mass is in fact secondary to splenomegaly. The sonographic appearance of a diffusely enlarged spleen is nonspecific and may be due to many diseases, including lymphoma, leukemia, and portal hypertension. Examination of the adjacent upper abdomen may reveal a likely cause, such as lymphadenopathy in lymphoma, or leukemia and a cirrhotic liver in portal hypertension.

A focal solid mass in the spleen can have a similar appearance to those in the liver.[1,2,3] It may be due to *lymphoma* or rarely *metastatic disease* from tumors of the lung or breast, or melanoma. These metastatic masses may be single or multiple. An old splenic *infarct* has the appearance of a focal echogenic mass. Cysts in the spleen are usually due to old trauma and frequently have calcification with acoustical shadowing in their wall. Trauma to the spleen is usually evaluated with a contrast-enhanced CT scan. However, a *hematoma* in or around the spleen can be visualized as an ill-defined complex echogenic area that becomes more organized and less echogenic as the clot lyses. *Calcified granulomata* are seen as punctate echogenic areas in the spleen which, when large enough, produce acoustical shadowing. These are usually secondary to prior histoplasmosis.

GALLBLADDER AND BILIARY TRACT

TECHNIQUE

Upper abdominal sonography.

INDICATIONS FOR EXAMINATION

(1) Suspected gallbladder stones.

(2) Jaundice.

(3) Palpable right upper quadrant mass; enlarged gallbladder.

Sonography is the procedure of choice to determine whether *gallbladder stones* are present. If abdominal radiographs have been taken, they should be reviewed, as calcified gallstones may be evident in approximately 10 per cent of cases, making an ultrasound examination unnecessary. Gallstones are identified as freely moving focal areas of echogenicity with acoustical shadowing in the gallbladder (Fig. 9-8A).[1,2,3] They may float in the bile or be adherent to the gallbladder wall (cholesterolosis). If the gallbladder is full of stones, acoustical shadowing will emanate from the entire gallbladder and no visible echo-free bile may be visualized. An oral cholecystogram is usually reserved for those patients who have a normal gallbladder sonogram but have a high clinical index of suspicion for gallstones.

In the fasting state, the thickness of the gallbladder wall should measure no more than 2 to 3mm. The presence of a thick gallbladder wall and gallstones denotes the presence of *acute and/or chronic cholecystitis*. Thickening of the wall, however, can be seen in ascites, hepatitis, hypoalbuminemia, acute pancreatitis, and renal disease. Although a technetium DISIDA (diisopropyliminodiacetic acid) nuclear medicine study is the most sensitive and specific for acute cholecystitis, false positive scans do occur when there is no exchange of bile

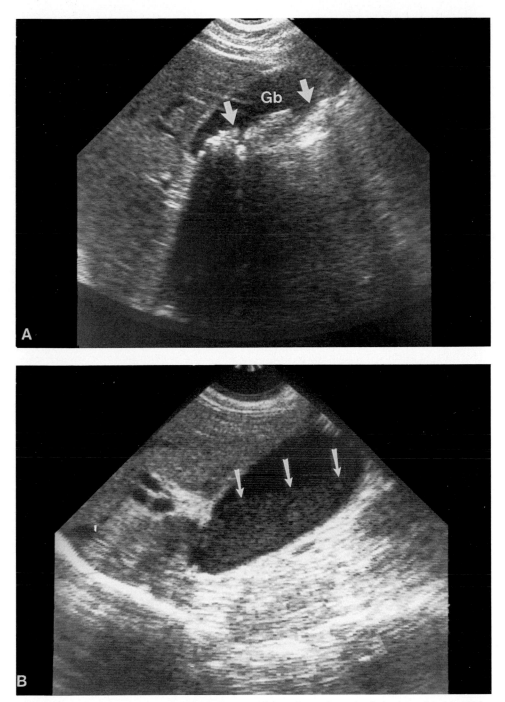

Figure 9-8.   A: Gallbladder stones. Multiple shadowing gallstones (arrows) are identified in the gallbladder (Gb).
B: Gallbladder sludge. Multiple low-level echoes (arrows) are seen in the dependent portion of the gallbladder.

between the common bile duct and gallbladder due to prolonged fasting or hyperalimentation.

The presence of *gallbladder sludge* is due to biliary stasis, where the bile salts have come out of solution, and unlike gallstones, this is a reversible process. Sonographically, sludge appears as an echogenic layer in the dependent portion of the gallbladder, and due to its viscous nature, it moves slowly with a change in patient position (Fig. 9-8B). It can be physiological due to prolonged fasting or be secondary to obstruction of the cystic or common bile duct. Its true nature may be assessed by reexamining the gallbladder and biliary tree after the patient has eaten.

The normal size of the gallbladder varies greatly. A globular appearance of the normally pear-shaped gallbladder suggests the diagnosis of *obstruction* of the cystic duct/common bile duct. This can be confirmed if the gallbladder is palpable. If this is the case, and if the gallbladder is filled with echoes, then *empyema of the gallbladder* should be suspected in the appropriate clinical setting. Fluid around the gallbladder may indicate that it has perforated.

A *gallbladder polyp* and focal thickening of the gallbladder wall due to *adenomyosis* can be identified sonographically. *Gallbladder carcinoma* presents as a focal or diffuse thickening of the gallbladder wall and gallstones are usually present (Fig. 9-9).[1,2,3] There may be direct invasion of the liver and/or porta hepatis by the tumor, rendering it surgically unresectable. Adjacent lymphadenopathy may also be seen.

The normal intrahepatic bile ducts cannot be identified sonographically, while the com-

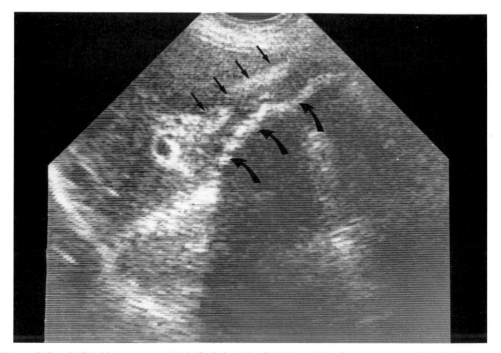

Figure 9-9. Gallbladder carcinoma. Markedly thickened gallbladder wall (small arrows) associated with multiple shadowing stones in the gallbladder (large arrows).

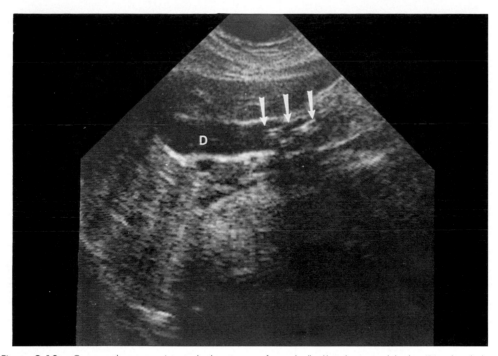

Figure 9-10. Common duct stones. Longitudinal sonogram of a markedly dilated common bile duct (D) with multiple shadowing stones at its lower end (arrows).

mon hepatic duct and common bile duct should not have an internal diameter exceeding 4 to 5mm and 5 to 6mm respectively. The nonobstructed common bile bile duct, however, can measure up to 10mm in patients who have had their gallbladder removed. If a patient has *obstruction of the biliary tree,* then dilatation can be identified sonographically in over 90 per cent of cases. If obstruction is early (i.e., less than 24 hours) or intermittent, then there may be no dilatation of the biliary tree.[1,2,3] Almost all patients, however, who have obstruction and clinical evidence of jaundice (scleral icterus) will have sonographically detectable dilatation of the biliary tree.

Once obstruction is detected, then its level and cause should be sought (Fig. 9-10). Obstructing stones in the common bile duct are difficult to identify sonographically in about half of the cases. These are usually associated with stones in the gallbladder, and other nonobstructing stones may be seen in the proximal dilated common bile duct. An obstructing mass in the porta hepatis is usually due to metastatic lymphadenopathy or a cholangiocarcinoma (Klatskin tumor), while an obstructing mass in the head of the pancreas may be due to pancreatic carcinoma, chronic pancreatitis, or a pancreatic pseudocyst (see Fig. 9-15).

If a dilated biliary tree is present, but the area of obstruction cannot be evaluated sonographically due to bowel gas, then an abdominal CT scan following the administration of oral and intravenous contrast should be performed. If a distally impacted stone in the common bile duct is suspected, oral contrast should not be given so that the obstructing calcified stone will stand out.

A *choledochal cyst* is sonographically identified as a cystic mass along the path of the common bile duct. It can be confused with a pseudocyst of the head of the pancreas. A technetium DISIDA nuclear medicine study will demonstrate its biliary origin.

PANCREAS

TECHNIQUE

Upper abdominal sonography.

INDICATIONS FOR EXAMINATION

(1) Detect complications of acute pancreatitis.
(2) Epigastric pain and weight loss. Rule out pancreatic carcinoma.

The head and body of the pancreas are usually easily seen by identifying the surrounding vascular landmarks, while the pancreatic tail is somewhat more difficult to visualize, as it lies behind the body of the stomach. If adequate visualization is not achieved sonographically, then an abdominal CT scan should be performed. The pancreas is as echogenic or more echogenic than the adjacent liver at the same depth. In older patients, the true outline of the pancreas may be difficult to identify, as its echogenicity blends in with that of the surrounding retroperitoneal peripancreatic fat.

In *acute pancreatitis* the gland appears normal in about 30 per cent of patients. The remaining patients will be equally divided between having diffuse or focal enlargement of the gland.[1,2,3] The involved area appears hypoechoic, and there may be dilatation of the pancreatic duct (internal diameter greater than 3mm) (Fig. 9-11). In 20 per cent of patients, the inflammation spreads outside of the gland, and an ill-defined hypoechoic mass may be seen *(phlegmonous pancreatitis)*.[4]

Other complications include pseudocyst formation (10 per cent), hemorrhage (3 per cent), and abscess (2 per cent). A *pancreatic pseudocyst* has fairly well-defined margins and is relatively echo-free, while areas of *abscess* or *hemorrhage* are less well-defined and tend to have more internal echoes (Fig. 9-12).[1,2,3] When clinically indicated, a percutaneous needle aspiration should be performed and the aspirate Gram-stained and cultured to determine whether a sonographically identified pancreatic cystic mass represents an abscess, a noninfected pancreatic pseudocyst, or an area of hemorrhage. Overall, CT is better than sonography in detecting the complications of acute pancreatitis, as the associated ileus precludes adequate sonographic evaluation. The phlegmonous changes resulting from acute pancreatitis can persist from weeks to months, long after the patient has made a full clinical recovery, so ultrasound should not be used to monitor the patient's recovery.

In *chronic pancreatitis* the gland can appear normal or be atrophied and difficult to identify. However, in about 30 per cent of patients there can be focal or diffuse enlargement.[1,2,3] When this is the case, pancreatic calcifications are usually present (90 per cent) and the pancreatic duct may be beaded and dilated (40 per cent) (Fig. 9-13). A pancreatic pseudocyst may also be seen (20 per cent). A mass due to chronic pancreatitis can usually be

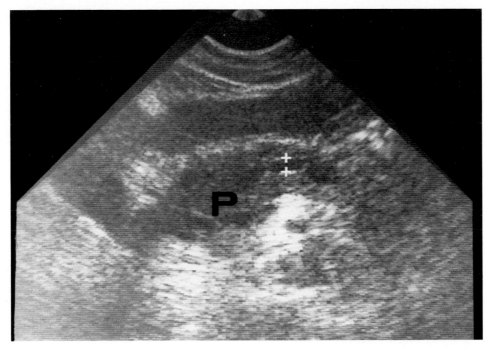

Figure 9-11.   Acute pancreatitis. Focal enlargement of the head of the pancreas (P) with a dilated pancreatic duct (+).

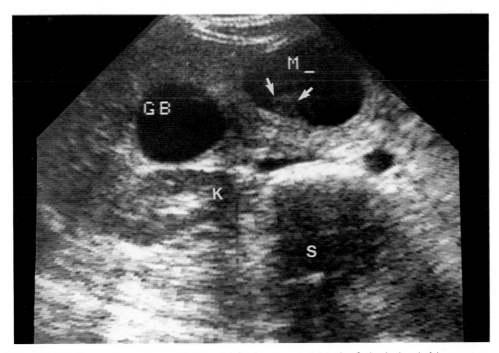

Figure 9-12.   Traumatic pseudocyst. A fairly well-defined cystic mass (M) is identified in the head of the pancreas. Echoes are identified in its dependent portion (arrows). Spine (S). Right kidney (K). Gallbladder (GB).

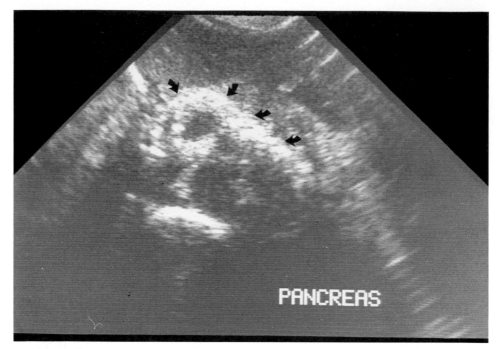

Figure 9-13.   Chronic pancreatitis with a diffusely echogenic pancreas (arrows) due to pancreatic calcifications.

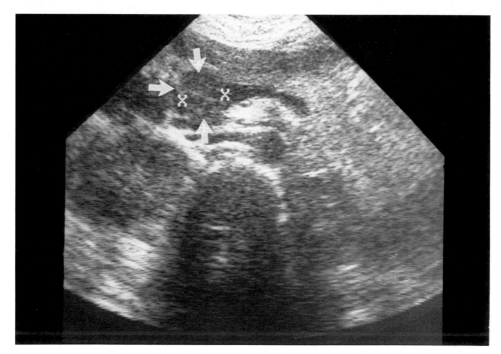

Figure 9-14.   Pancreatic carcinoma with a 3cm hypoechoic mass in the head of the pancreas (arrows).

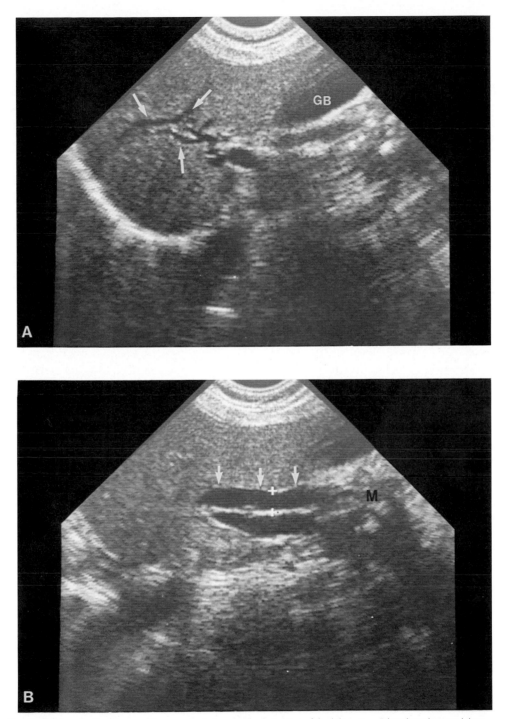

Figure 9-15. **A:** Carcinoma of the pancreatic head with obstruction of the biliary tree. Dilated intrahepatic biliary tree (arrows). Gallbladder (GB). **B:** Dilated common bile duct (arrows) down to the level of the mass (M) in the head of the pancreas.

distinguished from pancreatic carcinoma due to the presence of irregular punctate calcifications in the former, along with the absence of adjacent lymphadenopathy and liver metastasis.

Pancreatic carcinoma is better detected overall by CT in most cases (90 per cent). However, ultrasound can identify pancreatic carcinoma in 60 to 80 per cent of cases, especially in the thin, emaciated patient.[1,2,3] Carcinoma is usually hypoechoic, has irregular margins, and presents as a focal mass in the head, body, or tail of the pancreas, in 60, 20, and 10 per cent of cases, respectively (Fig. 9-14). It may, however, diffusely involve the entire gland. Carcinoma of the head of the pancreas tends to present earlier than those in the body or tail, as it obstructs the common bile duct, producing jaundice (Fig. 9-15). There may be obstruction of the pancreatic duct and adjacent lymphadenopathy along with liver metastasis. Echogenic tumor thrombus may be identified in the splenic or portal vein, and encasement of the superior mesenteric vessels may occur. These findings indicate surgical unresectability, and the diagnosis of carcinoma can be confirmed by ultrasound- or CT-guided fine needle aspiration of the mass.

Cystic neoplasms of the pancreas include *microcystic adenoma*, which is benign, and *cystadenocarcinoma*, which is malignant.[1,2,3] The cystic nature of the former may not be obvious sonographically as the cystic areas may only measure millimeters in diameter, while the multiloculated nature of the cystadenocarcinoma is easily seen sonographically. These tumors tend to arise in the pancreatic body and tail. Functioning *islet cell tumors*, because of their small size (1 to 3cm) at the time of clinical presentation, are difficult to locate in half the patients, as opposed to the nonfunctioning tumors which are larger in size. The malignant variety of these tumors may be inferred when adjacent lymphadenopathy along with liver metastases are seen.

URINARY TRACT

TECHNIQUE

Sonography of the kidneys, retroperitoneum, and bladder. Evaluate the liver for metastasis if a malignancy is present (e.g., hypernephroma).

INDICATIONS FOR EVALUATION

(1) Renal failure (parenchymal renal disease versus obstructive uropathy).

(2) Renal mass; nonfunctioning kidney seen on an intravenous urogram (IVU) or CT.

(3) Suspected abscess, urinoma, hematoma.

(4) Guidance for cyst aspiration; biopsy; nephrostomy.

Before performing a sonogram of the kidneys, all other studies that have been done should be reviewed, such as the site and location of a renal mass seen on an IVU. The sonographic size of both kidneys varies (9 to 13cm) and depends on the size of the patient. The thickness of the renal cortex and medulla is about 1.5 to 2.0cm. The cortex is more echogenic than the renal medulla which contains the hypoechoic renal pyramids (see Fig. 9-2D). The overall echogenicity of the renal parenchyma is less than that of the adjacent liver.[1,2,3,5] The pelvicalyceal echo complex is echogenic due to the presence of renal sinus fat. As the pelvis and calyces become distended with urine, they form a central echo-free area. In a *duplex kidney*, two separate pelvicalyceal echo complexes can be seen.

The normal nondistended ureters cannot be seen in the retroperitoneum. The bladder wall and lumen can be evaluated when it is distended with urine. If either one or both kidneys cannot be identified, then the lower abdomen and pelvis should be evaluated for a midline lower abdominal *horseshoe kidney* or *pelvic kidney(s)*. In *cross-fused ectopia* the upper pole of the kidney from one side fuses with the lower pole of the kidney on the opposite side. This condition can be identified sonographically.

In the patient presenting with renal failure, sonography can determine if it is due to parenchymal renal disease or obstructive uropathy. In *acute renal failure* due to parenchymal renal disease, the kidneys may appear normal sonographically or may be enlarged and echogenic, as with acute glomerulonephritis, drug toxicity, or bilateral vascular thrombosis (Fig. 9-16).[1,2,3,5] If, however, there is *endstage renal disease*, the kidneys will be small and more echogenic than usual, as in chronic glomerulonephritis. In *adult polycystic kidney disease*, the kidneys are large and contain numerous cysts of various size, from millimeters to centimeters, which entirely replace the normal architecture of the kidneys (Fig. 9-17).

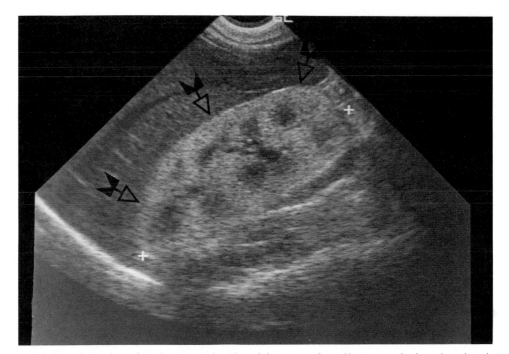

Figure 9-16.   Acute glomerulonephritis. Parenchymal renal disease as indicated by increased echoes throughout the right renal parenchyma (arrows).

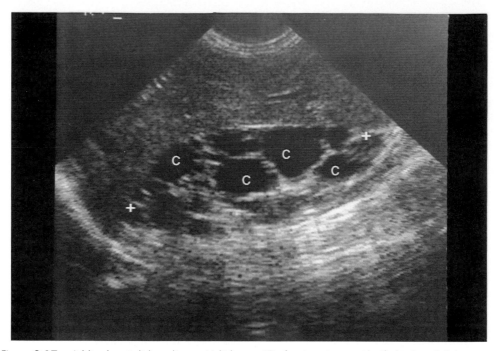

Figure 9-17. Adult polycystic kidney disease. Multiple cysts (C) of various sizes are identified in the right kidney.

There may be associated cysts in the liver in 60 per cent of patients, and in the pancreas as well.

If renal failure is due to *obstructive uropathy* there will be *hydronephrosis* of both kidneys. In such cases, the pelvis should be evaluated in the male to look for a distended bladder secondary to a large prostate (benign prostatic hypertrophy versus prostatic carcinoma), and in the female to identify a gynecological malignancy that has obstructed the ureters.[5,6] If neither is the case, then a bladder carcinoma or a retroperitoneal mass such as lymphadenopathy or retroperitoneal fibrosis should be suspected (Fig. 9-18). If sonography does not ascertain the cause of the hydronephrosis, then an abdominal CT scan should be performed. A percutaneous nephrostomy using ultrasound guidance can be done as the initial procedure to restore renal function in a patient with obstructive uropathy where ureteral stents cannot be inserted.

Renal sonography is not of much use in diagnosing acute pyelonephritis, as the kidney will only appear large and hypoechoic in a small percentage of cases. It is, however, of use in diagnosing *intrarenal* and *perinephric abscesses*. These can be identified as complex fluid-filled areas (Fig. 9-19).[1,2,3,5] In *xanthogranulomatous pyelonephritis* a large kidney is present, and the collecting system is filled with echogenic debris and stones with acoustical shadowing. Such kidneys often function poorly or not at all on an IVU.

Renal calculi are easily detected sonographically as focal areas of echogenicity in the pelvicalyceal system.[1,2,3,5] If a patient presents with renal colic due to passage of a stone into the ureter, the ureteric stone cannot be seen sonographically unless it is at the ureterovesical

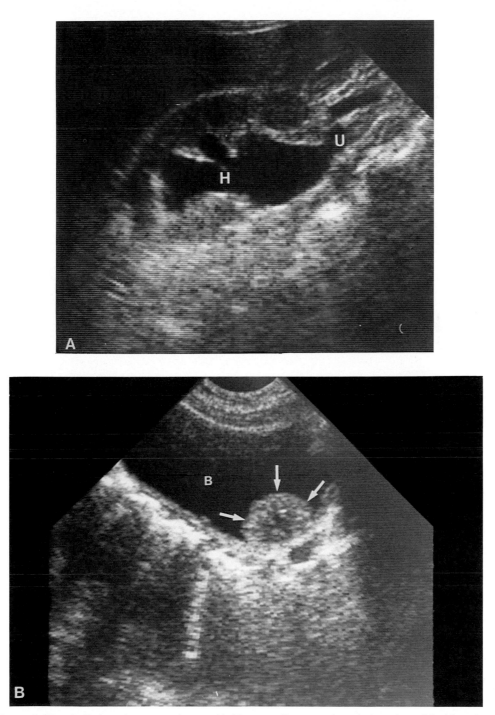

Figure 9-18.   A: Hydronephrosis secondary to a bladder tumor. There is moderate hydronephrosis (H) of the right kidney, and the visualized portion of the proximal right ureter (U) is dilated. **B:** A tumor (arrows) was identified in the bladder (B) at the right ureterovesical junction.

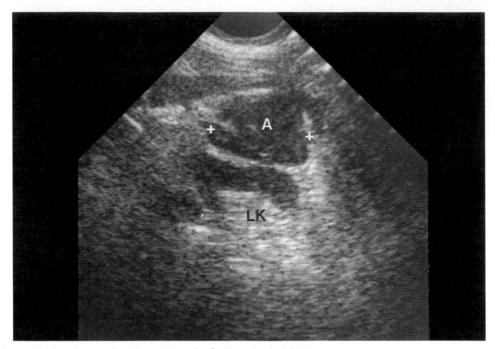

Figure 9-19.   A perinephric abscess (A) is identified lateral to the left kidney (LK).

junction or in the adjacent ureter (Fig. 9-20). Sonography is better than the IVU in diagnosing stones at the ureterovesical junction.

Renal trauma is usually best evaluated by a contrast-enhanced abdominal CT scan. Intrarenal or complex perinephric fluid collections secondary to hematoma can be identified. If there is no history of trauma, an underlying renal tumor (hypernephroma, angiomyolipoma) should be looked for to account for the hematoma. A *urinoma* usually appears as an echo-free fluid collection around the kidney and is secondary to extravasation of urine from an obstructing ureteric stone, or following trauma.

If a mass is identified on an IVU it cannot always be determined with certainty whether it represents a benign cyst or a hypernephroma. If a sonogram is to be performed, it is imperative that the IVU be used to identify the site and location of the mass, since (1) small hypernephromas can be easily missed on the sonogram, and (2) a small cyst adjacent to a hypernephroma may be mistakenly diagnosed as the mass. *Benign renal cysts* are extremely common and are found in about half of the population over 50 years of age. They may be single or multiple; however, if multiple they are countable and do not vary as greatly in size as in adult polycystic kidney disease. Sonographically they have well-defined, smooth, thin (2mm) walls, are echo-free, and have good through-transmission (Fig. 9-21).[1,2,3,5] On occasion, a small septum may be seen in the cyst, or there may be a minimal amount of echogenic debris in its dependent portion. If numerous internal echoes or septae are present, then a contrast-enhanced abdominal CT scan should be performed. Increased internal echoes can be secondary to pus or blood, and if it is the latter, this greatly increases the

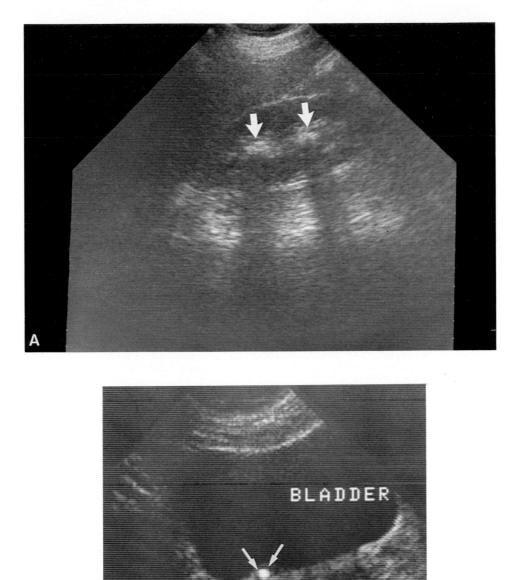

Figure 9-20. **A:** Renal stones with a stone at the right ureterovesical junction. Shadowing stones (arrows) are identified in the right pelvicaliceal system. **B:** A stone (arrows) was identified at the right ureterovesical junction by scanning through the full bladder.

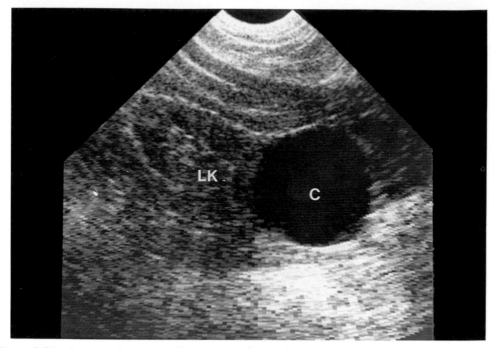

Figure 9-21. Benign renal cyst. A cyst (C) with a well-defined wall and an echo-free center is seen arising from the lower pole of the left kidney (LK).

likelihood of an underlying tumor, such as *cystic hypernephroma*. If there are numerous septae in the cyst, this could represent a *multilocular nephroma*. If this is the case, calcification may be present in the wall of the cyst. If there is a doubt regarding the etiology of a "cystic renal mass" and a noncontrast followed by a contrast-enhanced abdominal CT scan has not resolved the issue, then a renal angiogram can be performed if clinically indicated.

The most common solid renal mass is a *renal cell carcinoma* or *hypernephroma*. It may be hypoechoic, hyperechoic, or isoechoic with the renal parenchyma or may be a thick-walled irregular cystic mass.[1,2,3,5] Once the renal mass is identified, the renal vein and inferior vena cava (IVC) should be evaluated for tumor invasion. The opposite kidney should also be evaluated, and retroperitoneal adenopathy and liver metastases should be looked for (Fig. 9-22). Prior to surgery, a contrast-enhanced abdominal CT scan should be performed to fully stage the tumor.

An *angiomyolipoma* is a benign tumor that contains fat and is sonographically very echogenic. It usually presents as a solitary mass in a middle-aged female with hematuria; however, this tumor can be found in tuberous sclerosis in which case the masses may be multiple and bilateral. Other mass lesions that can be found in the kidney include *metastasis* (e.g., from lung carcinoma) and *lymphoma*.

A *transitional cell carcinoma* may be identified as a hypoechoic mass in the normally echogenic pelvicalyceal echo complex.[5,6] Such tumors are better seen on an IVU or retrograde pyelogram where they present as a lucent filling defect. These patients are often then

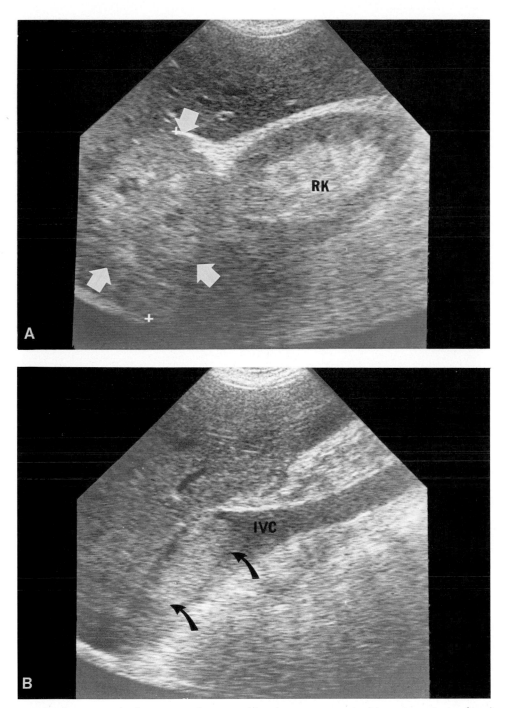

Figure 9-22.   A: Renal cell carcinoma with invasion of the inferior vena cava. A solid mass (arrows) arises from the upper pole of the right kidney (RK). **B:** Tumor (arrows) is identified in the adjacent portion of the inferior vena cava (IVC).

referred for a sonogram to rule out a radiolucent stone which sonographically would be echogenic and have acoustical shadowing.

Filling defects in the *urinary bladder* (carcinoma, polyps, or stones) can be evaluated in a similar manner with sonography (see Fig. 9-18). Although the *prostate* can be evaluated through the full bladder, transrectal sonography using a high frequency transducer provides better resolution and anatomic detail. It can determine when prostatic carcinoma has invaded through the capsule into the periprostatic fat and can detect a prostatic abscess.[5,6] Sonographically guided biopsies can be performed when prostate carcinoma is suspected.

Renal Transplants

Renal transplants are easy to evaluate due to their superficial location deep to the abdominal wall in either lower quadrant. Although sonography cannot make a definitive distinction between *acute tubular necrosis* versus *acute rejection*, it can determine whether transplant failure is due to *hydronephrosis*. It can also detect the presence of peritransplant and pelvic fluid collections (hematoma, urinoma, lymphocele, or abscess).[1,2,3,5] Using duplex Doppler sonography, the blood flow in and out of the kidney can be assessed, thus excluding a *vascular occlusion* as a cause for transplant failure.

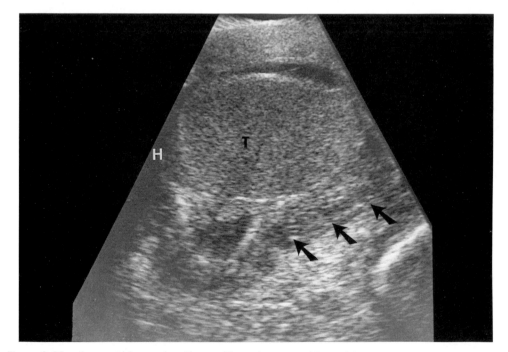

Figure 9-23.   Acute epididymo-orchitis. There is diffuse enlargement of the epididymis (arrows) and the testicle (T) is hypoechoic. There is an associated small hydrocele (H).

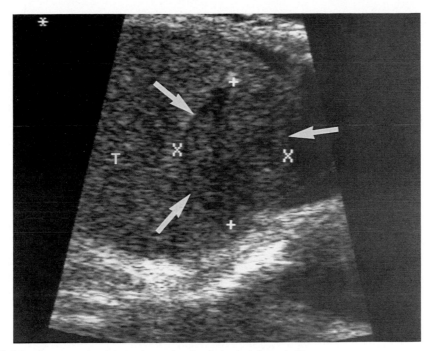

Figure 9-24.   Seminoma. A solid mass (arrows) is identified in the left testicle (T).

Scrotum

Sonographic examination of the scrotum is performed using a high frequency transducer with a short focal zone; the opposite normal hemiscrotum is a baseline for comparative evaluation.[5] A *hydrocele* is seen as an echo-free fluid collection surrounding the testis. It may be secondary to epididymitis or epididymo-orchitis, or it may be due to trauma. In *acute epididymitis* or *epididymo-orchitis*, the epididymis is enlarged and hypoechoic, as is the testis if it is also involved (Fig. 9-23). If a complex intratesticular mass is seen, then an *abscess* should be considered. Sonography can be used to determine if the testicle is ruptured following *trauma*, in which case surgery is indicated. A duplex Doppler sonogram can be used to evaluate for testicular *torsion*. However, a radionuclide flow study is probably more sensitive and specific. A *varicocele* is identified sonographically as multiple small tubular channels seen superior to the upper pole of the testis, and these enlarge in the upright position and with a Valsalva maneuver.

Sonography is very effective in determining whether a scrotal mass is cystic, solid, or complex and whether it is intra- or extratesticular. *Seminoma* and *embryonal cell carcinoma* are solid hypoechoic mass lesions of the testicle (Fig. 9-24). If such a mass is found, the retroperitoneum at the level of the kidneys should be evaluated for the presence of lymphadenopathy. Testicular *cysts* are uncommon and usually arise from the tunica albuginea. Most extratesticular masses are benign and cystic (spermatocele, epididymal cysts) and arise from the epididymis.

RETROPERITONEUM

TECHNIQUE

Sonography of the retroperitoneum. Evaluate upper abdominal organs if lymphadenopathy or mass is found.

INDICATIONS FOR EXAMINATION

(1) Suspected abdominal aortic aneurysm.

(2) Suspected retroperitoneal mass or adenopathy.

The retroperitoneum is divided into three spaces: (1) the anterior pararenal space, containing the pancreas, aorta, inferior vena cava, and ascending and descending colon; (2) the perirenal space, bounded by the anterior and posterior perirenal fascia (Gerota's fascia) which contains the kidney and perirenal fat; and (3) the posterior pararenal space.[4]

Sonography is the procedure of choice for evaluating the aorta for the presence of an *aneurysm*. If an aneurysm is found it should be traced superiorly to see if it involves the renal arteries and inferiorly to see if it involves the iliac arteries. Laminated clot, intimal flaps, and areas of dissection can also be identified sonographically.[1,2,3] The maximum anteroposterior diameter of the aneurysm from outer wall to outer wall should be measured for future reference (Fig. 9-25). The inferior vena cava is usually seen in the upper abdomen at and above the level of the head of the pancreas. It may be involved with thrombus or be displaced by a mass (lymphadenopathy, adrenal mass, or primary retroperitoneal mass). If *thrombus* is identified in the inferior vena cava, its etiology should be determined: hypernephroma, hepatoma, or extension from the pelvis or lower limbs (see Fig. 9-22).

Retroperitoneal *lymphadenopathy* may be secondary to lymphoma or metastasis, from breast, lung, kidney, prostate, bladder, gynecological, or testicular carcinoma (Fig. 9-26).[1,2,3] Such adenopathy is usually screened with and followed by abdominal CT, but it may be initially detected by sonography. Primary retroperitoneal masses are usually *sarcomas*, (e.g., liposarcoma or mixed mesenchymal sarcomas) and are often large when first discovered. Retroperitoneal fluid collections are usually abscesses or hematomas. A *hematoma* may be secondary to trauma or an underlying tumor. It can occur secondary to anticoagulant therapy, in which case it usually arises in the posterior pararenal space and displaces the kidney anteriorly. Retroperitoneal *abscesses* may arise from rupture of a renal abscess or may occur in the psoas muscle due to spread from an infection of an intervertebral disc space. They may also occur from a posterior perforation of a duodenal ulcer or rupture of a diverticular abscess of the ascending or descending colon.

Adrenal Gland

The adrenal gland is usually evaluated by CT. However, an adrenal mass may be discovered incidentally during a sonographic examination. It may be *cystic* or *solid*. A solid mass may be a nonfunctioning or functioning adenoma, metastasis, pheochromocytoma, or adrenal carci-

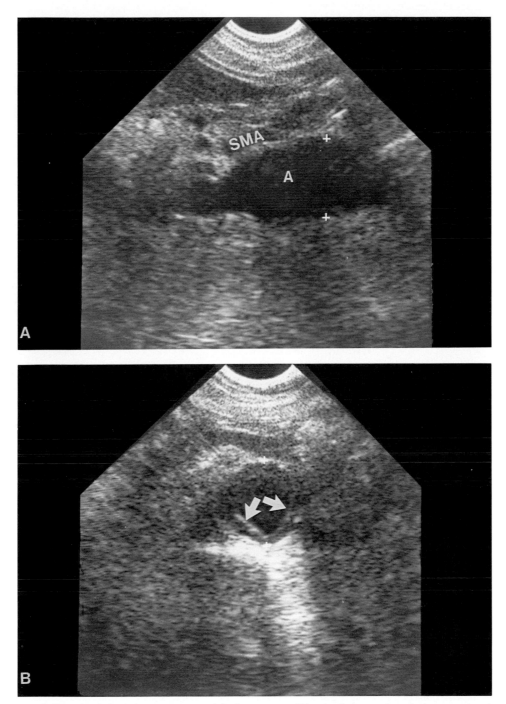

Figure 9-25.   A: Abdominal aortic aneurysm. A fusiform aneurysm (A) is identified arising from the lower portion of the abdominal aorta. The superior mesenteric artery (SMA) can be identified anterior to the aneurysm. **B:** A transverse sonogram of the aneurysm shows clot (arrows) within the lumen of the aneurysm.

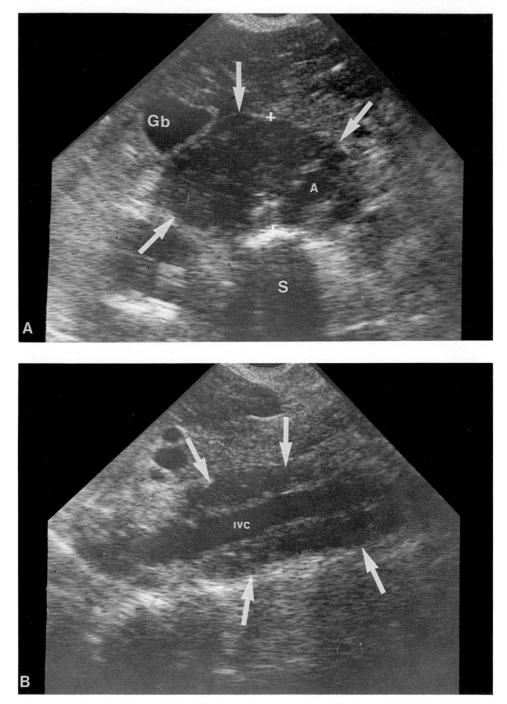

Figure 9-26.   **A:** Prostatic carcinoma with diffuse retroperitoneal adenopathy (arrows) encasing the aorta (A). Spine (S). Gallbladder (Gb). **B:** Longitudinal sonogram of the inferior vena cava (IVC) surrounded by adenopathy (arrows).

noma. Retroperitoneal adenopathy should be looked for, along with invasion of the inferior vena cava, so as to determine whether the mass is possibly malignant.[1,2,3]

Intra-abdominal Fluid Collections

Patients are often referred for a sonogram following abdominal or pelvic surgery to rule out an *abscess*. Before such a study is performed, the abdominal radiographs should be reviewed as the abscess may be gas-containing and be obvious on the radiograph. Such gas-containing abscesses are often difficult or impossible to identify by sonography. Small *serous fluid collections* can be found in the abdomen following surgery; however, these usually resolve within 10 to 14 days. They should never increase in size, and if this occurs, then an abscess should be suspected.[1,2,3,4] The areas that should be evaluated include the site of surgery, the liver, both paracolic gutters, and the pelvis. To prove that a fluid collection is an abscess, an ultrasound-guided percutaneous aspiration can be performed, followed by a gram stain and culture. If the sonogram is negative for an abscess then a CT scan should be done, as it can better detect abscesses in the left upper quadrant, in the retroperitoneum, and among loops of intestine.

Abdominal Wall

If a mass is palpated in the wall of the abdomen, a sonogram can help determine whether it represents a *hernia*, *abscess*, or rectus sheath *hematoma*.[1,2,3] It can also help determine whether the mass is due to an inflammatory (Crohn's disease) or neoplastic (colon carcinoma) process arising in the abdomen and involving the abdominal wall.

GYNECOLOGICAL ULTRASOUND

TECHNIQUE

Sonography of the pelvis, include both kidneys and the lower abdomen. Abdominal and retroperitoneal evaluation should be performed when a gynecological malignancy is suspected.

INDICATIONS FOR EXAMINATION

(1) Evaluate a pelvic mass or abscess.
(2) Locate an intrauterine contraceptive device.

Sonographic evaluation of the pelvis should include the lower abdomen, as the full bladder may displace a pelvic mass into either lower quadrant. The kidneys should also be evaluated, as a pelvic mass can obstruct the kidney (carcinoma of the cervix), while a pelvic kidney or horseshoe kidney can be mistaken for a lower abdominal or pelvic mass. Pelvic sonography helps determine the origin of the mass (uterus versus ovary) and whether the mass is cystic, solid, or complex.

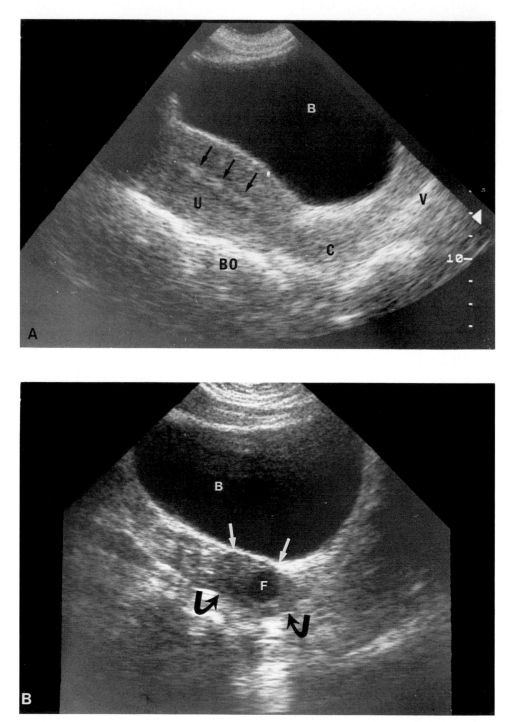

Figure 9-27.   A: Longitudinal sonogram of the normal uterus (U), cervix (C), and vagina (V). Note the linear echogenic line representing the endometrium (arrows). Bladder (B). Bowel (BO). **B:** Normal appearing ovary (arrows) containing a 1.5 cm follicle (F). Bladder (B).

Uterus

The normal uterus of an adult woman measures 6 to 8cm long, 3 to 5cm in its anteroposterior diameter, and 3 to 5cm in its lateral diameter. Its size decreases after the menopause. The uterus has a homogeneous echo pattern and a smooth outline, while the endometrial cavity is delineated by a linear echogenic line that varies in thickness (millimeters) during the menstrual cycle (Fig. 9-27A).[1,3,7]

A *fibroid uterus* is denoted by the presence of a single or multiple inhomogeneous hypoechoic mass(es) in the uterine wall, some of which may be pedunculated (Fig. 9-28). Calcification may be present within some or all of these fibroids. Sarcomatous degeneration is rare but should be suspected when a postmenopausal "fibroid uterus" enlarges. *Carcinoma of the endometrium* produces thickening of the endometrial echoes, and with invasion of the wall the uterus becomes enlarged and its echo pattern becomes inhomogeneous. In *carcinoma of the cervix*, the cervix may appear large, and there may be obstruction of one or other of the ureters and/or invasion of the bladder and sidewall of the pelvis. Such patients, if discovered sonographically, should be further evaluated with an abdominal/pelvic CT scan.

Sonography can diagnose uterine malformations such as a *bicornuate uterus* and also a *T-shaped uterus* in women exposed to diethylstilbesterol in utero (Fig. 9-29).[7] *Hematometra* is due to obstruction of the uterus with a buildup of blood and secretions in the endometrial cavity. In a child this is usually due to an imperforate hymen hematometrocolpos. In the adult it may be due to carcinoma of the cervix or pelvic irradiation.

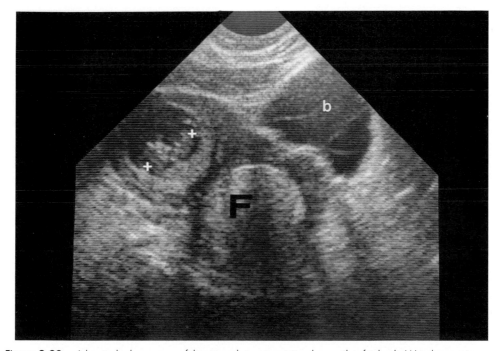

Figure 9-28. A longitudinal sonogram of the uterus shows a gestational sac with a fetal pole (+) in the superior portion of the uterus. A 5cm echogenic fibroid (F) is identified in the lower portion of the uterus. Bladder (b).

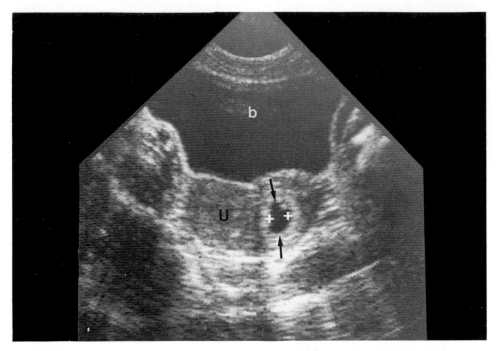

Figure 9-29.   Bicornuate uterus with a five week gestational sac (arrows) in the left horn. Right uterine horn (U). Bladder (b).

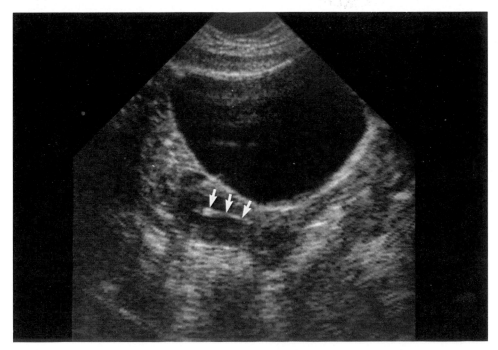

Figure 9-30.   A centrally placed intrauterine contraceptive device (arrows) is present in the endometrial cavity of the uterus.

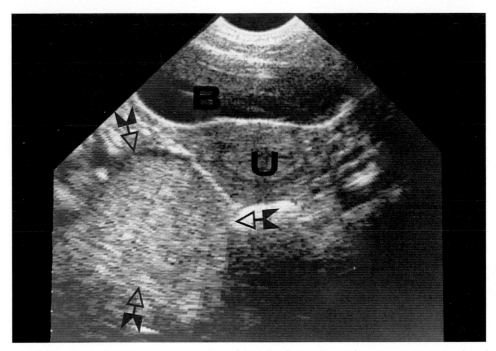

Figure 9-31. Dermoid cyst. A transverse sonogram of the pelvis shows a large echogenic mass (arrows) to the right of the uterus (U). Bladder (B).

An *intrauterine contraceptive device* can be identified in the endometrial cavity or, if it is abnormally placed, in the wall of the uterus (Fig. 9-30).[1,3,7] It cannot be identified if it is outside of the uterus as it is usually hidden by bowel gas. If this is suspected following a normal pelvic sonogram, an abdominal/pelvic radiograph should be obtained to see if it is in the abdomen or pelvis.

Ovaries

The normal ovary in an adult woman measures 3cm by 2cm. *Follicles* within the ovary are identified as small unilocular cystic areas along the periphery of the ovary that usually do not exceed 20 to 25mm in diameter (see Fig. 9-27B).[1,3,7] Their size increases until the time of ovulation when they should involute. Follicles may be multiple and bilateral when the ovaries are being stimulated with clomiphene or human menopausal gonadotropin for in vitro fertilization. The ova from such follicles can be retrieved using ultrasound-guided needle aspiration via the vagina or bladder. If a follicle persists after ovulation, a *follicular cyst* is said to be present and this usually measures no more than 3 to 4cm. These cysts usually disappear following estrogen suppression. They can present with acute pain due to hemorrhage or torsion.

A *dermoid cyst* is the most common ovarian neoplasm in young women. It may be entirely cystic but usually contains some solid elements and may be entirely echogenic due to the presence of fat, hair, and sebum in the cyst (Fig. 9-31).[1,3,7] Foci of calcification with acoustical shadowing may also be seen. The presence of septae in an adnexal cyst should

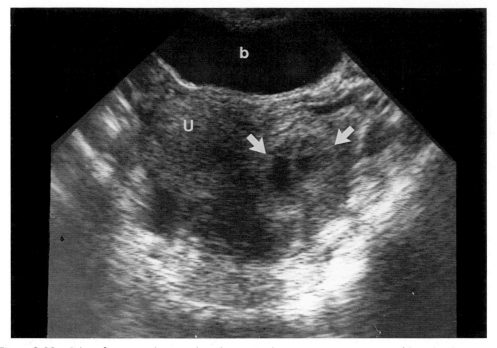

Figure 9-32.   Pelvic inflammatory disease with a tuboovarian abscess. Transverse sonogram of the pelvis shows a complex process in the left adnexa (arrows) representing a tuboovarian abscess with fluid posterior to the uterus (U) in the cul-de-sac. Bladder (b).

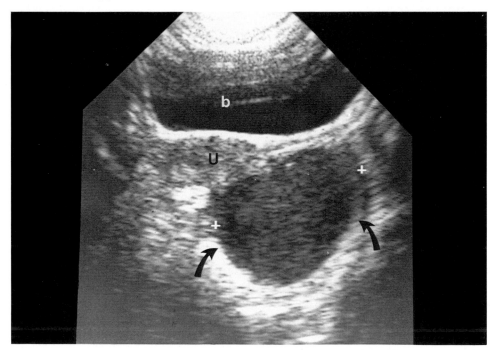

Figure 9-33.   Endometrioma (arrows) in the left adnexa. This cystic mass has low-level internal echoes. Uterus (U). Bladder (b).

suggest the presence of an *ovarian cystadenoma* or *cystadenocarcinoma*. A solid mass in the ovary can be benign (fibroma) or malignant (adenocarcinoma). The latter category would be indicated by the presence of direct spread of tumor beyond the ovary itself along with the presence of ascites.

Pelvic Inflammatory Disease

A sonogram is usually normal in *pelvic inflammatory disease* and should only be performed if the patient fails to respond to medical treatment. Multiple microabscesses may be seen in the cul-de-sac and/or adnexa, or there may be a dominant adnexal *tuboovarian abscess* (Fig. 9-32).[1,3,7] As a result of pelvic inflammatory disease, a dilated tubular cystic adnexal structure due to a *hydrosalpinx* may be seen.

Endometriosis

The pelvic sonogram in most patients with *endometriosis* appears normal, as the endometrial implants are too small to be seen sonographically. Sonography helps to evaluate an adnexal mass in a patient with endometriosis. Single or multiple cul-de-sac and/or adnexal masses with diffuse low level echoes may be found, such as the *endometrioma* shown in Figure 9-33.[1,3,7] The uterus may also be mildly enlarged and irregular due to endometrial implants.

OBSTETRICAL SONOGRAPHY

TECHNIQUE

Sequential longitudinal and transverse scans are performed to document fetal anatomy, the amount of amniotic fluid, and placental position, while appropriate measurements are made to estimate the gestational age.

INDICATIONS FOR EXAMINATION

(1) Estimate the gestational age of the fetus if fundal height does not correspond to the date of the last menstrual period.

(2) Evaluate for multiple pregnancy.

(3) Vaginal bleeding in pregnancy.

(4) Confirm fetal growth and fetal viability.

(5) Assess for fetal anomalies.

A *gestational sac* can be sonographically identified in the uterus at about 5 weeks after the first day of the last menstrual period, approximately three weeks after conception (see Fig. 9-29).[1,3,7] The average size of the sac is used to estimate the gestational age. By about the sixth or seventh week, a fetal pole with heart motion should be seen, thus indicating the presence of a viable intrauterine gestation (Figs. 9-34, 9-35). Beyond that date and up to the tenth or eleventh week, the crown-rump length of the fetus is used to estimate the gestational age. By now a fetal head, fetal trunk, and fetal limbs can be sonographically identified (Fig. 9-36).[7,8] The fetal age can now be estimated by (1) the biparietal diameter of the fetal head,

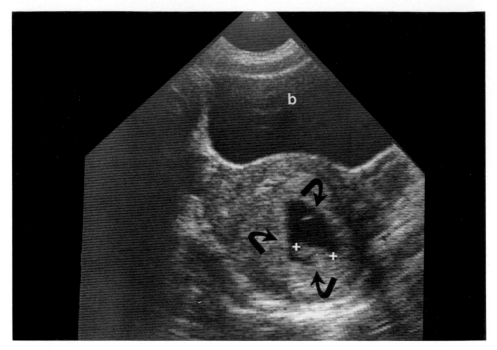

Figure 9-34. Eight-week gestational sac (arrows) in the uterus with a fetal pole (+). Fetal heart motion was seen on real-time scanning. Bladder (b).

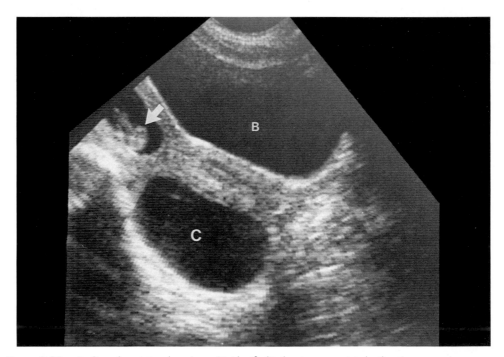

Figure 9-35. An 8-week gestational sac (arrow) is identified in the uterus associated with a 6cm corpus luteum cyst (C) in the cul-de-sac. Bladder (B).

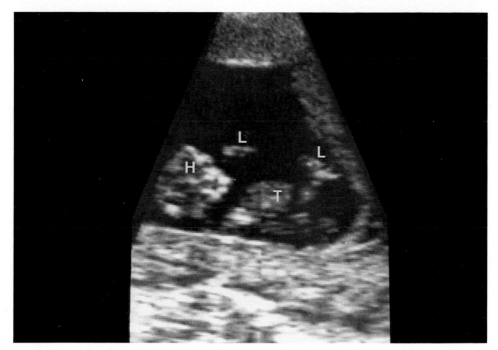

Figure 9-36.   Ten-week intrauterine gestation. A fetal head (H), fetal trunk (T), and fetal upper and lower limbs (L) can be identified.

(2) the circumference of the fetal trunk at the level of the liver, and (3) the length of the fetal femur. The average of these numbers gives the estimated gestational age. The fetal weight can be calculated from the biparietal diameter and abdominal circumference. The presentation of the fetus along with the position and maturity of the placenta is noted, as is the amount of amniotic fluid. Placental maturity is graded (0 to 3) based on the location of the calcifications in the placenta.

The optimal time to assess fetal anomalies is around 16 to 18 weeks gestation, as this allows time for genetic amniocentesis and for an abortion to be performed if necessary.[1,3,7] The fetus should be screened sonographically for an anomaly if the age of the mother is 35 years or greater, there is a family history of a genetic disorder or a previously abnormal fetus, or elevation of the maternal serum alpha fetoprotein.

A sonographic evaluation should include:

(1) Examination of the fetal brain and spine.

(2) Evaluation for a four-chambered heart in the left chest with the aortic arch on the left and the aorta descending to the left of the spine.

(3) Determination of normal abdominal situs with the liver in the right upper quadrant and the fluid-filled stomach in the left upper quadrant.

(4) Evaluation of the kidneys and the urine-filled bladder.

(5) Assessment of the fetal skeleton and limbs.

(6) Determination of the amount of amniotic fluid and whether it is normal, increased (polyhydramnios), or decreased (oligohydramnios) (Fig. 9-37).[1,3,7,8]

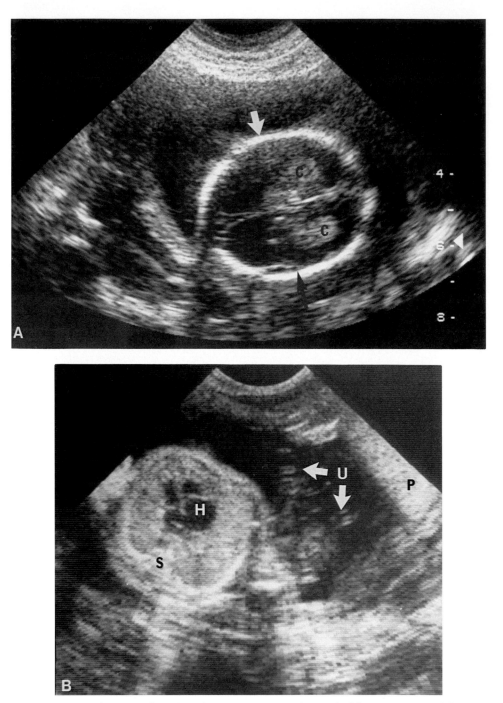

Figure 9-37.   Normal anatomy of an 18-week intrauterine gestation showing the following: **A:** Biparietal diameter of the fetal head (arrows). Echogenic choroid plexus (C). **B:** Normal fetal anatomy (cont.): A four-chambered view of the fetal heart (H). Fetal spine (S). Placenta (P). Umbilical cord (U).

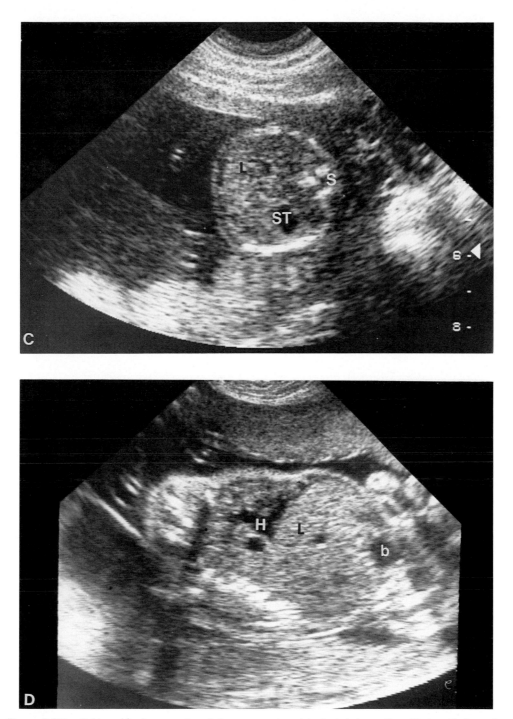

Figure 9-37. **C:** Normal fetal anatomy (cont.): A transverse view of the fetal abdomen. Spine (S). Liver (L). Stomach (ST). **D:** Normal fetal anatomy (cont.): Longitudinal view of the fetal trunk. Heart (H). Liver (L). Urinary bladder (b).

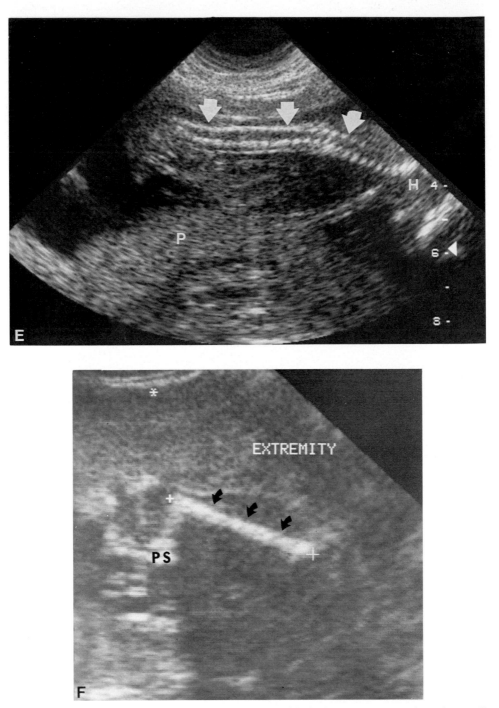

Figure 9-37. **E:** Normal fetal anatomy (cont.): Longitudinal view of the fetal spine (arrows). Head (H). Placenta (P).
F: Normal fetal anatomy (cont.): Measurement (+) of the fetal femur (arrows). Side wall of bony pelvis (PS).

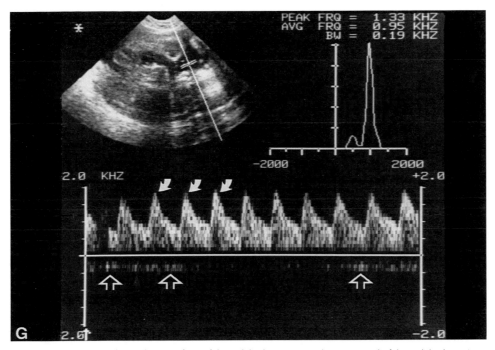

Figure 9-37. **G:** Normal Doppler waveform of the umbilical artery (curved arrows), and of the umbilical vein (open arrowheads).

As the fetus grows, it does so symmetrically, and all of the fetal measurements should increase in unison. Up to about 32 weeks of gestation the sonographic assessment of fetal age is fairly accurate to within 7 to 10 days of the true gestational age. After this, however, the accuracy of sonography in estimating fetal age decreases as the incremental growth of the fetus decreases. As one nears term, the sonographic evaluation of fetal age can be off by as much as 4 weeks.

Sonography in the Evaluation of the Complications of Pregnancy

When a patient is bleeding early in pregnancy, (7 to 8 weeks), a sonogram is usually performed to assess fetal viability. If there has been an *abortion*, there may be sonographic evidence of residual tissue in the uterus (incomplete abortion), or the uterus may be empty (complete abortion) (Fig. 9-38).[1,3,7] Around 10 to 12 weeks of gestation the placental position can be determined. Most *placenta previas* diagnosed before 20 weeks of gestation do not persist to term. If a placenta previa is found beyond this time, a repeat examination should be performed at 36 weeks of gestation to see if it is still present so that appropriate obstetrical management can be planned (Fig. 9-39). In most cases of *placental abruption*, the abrupted area cannot be identified sonographically. Sometimes there may be evidence of separation of the membranes from the lower uterine segment or cervix by the blood; however, it is uncommon to see a retroplacental hematoma.

A diagnosis of *intrauterine growth retardation* (IUGR) is usually made on serial stud-

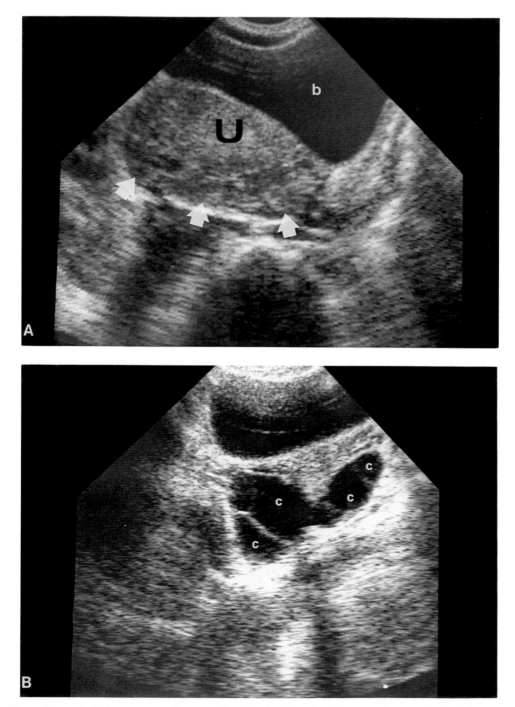

Figure 9-44.   A: Molar pregnancy. The uterus (U) is diffusely enlarged and has a complex internal echo pattern (arrows). Bladder (b). **B:** Transverse sonogram of the pelvis revealing the presence of bilateral theca luteum cysts (C).

Dermoid cysts and *cystadenoma* of the ovary can also be found in pregnancy (see Fig. 9-31). Multiple, bilateral ovarian cysts called *theca luteum cysts* can occur in clomiphene-induced pregnancy, in multiple pregnancy, and also with molar pregnancy (Fig. 9-44).

Molar Pregnancy

A *molar pregnancy* can have the appearance of an incomplete abortion with a complex echo pattern in the endometrial cavity of an enlarged uterus. Bilateral theca luteum cysts should be looked for (see Fig. 9-44).[1,3,7] The diagnosis can be confirmed by a quantitative serum beta human chorionic gonadotropin (HCG) level, followed by pathological examination of the evacuated uterine contents. Rarely a viable fetus can be found with partial molar degeneration of the placenta or a mole may arise from one twin of a twin gestation.

Ectopic Pregnancy

The presence of a gestational sac with a fetal pole and fetal heart motion in the uterus virtually excludes an *ectopic pregnancy*. It is uncommon to have such a finding outside of the uterus where one can make a specific diagnosis of ectopic pregnancy.[1,3,7] A gestational sac should be seen in the uterus when the serum beta HCG level is 6500mIU/ml or greater. If a well-formed gestational sac is seen in the uterus, a transvaginal sonogram may show a yolk sac or a fetal pole with heart motion which was not seen with the abdominal approach. A follow up pelvic sonogram could also be done to determine that a 6 week size sac, truly

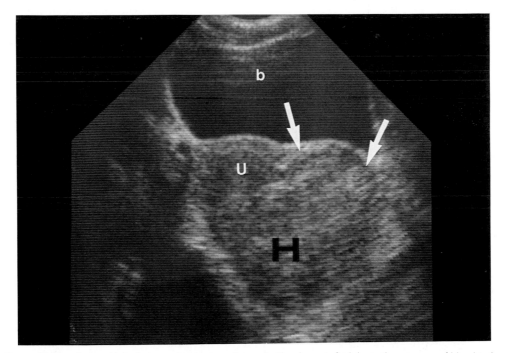

Figure 9-45.   Ruptured left tubal ectopic pregnancy (arrows) with echogenic fluid due to the presence of blood in the cul-de-sac (H) posterior to the uterus (u). Bladder (b).

represents an ongoing viable intrauterine gestation, as a fetal pole with fetal heart motion should develop in seven to ten days. If the sac seen in the uterus is irregular and does not contain a fetal pole, it could be a *blighted ovum, incomplete abortion,* or *decidual reaction* from an ectopic pregnancy that cannot be sonographically identified. If the uterus is empty or if cul-de-sac fluid or a complex adnexal mass is present, these are nonspecific signs for ectopic pregnancy that need to be correlated with a quantitative serum beta HCG (Fig. 9-45). If the serum pregnancy test indicates that a gestational sac should be seen in the uterus, and one is not present and the patient has not bled, then an ectopic pregnancy has to be strongly considered.

A large echogenic solid-looking pelvic mass may be seen in the pelvis with a chronically ruptured ectopic pregnancy. An *abdominal pregnancy* can be difficult to diagnose sonographically.

MISCELLANEOUS USES OF SONOGRAPHY

A *chest* sonogram can be used to determine if an area of pleural thickening on a chest radiograph represents fluid. It can also be used to choose an appropriate site for thoracentesis.[1,3] Sonography of the *breast* can determine whether a mass seen on a mammogram is cystic or solid. If the mass is solid, however, sonography cannot consistently determine whether the mass is benign or malignant. Sonography can determine whether a *thyroid* abnormality is focal or diffuse. A nonfunctioning nodule on a nuclear medicine study can be classified sonographically as cystic, solid, or complex and sonography can be used to guide a needle aspiration if the mass is not clinically palpable. However, sonography cannot be used to differentiate benign from malignant masses.

BIBLIOGRAPHY

1. Fleischer AC, James AE: *Real Time Sonography.* Norwalk, Appleton-Century-Crofts, 1984.
2. Goldberg BB: *Abdominal Sonography,* ed 2. New York, John Wiley & Sons, 1984.
3. Sanders RC: *Clinical Sonography: A Practical Guide.* Boston, Little Brown & Company, 1984.
4. Meyers MA: *Dynamic Radiology of the Abdomen: Normal and Pathological Anatomy,* ed 2. New York, Springer-Verlag, 1982.
5. Resnick MI, Sanders RC: *Ultrasound in Urology,* ed 2. Baltimore, Williams and Wilkins, 1984.
6. Rifkin MD: *Diagnostic Imaging of the Lower Genitourinary Tract.* New York, Raven Press, 1985.
7. Sanders RC, James AE: *The Principles and Practice of Ultrasonography in Obstetrics and Gynecology,* ed 2. New York, Appleton-Century-Crofts, 1980.
8. Bowerman RA: *Atlas of Normal Fetal Ultrasonographic Anatomy.* Chicago, Year Book Medical Publishers, 1986.

CHAPTER 10

NEURORADIOLOGY

Thomas S. Dina

The need for communication between referring physician and radiologist is especially true in neuroradiology. The term "routine exam" has almost no application. Specifics of the clinical history with details of symptoms and physical findings not only determine the appropriate study and details of its execution, but also play a vital role in avoiding undue risk to the patient. Risks range from potential worsening of the patient's condition to life-threatening complications and permanent neurologic deficit. All examinations must be warranted and risks justified; the study must be in the patient's overall best interest. Lack of information or communication can result in an inappropriate or incomplete examination, increased morbidity, inefficiency, and unnecessary cost.

In this chapter, neuroradiologic diagnosis will be presented in the context of clinical case presentations. This will include cranial and spinal symptomatology with presentations as acute, progressive, chronic, or traumatic. Most imaging modalities are briefly discussed in the case section in which their application is most appropriate clinically. Cerebrovascular imaging is presented in a separate section.

THE SKULL AND BRAIN

THE EMERGENCY ROOM PATIENT—THE NEUROLOGIC "EMERGENCY"

"Emergency" for discussion purposes includes not only those patients whose neuropathology demands immediate attention (the true medical emergency), but also those patients in whom the onset of symptoms is sufficiently rapid or the severity sufficiently great to seek immediate attention. Such patients will most often present to the hospital emergency room or as urgent same-day office or clinic visits.

CASE NUMBER 1: ACUTE ONSET SEVERE HEADACHE

A 38-year-old woman complains of the fairly rapid onset of a severe headache, "the worst headache of her life," beginning approximately 24 hours ago. She now also notes mild weakness of her left arm and mild lethargy. To others, she has appeared slightly confused at times during that day.

The major diagnostic considerations include cerebritis/meningitis and intracranial hemorrhage, either subarachnoid or intracerebral. The presence of left upper extremity weakness indicates the possibility of a cerebral hemisphere mass or at least unilateral mass effect. Unilateral edema, for example, would increase the risk of herniation following lumbar puncture for cerebrospinal fluid examination. After completion of a history and physical examination, including a search for signs of infection, trauma, bleeding diasthesis, and other clues, and even while supportive laboratory work is pending, radiologic examination is in order.

The radiographic examination of the skull is a simple, inexpensive study of limited usefulness. It is primarily a study of osseous structures only. It will only rarely provide meaningful information in the acute situation (e.g., unsuspected fracture). Displacement of the calcified pineal gland is an important observation, but this is superseded by the more informative and often definitive information provided by computed tomography.

The initial procedure of choice, therefore, is computed tomography (the CT scan). The scan is performed in the supine position and requires little active patient cooperation with the exception of lack of movement for about a ten-minute period. From the skull base to the vertex, a series of ten to fifteen 10mm thick scans are usually necessary for a complete CT examination. Intravenous contrast material is not injected, since one of the main purposes of the examination is to detect intracranial hemorrhage, the hyperdense (white) appearance of which might not be distinguishable from contrast-enhanced tumor or inflammatory processes.

Subarachnoid Hemorrhage (SAH)

The great majority of subarachnoid hemorrhages will be detected by computed tomography. On a normal noncontrast-enhanced CT, the CSF-filled basilar cisterns and ventricles afford less x-ray attenuation and, therefore, appear relatively black or hypodense as compared to normal adjacent brain. Recent hemorrhage, especially with clot formation, will appear white or hyperdense. The subarachnoid blood may diffuse throughout the subarachnoid space or may collect in a single or prominent larger focus that may provide a clue as to the site of hemorrhage. When SAH is confirmed on CT, CSF examination is no longer necessary. A normal CT scan, however, does not exclude the possibility of subarachnoid hemorrhage. Lumbar puncture then becomes necessary. If SAH is confirmed, cerebral angiography must be considered next, since the most common etiology of nontraumatic SAH is rupture of a berry aneurysm. Hypertension and vascular malformations are other common etiologies of SAH, although intracerebral or intraventricular hemorrhage is usually the predominant CT finding.

Figure 10-1 illustrates anatomic structures seen by CT. Note the basilar cisterns or subarachnoid spaces at the skull base, especially the larger suprasellar area, (suprasellar cistern), which extends laterally to the sylvian cisterns and anteriorly to the interhemispheric fissure. These spaces are slightly better seen in this patient with mild cerebral atrophy. Intravenous contrast material enhances normal vessels (arteries and veins) within the suprasellar and sylvian cisterns. White/gray matter differentiation is also enhanced. This appearance can be contrasted to that of Figure 10-2, which shows an example of recent subarachnoid hemorrhage.

Intracerebral Hematoma (ICH)

An acute intracerebral hematoma will be quite apparent on CT (see Figure 10-3). They tend to be of moderate to large size and occasionally burst into the ventricular system. Such patients are usually more obtunded and exhibit greater neurologic deficit depending on the relative size and location of the hemorrhage. The differential diagnosis of nontraumatic ICH includes a hypertensive bleed, by far the most common etiology. Past medical history is of utmost importance since the patient may be acutely hypertensive secondary to an increase in intracranial pressure. Rupture of an arteriovenous malformation (AVM) will account for less than 10 per cent of intracerebral hematomas, hemorrhage within or adjacent to a tumor accounts for a few per cent, and approximately 30 per cent of ruptured aneurysms will have an associated ICH. Angiography may be necessary, especially if surgical evacuation is considered.

Cerebritis and Meningitis

Early in their course and especially if uncomplicated, acute infectious processes usually have normal CT examinations. With the knowledge of a normal CT study, however, one can safely proceed to lumbar puncture for CSF analysis. If the diagnosis of an acute bacterial meningitis is confirmed, or viral meningitis or cerebritis is strongly supported clinically, further radiologic diagnostic procedures might not be necessary. CT is used to evaluate a poor clinical response, or to search for a subdural empyema or intracerebral abscess. Late CT follow-up may be appropriate to exclude secondary communicating hydrocephalus.

CASE NUMBER 2: ACUTE ONSET NEUROLOGIC DEFICIT

A 64-year-old man was in seemingly good health until that morning when he noted the sudden onset of slurred speech and the rapid progression of weakness of his right side, upper extremity greater than lower. On physical examination, the patient was normotensive, aphasic with a right central facial palsy and right hemiparesis.

The need for radiologic studies is generally determined by the clinical course during the first few to 24 hours. The working diagnosis will fall into the general category of *cerebrovascular accident* (CVA) but with its full extent or permanence as yet unknown. The *transient*

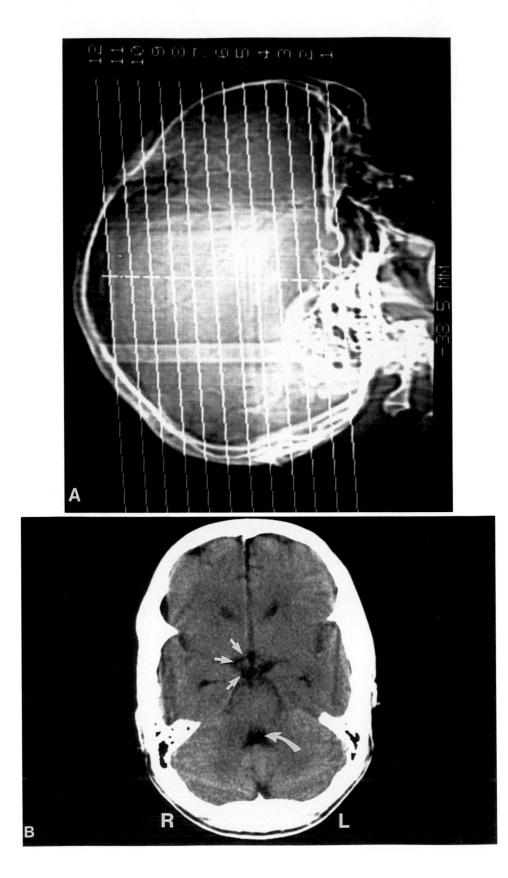

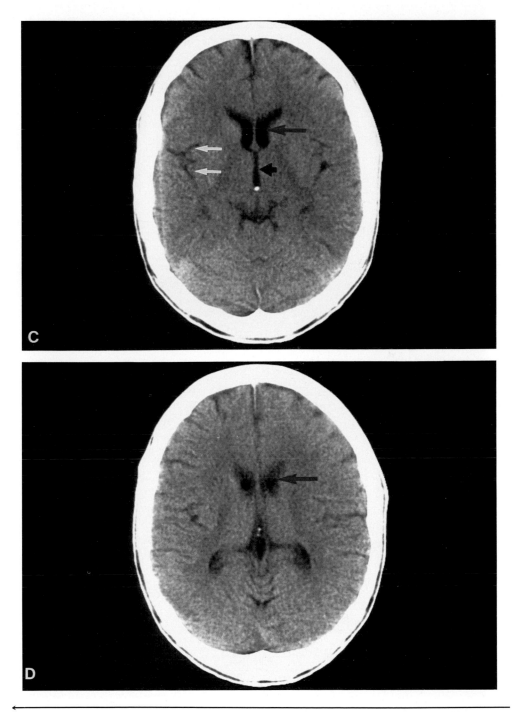

Figure 10-1. Computed tomography of the brain. Localization view **(A).** Nonenhanced scans **(B, C, D).** Normal contrast-enhanced scans **(E, F).** The localization view (A) illustrates the levels of the axial scans in a patient with mild cerebral atrophy; scan numbers 3, 4, and 6 are seen in B, C, and D. In B, note the cerebrospinal fluid-filled (black) basilar cisterns (small white arrows) and fourth ventricle (curved white arrow). In C and D, note the sylvian cistern (larger white arrows), third ventricle (short black arrow), and left lateral ventricle (black arrow).

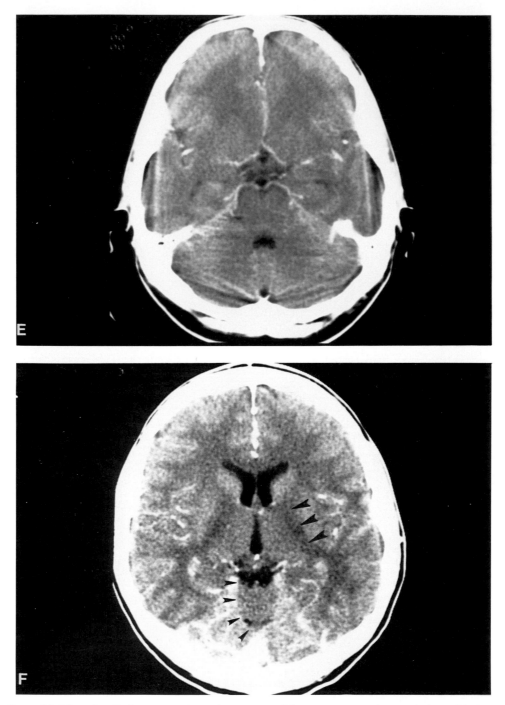

Figure 10-1 (cont.).   On the contrast enhanced scans, note in E the serpiginous vasculature at the base of the brain and in F the improved demarcation of the internal capsule (larger black arrowheads) with the basal ganglia laterally and thalamus medially and edge of the tentorium (small black arrowheads). Note that the patient's right side is on the reader's left as will be the convention throughout this chapter unless otherwise indicated.

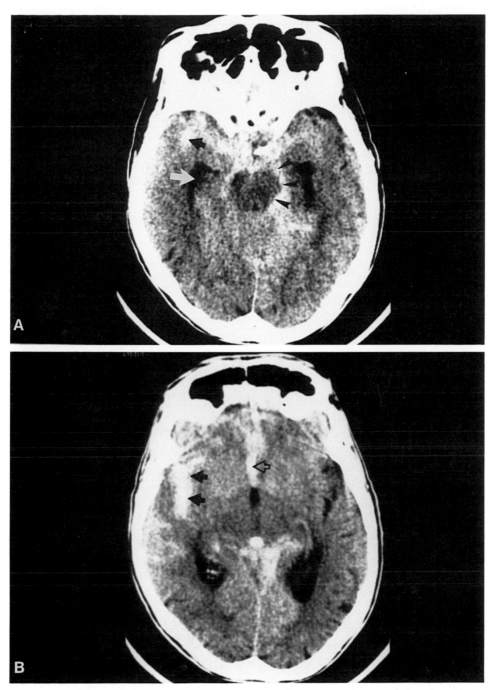

Figure 10-2. Subarachnoid hemorrhage. Nonenhanced CT scans of the base of the brain **(A)** and next level higher **(B).** The blood-containing CSF spaces at the base of the brain are white (hyperdense). These compartments are contiguous, outlining the brainstem (black arrowheads) and extending well into the sylvian cistern on the right (black arrows) and interhemispheric fissure anteriorly (open black arrow). The temporal horns of the lateral ventricles are dilated (white arrow).

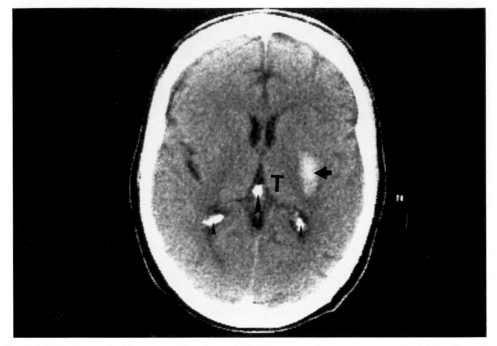

Figure 10-3.   Intracerebral hematoma. Nonenhanced CT. A hyperdense hematoma is seen in the left basal ganglia (small black arrow) lateral to the posterior limb of the internal capsule which lies between the hematoma and the thalamus (T). There is compression of the left Sylvian cistern which is consequently less well seen than the right. Note also the normal findings of a calcified pineal gland (large black arrowhead) and calcified choroid plexus (small black arrowheads).

ischemic attack (TIA) will usually have completely resolved by the time the patient is seen, while the patient with a *reversible ischemic neurologic deficit* (RIND) may be in the process of recovering if seen within a few hours of the initial event. CT may be in order if more active treatment such as anticoagulation therapy is felt to be appropriate or additional diagnostic studies such as duplex carotid sonography and angiography are planned.

If the neurologic deficit appears complete and stable, emergency CT is usually not necessary. Cerebral infarcts are less likely to be apparent in the first 24 hours and the confirmation of an infarct adds little to acute patient management. In many patients, however, the presentation is not clear-cut or their neurologic status continues to deteriorate, in which case other diagnostic possibilities enter into the differential. CT then assumes an urgent or emergency role in excluding other etiologies, such as intracranial hemorrhage or unsuspected trauma in the case of inaccurate or unavailable medical history.

Figure 10-4 is an example of an acute infarction in the distribution of the left middle cerebral artery. The hypodensity within the temporal lobe, frontal and parietal opercular areas is a reflection of vasogenic edema, an early structural change in acute infarction. These changes become much more apparent several days after the acute event. There is relatively little mass effect (displacement of structures from their normal position) considering the volume of brain involved. There is but mild compression of the frontal horn of the left lateral

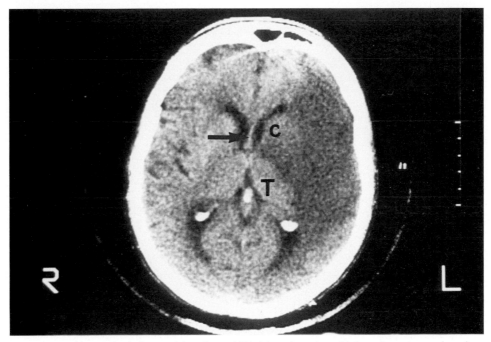

Figure 10-4. Acute cerebral infarction. Nonenhanced CT. A large hypodense (dark gray) area is seen throughout much of the left cerebral hemisphere lateral to the internal capsule, with relative sparing of the thalamus (T) and head of the caudate nucleus (C). Note minimal displacement of the septum pellucidum to the right (arrow).

ventricle, minimal displacement of midline structures (third ventricle and septum pellucidum) to the contralateral side, and effacement of cortical sulci.

Soon after an acute infarction, CT is performed without the intravenous infusion of contrast material. There is a statistically potential risk of worsening the clinical outcome by performing contrast-enhanced CT in the acute stage of infarction. Contrast enhancement is therefore reserved for situations in which the baseline CT scan is indeterminate, suggesting other diagnoses such as primary or metastatic tumor.

The need for follow-up examination is usually determined by the clinical course. Unexpected deterioration usually warrants CT reexamination. A greater than expected degree of edema or mass effect may be present or, in the case of sudden marked deterioration, hemorrhage within the site of infarction may have taken place. In another patient shown in Figure 10-5, the early changes of infarction are similar to that in Figure 10-4 but are much more subtle and are barely discernible. Following rapid deterioration two days later, the area of hypodense infarction is much better defined (Fig. 10-5B), but there is also a large area of acute hemorrhage centrally which has extended into the frontal horn of the left lateral ventricle and caused considerable mass effect with displacement of midline structures to the right.

Angiography is usually not appropriate in the acute or subacute setting since the risk of complication is greater and the information gained will not usually alter treatment in the

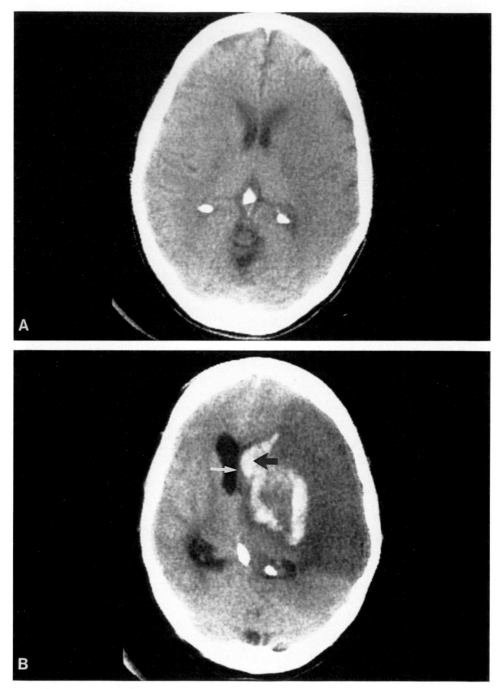

Figure 10-5.   Acute cerebral infarction with hemorrhage. Nonenhanced CT **(A)** and follow-up two days later **(B).** The acute change of hypodensity in A is similar, though more subtle, than that in Figure 10-4. Two days later (B), the infarct is better defined. There is central hemorrhage with blood extending into the frontal horn of the left lateral ventricle (black arrow) and marked displacement of the septum pellucidum to the right (white arrow).

acute situation. The controversial exception may be the emergency endarterectomy in the patient with RIND or multiple repeated TIA's in a short period of time.

CASE NUMBER 3: HEAD TRAUMA

A 20-year-old, having been in an auto accident an hour earlier, arrives in the emergency room in a semiconscious state with findings of obvious head trauma, a dilated right pupil, and left hemiparesis.

Epidural Hematoma

When the presentation of acute head trauma is obvious and severe, only the essential life-support procedures should be undertaken along with a determination, as much as possible, of the full extent of serious injury (especially cervical spine injury associated with head trauma). Computed tomography is the emergency procedure of choice. Unless there is evidence of a penetrating skull injury or depressed fracture, the skull x-ray series will not add meaningful information. While it is true that the presence of a fracture crossing a meningeal arterial groove indicates the possibility of an *acute epidural hematoma* (EDH), the definitive diagnosis is made by CT. The exclusion of a skull fracture does not allow one to relax, since significant intracranial injury secondary to trauma is equally as common with or without a nondepressed fracture.

The lateral projection of the skull in Figure 10-6A reveals two sharp linear lucencies (fractures) crossing the groove of the middle meningeal artery and vein. The fractures are not seen on the frontal projection (Fig. 10-6B), but there is a shift of the calcified pineal gland to the left of the midline of 10mm, the upper limit of normal being 2mm. Although the fracture may be seen on either right or left lateral projection, it is sharper on the "right" labeled lateral, because that side is closest to the film.

The patient with an EDH may present with a brief lucid period followed by rapid deterioration due to the usual origin of the hematoma as an arterial injury. Since the dura is closely adherent to the inner table of the skull, dissection of the hematoma along the inner surface of the calvarium is somewhat confined, accounting for the increasing central thickness and focal mass effect. An acute EDH is illustrated in Figure 10-7.

Subdural Hematoma

The more common extraaxial traumatic lesion is the subdural hematoma (SDH). This usually occurs as a result of disruption of bridging veins in the subdural extraarachnoid space. The extravasated blood can more readily dissect through the potential subdural space. Such collections tend to be less confined, extending from front to back, vertex to base. This extent, over an entire hemisphere, accounts for the overall greater mass effect than one might expect from the relatively "thin" sheet of hematoma.

Figure 10-8 shows an acute left SDH manifest as a rim of hyperdensity adjacent to the inner table of the skull, effacement of underlying cortical sulci, compression of the left lateral ventricle, and moderate displacement of midline structures to the right. There is also white matter edema of contusion posteriorly.

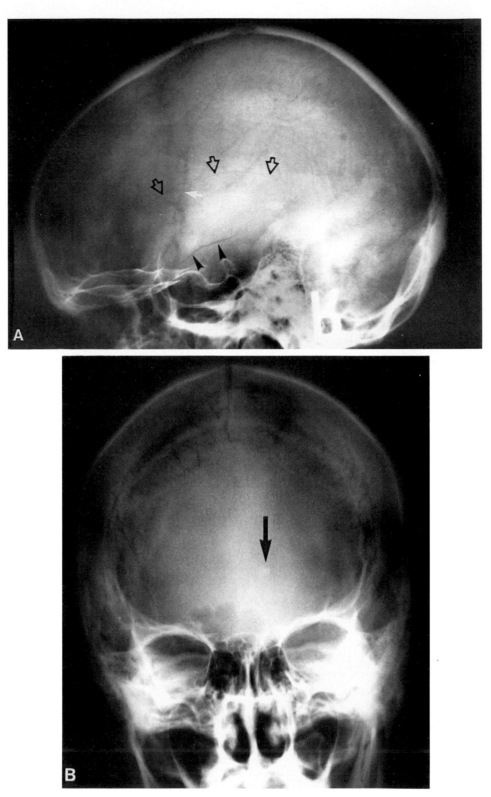

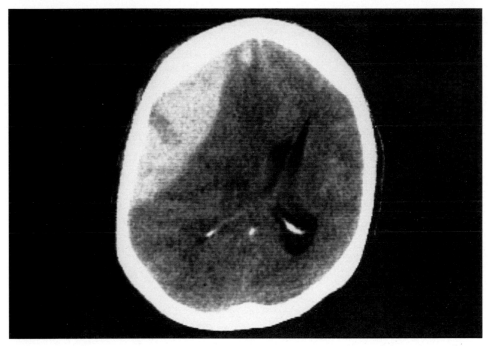

Figure 10-7. Epidural hematoma. A nonenhanced axial CT scan demonstrates a large right hyperdense collection of blood compressing brain and markedly displacing midline structures to the left.

CASE NUMBER 4: NEW ONSET SEIZURES

A young adult experiences a sudden loss of consciousness followed by generalized tonic and clonic spasms and urinary incontinence. The patient is brought to the emergency room while still recovering from the postictal state.

A patient having experienced his or her first focal or generalized seizure will often be brought to the emergency room, by a friend, while still recovering from the postictal state. The need for radiologic work-up depends on the clinical state at the time. The evaluation of the patient who is completely recovered is less urgent than that of the patient with focal neurologic findings or constitutional symptoms. Approximately half of patients without focal findings will have idiopathic epilepsy and a normal radiologic examination. The list of other etiologic possibilities is long and includes toxic/metabolic states (especially alcoholism), infarction, hemorrhage, trauma, and neoplasm. The patient's clinical condition will determine the need for CT or magnetic resonance imaging (MRI) and the degree of urgency.

Figure 10-6. Skull fracture. The right lateral radiograph **(A)** shows a faint sharp curvilinear fracture (open arrow) crossing the groove of the middle meningeal artery (white arrow) and a second more prominent fracture inferiorly (arrowheads). In the frontal projection **(B),** the faintly visualized calcified pineal gland is seen displaced to the left of midline (black arrow).

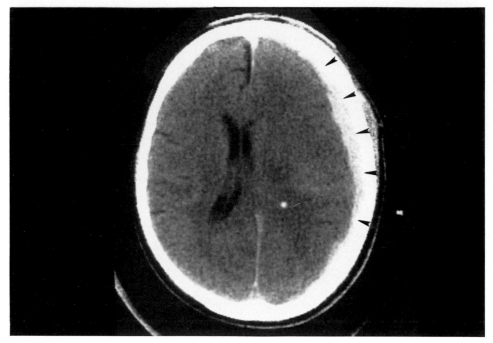

Figure 10-8. Subdural hematoma. A nonenhanced axial CT scan demonstrates a hyperdense rim of blood extending from anterior to posterior along the inner table of the skull (arrowheads), obliterating sulci and displacing midline structures to the right.

NONACUTE NEUROLOGIC PRESENTATIONS

CASE NUMBER 5: SLOWLY PROGRESSIVE NEUROLOGIC DEFICIT

A 50-year-old gives a history of increasing headache over the past few months, difficulty finding words, and weakness of his right upper extremity. He experienced an episode of seizure-like activity of which his recollection is vague.

Clinically, such patients may be the most difficult to evaluate. Initial signs and symptoms may be very subtle and go unnoticed by both patient and physician. Slowly expanding mass lesions may attain great size if they start in relatively silent areas. Strategically located lesions that cause increased intracranial pressure by ventricular obstruction may have even more vague presentations. Only the most subtle findings may be present on neurologic exam. Other times, the physical examination can be quite precise in locating a lesion anatomically.

Intraaxial Neoplasm

Primary intracranial neoplasms vary considerably in clinical presentation and radiologic appearance. Only generalizations may be made and characteristic findings described. Few are specific and none pathognomonic.

Less well-defined and more varied appearances are seen in intraaxial (intraparenchymal) lesions as opposed to those involving dura, the arachnoid space, peripheral cranial nerves, or the pituitary gland. Even though many tumors are highly infiltrative, most make their presence known through the specific structures involved and the mass effect produced. Surrounding structures are displaced or compressed either by the neoplasm itself or adjacent edema which is almost invariably present.

There is a greater tendency for benign lesions to contain calcification or have a cystic component. The more benign cystic tumors tend to have well-defined thin walls over much of the cyst, the classic example of which is the cystic cerebellar astrocytoma seen in childhood. Unfortunately, most primary intraaxial tumors tend to contain a mixture of grades of neoplastic activity, and with time (months to years) the more malignant cells become the dominant cell type.

The less critically ill the patient at presentation, the more appropriate is magnetic resonance imaging (MRI) as the initial diagnostic procedure. The need for patient cooperation is more stringent with MRI than CT. The patient must be free of ferromagnetic objects or devices including life-support apparatus. A full head examination in one plane may take ten minutes or longer, during which time the patient must be motionless. Lack of movement is more critical since a "block" of images are imaged at one time and one cannot simply rescan the single image degraded by movement as might be done with CT.

While many MRI findings remain nonspecific, the superior sensitivity of MRI provides improved yield in demonstrating lesions and multiplicity of lesions. This sensitivity also accounts for the improved definition of normal anatomic structures. T1-weighted images (short TE and short TR) tend to give improved anatomic detail as illustrated by the midsagittal image in Figure 10-9A and the coronal image in B. For greater sensitivity in demonstrating intraaxial lesions, an intermediate and T2-weighted imaging sequence is usually obtained (short and moderately long TE with long TR spin-echo sequence). This sequence also provides improved white/gray matter differentiation as illustrated in Figures 10-9C and D.

While precise tumor location has been greatly improved with MRI, a limitation remains in the differentiation of tumor margin and surrounding edema. Part of this difficulty, of course, lies in the inherent lack of precise tumor margins pathologically.

A *glioma* in the suprasylvian area of the left parietal lobe is well localized on the sagittal and coronal T1-weighted images in Figures 10-10A and B. There is diminished signal intensity at the tumor site. On an axial T2-weighted image (Fig. 10-10C), there is increased signal intensity (whiteness) at least in part due to surrounding edema.

On CT, a *glioblastoma* usually appears as an irregularly shaped mass with inhomogeneous enhancement and often a central lucency. This central lucency may represent necrotic tumor, cyst, or merely a poorly vascularized central area that would enhance if given a higher dose of contrast material and a delay before scanning. The nonenhanced scan in Figures 10-11A and B shows white matter edema (hypodensity and mass effect), while intravenous contrast material greatly enhances the tumor margins leaving a relatively hypodense center and surrounding edema (Figs. 10-11C and D).

Extraaxial Neoplasm

One truly benign neoplasm whose specific cytologic group can be strongly suggested is the *meningioma*. With the rare exception of an intraventricular location, these are extraaxial and

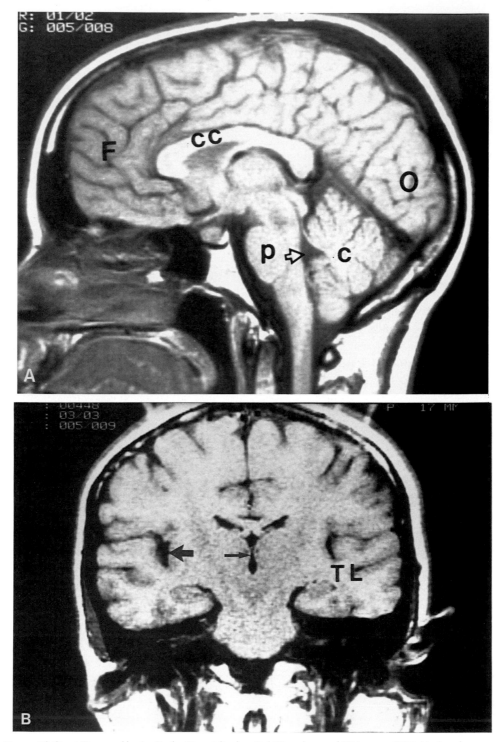

Figure 10-9. MRI, normal brain. On the T1-weighted sagittal **(A)** and coronal **(B)** images, CSF is black and anatomic detail is well delineated.

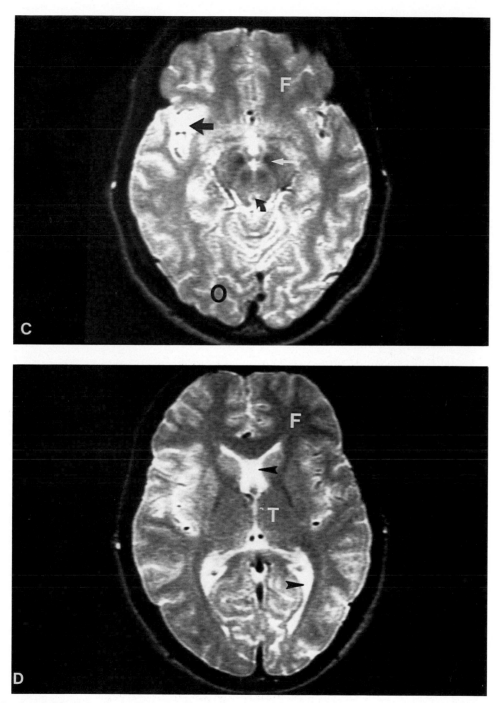

Figure 10-9 (cont.). On the T2-weighted axial images **(C and D),** CSF is white and white/gray matter differentiation is enhanced. Note the labeled major structures: cerebellum (C), corpus callosum (CC), pons (P), frontal lobe (F), occipital lobe (O), fourth ventricle (open black arrow), third ventricle (thin black arrow), left lateral ventricle (black arrowheads), sylvian cistern (wide black arrow), temporal lobe (TL), thalamus (white T), substantia nigra (white arrow), cerebral aqueduct (curved black arrow).

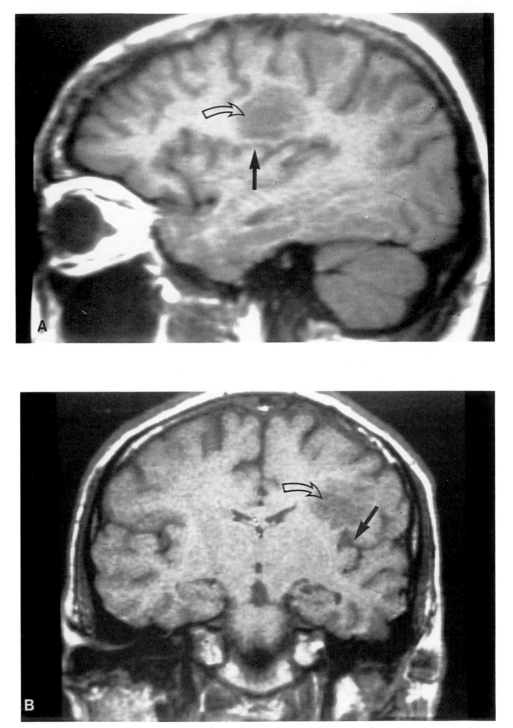

Figure 10-10.   Glioma, MRI. On T1-weighted sagittal (**A**) and coronal (**B**) images, the low signal intensity of the tumor (curved open arrow) is seen above the sylvian cistern depressing it inferiorly (black arrow).

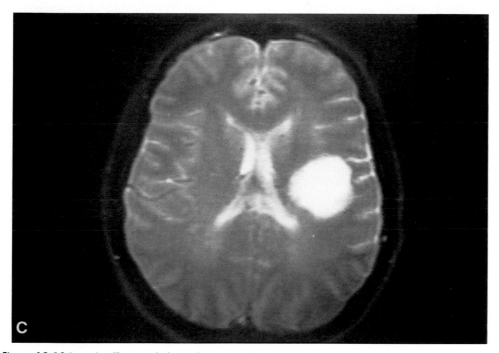

Figure 10-10 (cont.). There is a high signal intensity on the T2-weighted axial image **(C)** similar to CSF within the lateral ventricles.

often readily accessible surgically. The displacement of normal overlying brain and a broad-based dural origin can be readily appreciated with the appropriate plane of MRI. With high field-strength magnet imaging (e.g., 1.5 Tesla), they tend to have similar signal intensity to that of normal brain on T1-weighted images and a relatively less intense signal on T2-weighted spin-echo sequences. The delineation of white and gray matter and the thin rim of cerebrospinal fluid or overlying veins help define its location. The brain often appears to have "remodeled" or "invaginated" to accommodate the slow-growing tumor. They may attain great size or stimulate edema in adjacent brain before becoming clinically manifest. The overall edema is well seen on T2-weighted MR images.

On CT, meningiomas typically enhance homogeneously. They should abut a dural surface. Although the appearance may be strongly suggestive, other lesions such as lymphoma and metastatic tumors may mimic meningioma.

Figure 10-12A is that of a large posterior fossa meningioma seen on a T1-weighted image just below the torcula and markedly compressing the cerebellum. There is ventricular obstruction at the fourth ventricle resulting in enlargement of the third and lateral ventricles. The signal intensity is similar to that of normal supratentorial brain. An axial T2-weighted image (Fig. 10-12B) shows the tumor to be to the right of midline, "invaginating" the cerebellum, and of low signal intensity relative to cerebellum and CSF. A contrast-enhanced CT scan of another patient (Fig. 10-13) shows a homogeneously enhancing meningioma in the left parietal area with relatively little mass effect.

The other common extraaxial tumors occur in the cerebellopontine angle cistern (primar-

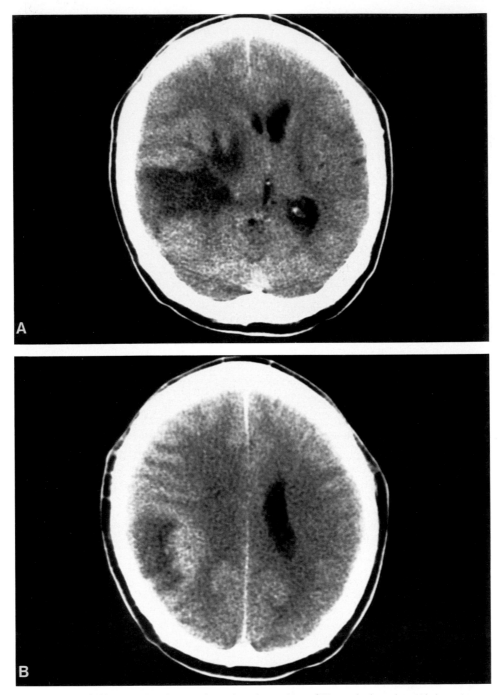

Figure 10-11. Glioblastoma, CT. The nonenhanced axial scans (**A and B**) reveal a hypodense (dark gray) area within white matter and cortex of the posterior right temporal lobe extending into the parietal lobe, compressing the right lateral ventricle and displacing midline structures to the left.

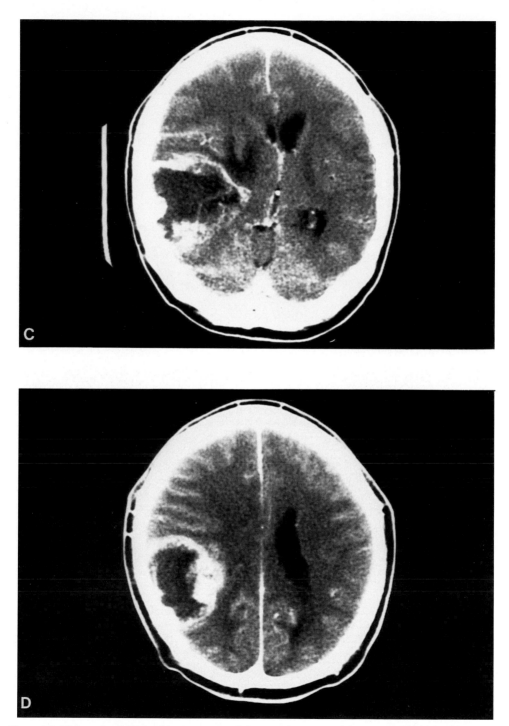

Figure 10-11 (cont.). Following IV contrast material, there is enhancement of the tumor periphery **(C and D)**.

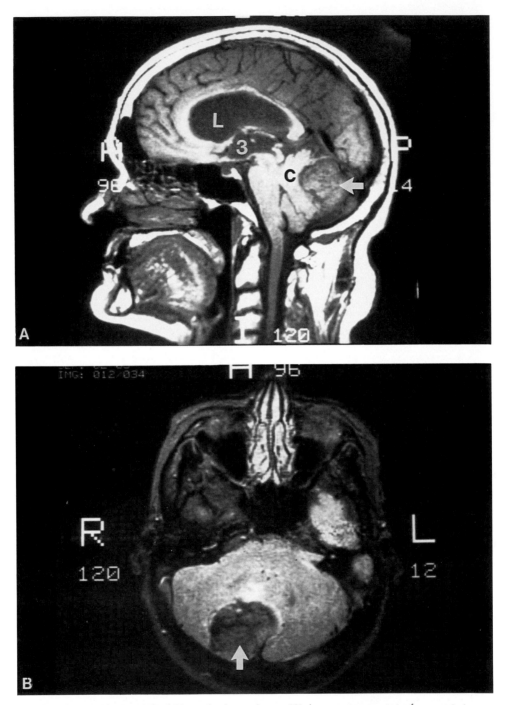

Figure 10-12.   Meningioma, MRI. A T1-weighted sagittal image **(A)** demonstrates a posterior fossa meningioma (white arrow) markedly compressing the cerebellum (C) and causing ventricular obstruction with enlargement of the third (3) and lateral (L) ventricles. The axial T2-weighted image **(B)** shows the cerebellum compressed by the low signal intensity tumor (white arrow).

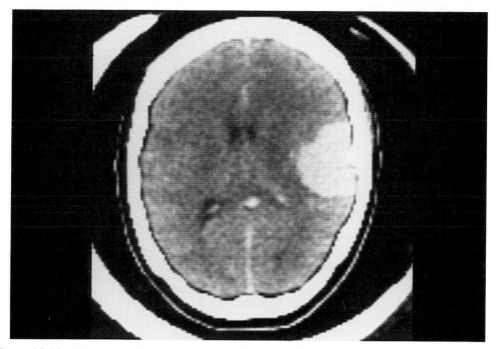

Figure 10-13. Meningioma. Contrast-enhanced axial CT. The broad-based homogeneously enhancing mass abuts the calvarium and causes relatively little compression of the left lateral ventricle.

ily acoustic neuromas and less commonly meningiomas) and the area of the sella turcica (see Case Number 7).

Infectious Disease

With more rapid (subacute) progression of symptoms, inflammatory processes must be considered. These include acute infection, such as *pyogenic abscess* and the more indolent *fungal* or *parasitic* infestations seen usually in the immunocompromised host. Occasionally neoplasms appear to present with a relatively short history due to their strategic location and attainment of a critical mass in terms of compression or involvement of key structures. Metastatic tumors may occasionally act in this manner as well.

Pyogenic infections do not necessarily present acutely in an obviously septic patient. It is not unusual for an abscess to remain relatively silent for weeks or even months. Initially, symptoms may be few and only slowly progressive. The clinical course may mimic that of tumor. Such lesions will usually be beyond the diffuse inflammatory cerebritis stage and have a well-formed cavity. The "walls" tend to be thin and regular, helping to differentiate its abscess cavity from the necrotic center and irregular walls of tumor.

The pyogenic *(Staphylococcus aureus)* abscess seen on CT in Figure 10-14 appears as a hypodense cavity surrounded by an enhancing rim, which consists of the inflammatory, macrophage-laden margin where the blood-brain barrier breakdown is greatest. In this case, the rim is somewhat thick and irregular.

The axial CT scans in Figure 10-15 illustrate multiple enhancing nodules with cavitation

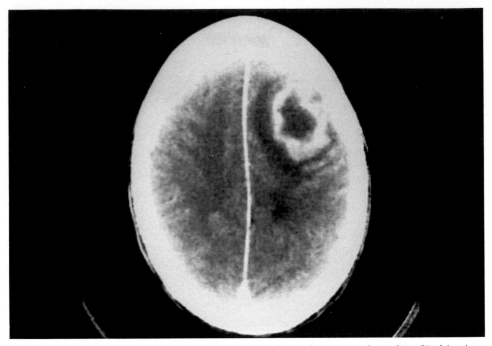

Figure 10-14. Abscess. Contrast-enhanced axial CT. The slightly irregular contrast-enhanced "wall" of the abscess cavity is seen in the posterior left frontal lobe surrounded by low-density edema.

that are typical of *Toxoplasma gondii encephalitis*. In another patient (Fig. 10-16), innumerable lesions are seen on T2 weighted MR images. MRI has been shown to be more sensitive in demonstrating a multiplicity of lesions and is therefore the imaging procedure of choice if the patient is able to cooperate. Toxoplasma is the most common etiology of focal inflammatory mass lesions seen in patients with the acquired immunodeficiency syndrome (AIDS). The presentation in such patients is typically subacute, often with mental status changes before structural lesions are demonstrated with either CT or MRI. The presence of the Human Immunodeficiency Virus (HIV) within brain itself may account for the mental changes. Imaging studies may remain normal or show brain shrinkage. Innumerable other infectious organisms have been demonstrated in the AIDS patient. A partial list of the most common include cytomegalovirus, progressive multifocal leukoencephalopathy (papovavirus), cryptococcosis (usually meningeal), candidiasis, and tuberculosis. Care must be taken to differentiate these infectious etiologies from Kaposi's sarcoma and lymphoma which also occur with increased frequency in AIDS.

CASE NUMBER 6: VARIABLE CNS SYMPTOMATOLOGY

A 33-year-old woman presents with a history of loss of visual acuity, unilateral upper extremity weakness, and clumsiness which initially improved but was then followed by bilateral leg weakness. These symptoms have recently recurred with an increase in severity as well.

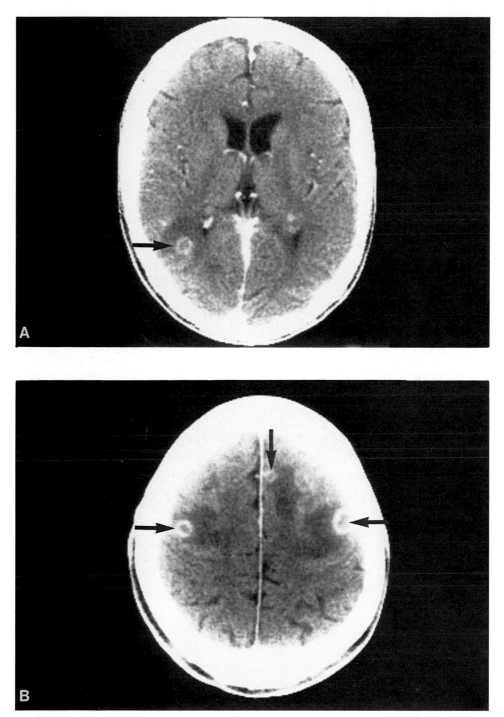

Figure 10-15. Toxoplasmosis. Contrast-enhanced axial CT. In the right posterior temporal lobe in **(A)** and bilateral posterior frontal/parietal lobes in the same patient at a higher level **(B)** are seen multiple ring-like areas of enhancement (arrows) with surrounding low-density edema. These are typical of cerebral toxoplasmosis in the AIDS patient.

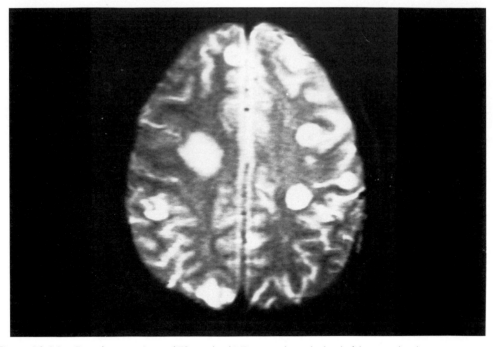

Figure 10-16.   Toxoplasmosis. An axial T2-weighted MR image above the level of the ventricles demonstrates multiple rounded lesions of high signal intensity (imaged white, similar in intensity to the CSF seen within cortical sulci in this example). Both the lesions and surrounding edema contribute to the high signal intensity.

Demyelinating and Related Diseases

The more variable the symptomatology, the more difficult can be the clinical localization of a lesion. Symptoms might vary in severity and extent and also in location. In the younger adult population, the concern may be that of demyelinating disease, most commonly *multiple sclerosis* (MS). Although nonspecific, MRI can be highly suggestive of the diagnosis. The MS plaques are well seen, especially on T2-weighted images, as areas of increased signal intensity within white matter, especially periventricular and centrum semiovale in location. Lesions may also be seen in the brainstem, cerebellum, and spinal cord. Again, the importance of conveying the clinical history or at least the clinical suspicion to the radiologist monitoring the examination cannot be overemphasized.

While the MRI findings may be consistent with the diagnosis and be supportive, they remain nonspecific. An important part of the usefulness and necessity of the examination is the exclusion of other lesions, especially in the area of the foramen magnum, a strategic location where a meningioma, for example, might mimic MS clinically. MRI is especially valuable in studying the posterior fossa/foramen magnum area due to the ease of obtaining sagittal images (see Fig. 10-9A).

Multiple high-signal plaques are seen on the intermediate T2-weighted image in Figure 10-17. On CT, plaques are seen as hypodense white matter changes, occasionally with foci of enhancement. CT, however, will be abnormal in only about 25 per cent of patients with positive MR images.

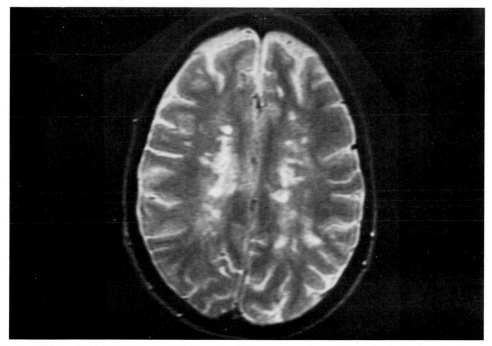

Figure 10-17. Multiple sclerosis. An axial T2-weighted MR image just above the lateral ventricles demonstrates multiple foci, both separate and confluent, of high signal intensity (white) areas within white matter. Although nonspecific, these findings are typical of MS.

Variable Symptomatology of Miscellaneous Etiologies

Other etiologies to be considered in the case of multifocal variable symptomatology include *vasculitis* and *systemic diseases* that have CNS manifestations. Such manifestations are often due to ischemia. In the elderly, subcortical arteriosclerotic encephalopathy (Binswanger's disease) and multiinfarct dementia may be seen as patchy white matter hypodensities on CT and as areas of increased signal intensity on MRI.

In the immumocompromised patient, symptoms may be due to the disease process itself or superimposed (usually multifocal) opportunistic infection. In the AIDS patient for example, the likely presence of HIV retrovirus within brain tissue may account for mental status changes and other ill-defined neurologic findings, while CT and MRI demonstrate only "atrophy." Commonly occurring cryptococcal meningitis will most likely be manifest radiologically by the complication of hydrocephalus. Other CNS opportunistic infections such as toxoplasmosis are discussed above (see Case Number 5, Infectious Disease).

Normal pressure hydrocephalus (NPH) is included here because symptoms also vary in intensity and the predominant symptom will determine the chief complaint. The diagnosis based on the presence of the classic triad of dementia, ataxia, and incontinence is difficult, since these symptoms are in themselves nonspecific and not uncommon in the older population. MRI and CT add little to the diagnosis with the exception of excluding other etiologies. The difficulty usually lies in the differentiation of NPH from atrophy. In the case of NPH, look for ventricular enlargement, especially temporal horn enlargement, out of

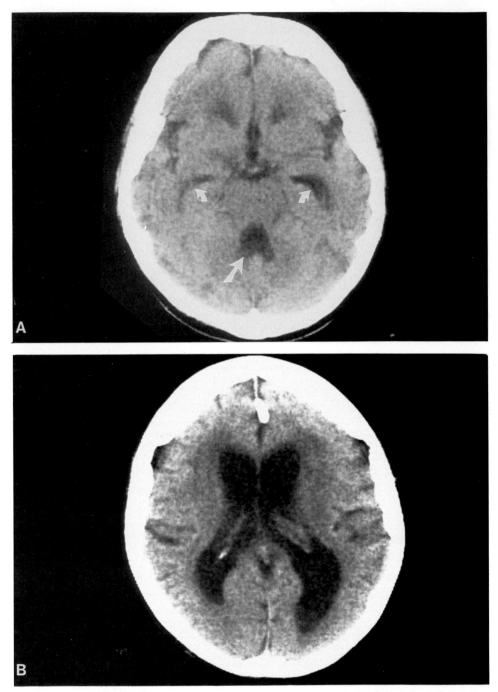

Figure 10-18.   Normal pressure hydrocephalus (NPH). Nonenhanced axial CT scans at the base of the brain **(A)** and the lateral ventricles **(B)** demonstrate an enlarged fourth ventricle (white arrow), temporal horns of the lateral ventricles (curved white arrows), and moderately enlarged lateral ventricles (B). Cortical sulci are not especially prominent for this 70-year-old patient. Contrast this CT scan with that in Figure 10-19.

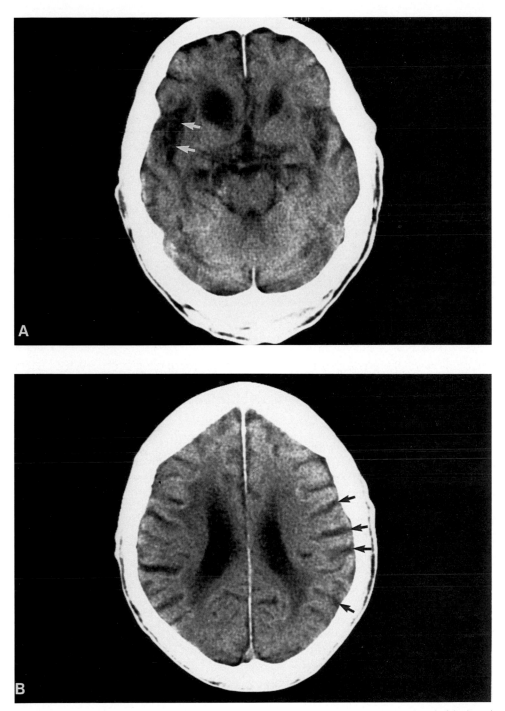

Figure 10-19. Cerebral atrophy. Nonenhanced axial CT scans at the base of the brain **(A)** and roof of the lateral ventricles **(B)** demonstrate enlargement of the CSF spaces at the base of the brain, including the sylvian cisterns (white arrows point to the right sylvian cistern). Cortical sulci are diffusely widened, some of which are labeled with black arrows.

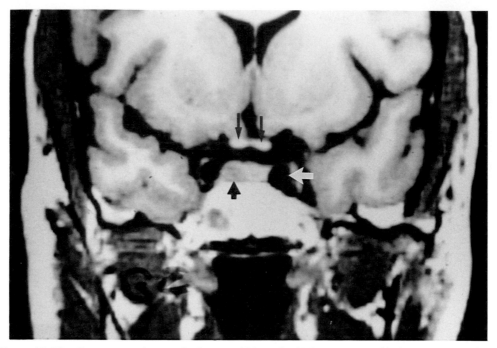

Figure 10-20. Pituitary microadenoma. On this coronal T1-weighted MR image a mass (black arrow) is seen within the sella turcica on the right having a lower signal intensity than that of the adjacent pituitary gland. Note also the internal carotid arteries (low signal intensity appearing black) adjacent to the sella, within the cavernous sinus (white arrow points to left ICA). The optic chiasm (thin black arrows) is separated from the pituitary and adenoma by a CSF-filled space.

proportion to the width of sulci, and enlargement of basilar cisterns. Radionuclide cisternography may aid in the diagnosis. Figures 10-18 and 10-19 illustrate these characteristic differences as seen on CT.

CASE NUMBER 7: SELLA TURCICA REGION SYMPTOMS

A 30-year-old woman has noted a steady decrease in menstruation and an increase in lactation. Serum prolactin levels average greater than 150 ng/ml. She also complains of mild headache. Visual fields are normal.

A specific history that alerts one to suspect a pituitary abnormality must be conveyed to the radiologist. The examination must be monitored and occasionally tailored during its course. A *microadenoma* (less than 10mm in diameter) is best seen on coronal, thin slice (3mm or less), contrast-enhanced CT or T1-weighted MRI. The coronal T1-weighted image in Figure 10-20 illustrates a microadenoma of low signal intensity slightly increasing the height of the pituitary gland on the right. If a nonsecreting adenoma is suspected, additional information would become even more important. This includes the status of the patient's visual fields and cranial nerve function. In such cases, a preliminary sagittal localization MRI might be reviewed first to look for extrasellar extension of tumor. This then may dictate the

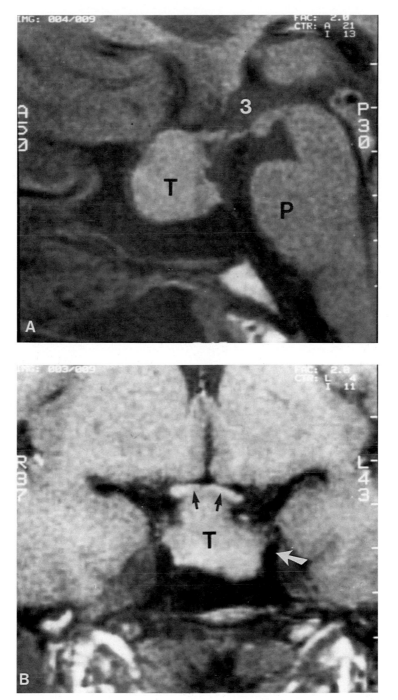

Figure 10-21. Pituitary adenoma. T1-weighted sagittal **(A)** and coronal **(B)** MR images illustrate a pituitary adenoma (T) that has enlarged the sella turcica and extended above the sella, compressing and elevating the optic chiasm (black arrows). Note the partially visible (black) left internal carotid artery within the cavernous sinus displaced laterally (white arrow). Pons (P). Anterior third ventricle (3).

need for thin or thicker coronal images and possibly axial images, as well as a T2-weighted spin-echo sequence. Pituitary tumors need extend only minimally above the diaphrama sellae to impress upon the optic chiasm. They can be quite aggressive, extending laterally to the cavernous sinus, into the middle fossa, and posteriorly beyond the dorsum.

A *pituitary macroadenoma* is seen in sagittal and coronal planes (Fig. 10-21A and B) to extend upward into the suprasellar cistern elevating the optic chiasm and laterally to compress the left cavernous sinus.

If the primary symptoms are those of a visual field cut, other parasellar lesions enter into the differential diagnosis. Meningiomas are seen to arise from the planum sphenoidale, craniopharyngiomas sit just above the sella and may extend into it, and even carotid artery aneurysms can project medially into the sella resulting in pituitary insufficiency. Craniopharyngiomas tend to contain calcification as well as cystic areas.

CEREBROVASCULAR IMAGING

Since cerebrovascular disease and stroke rank so high on the list of causes of death, a great deal of medical attention has focused on all aspects of its manifestations including etiology, diagnosis, treatment, and prevention. A history of risk factors, recent premonitory symptoms, and physical findings such as a bruit heard over the common carotid artery bifurcation can suggest the possibility of arterial disease. The confirmation of this diagnosis can be difficult and not without significant risk to the patient. A completely noninvasive, risk-free imaging modality has long been sought. The problem is compounded by the fact that considerable debate remains over what to do with the information once it is known: surgical intervention versus medical management versus the natural course of the disease. The focus of attention is the prevention of stroke and, therefore, when there is a clinical suspicion of risk or premonitory stroke symptoms have occurred, the quest is for the most definitive diagnostic study with the lowest risk and cost.

IMAGING MODALITIES

DUPLEX CAROTID SONOGRAPHY (DCS)

Using relatively recently refined technology, real-time sonography can produce a sharp accurate image of the cervical common carotid artery, its bifurcation, and the proximal internal and external carotid arteries. With the skill gained from experience and a knowledge of the variable normal anatomy, one can image these vessels and, more importantly, by means of "simultaneous" pulsed Doppler, analyze the flow pattern at specific points along and within each vessel. An ultrasound wave of known frequency is reflected off moving red blood cells. These reflected waves have a measurable slightly different frequency (a frequency shift) which, when coupled with the angle of incidence to the flow of blood, can be used to calculate the velocity of the red blood cells. The peak frequency shift (and velocity) increases through a stenotic area and the spectrum of frequencies of echoes increases

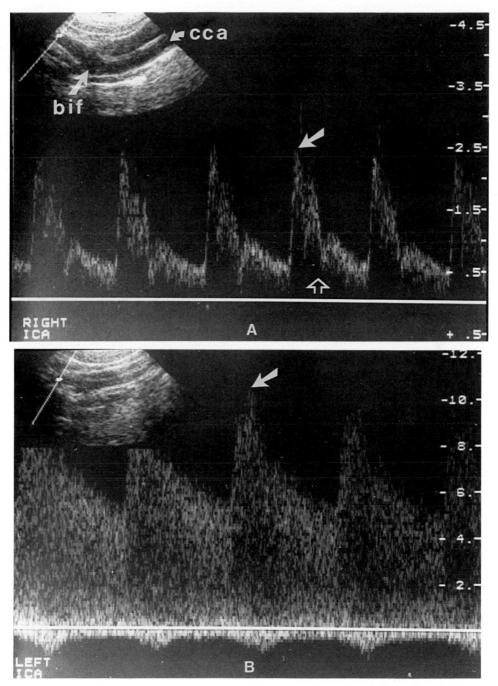

Figure 10-22. Duplex carotid sonography (DCS). Normal internal carotid artery **(A).** Internal carotid artery stenosis **(B).** The image in the left upper corner displays the point of Doppler sampling, the proximal ICA in example A. The spectral wave of flow at this point is plotted continuously at the bottom of the illustration. The systolic peak frequency shift (white arrow) is noted relative to the scale on the right as well as the wave form and the appearance of the clear space or "window" beneath the wave (open arrow). Common carotid artery (cca). Common carotid bifurcation (bif). In example B the wave form is markedly abnormal with an increase in peak frequency shift (white arrow) and spectral broadening as seen by the filling in of the space or window beneath the wave. This is indicative of a high grade stenosis of the ICA origin.

(broadens) with turbulence beyond a plaque or stenosis. Such duplex examinations (real-time imaging and Doppler ultrasound spectral analysis) are quite accurate in screening for cervical carotid artery disease.

Duplex carotid sonography is especially useful when the clinical history is uncertain or an incidental bruit is heard. Less than one-half of audible bruits are associated with significant stenotic disease. A limitation of the DCS examination is that neither the proximal carotid artery (its origin) nor its distal intracranial portions are included. If surgery is contemplated or the area of interest is the intracranial circulation, invasive studies may be necessary. The term "invasive" applies to procedures that "invade" at least by venipuncture with the injection of contrast material or more commonly by catheterization of an upper extremity vein or artery or femoral artery for the selective catheterization and injection of cerebral arteries. The role of MRI in assessing carotid disease is promising but still being evaluated.

Figure 10-22A is a combined static image taken during real-time imaging filmed simultaneously with the spectral wave tracing from the internal carotid artery just distal to the carotid bulb. The common carotid and internal carotid arteries are imaged as normally patent. The systolic peak and continuous blood flow in diastole are typical of internal carotid artery flow. In another patient (Fig. 10-22B), one can see a markedly abnormal wave form with a marked increase in peak frequency shift and spectral broadening as evidenced by filling in of

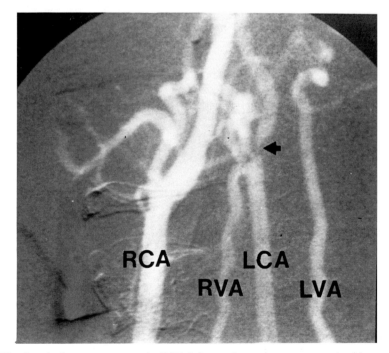

Figure 10-23.   Digital subtraction arteriography (DSA). Left internal carotid artery stenosis. An oblique projection of the cervical portion of the cranial arteries in the same patient whose DCS is illustrated in Figure 10-22B, demonstrates both the normal right common carotid artery bifurcation and normal right internal carotid artery and the markedly stenotic left internal carotid artery origin (arrow). The right vertebral artery partially overlaps the left external carotid artery. Right common carotid artery (RCA). Right vertebral artery (RVA). Left common carotid artery (LCA). Left vertebral artery (LVA).

the normally clear "window" under the wave by echoes of multiple frequencies. This is indicative of a tight stenosis at the internal carotid artery origin.

DIGITAL SUBTRACTION ANGIOGRAPHY (DSA)

DSA refers to a technology of imaging. A digitalized video image of the area of interest is recorded, reversed (black to white, etc.), and used to subtract the background from subsequent images while contrast material flows through the vessels in the field. This occurs in almost real-time at a predetermined frame-per-second rate. The images can then be recorded on transparent film for viewing on standard x-ray viewboxes.

Patient cooperation is essential because any patient movement (especially swallowing) will not allow proper subtraction. This is especially true with venous injections, since the contrast material must first travel through the pulmonary circulation and the heat sensation felt in the chest and upper body can be alarming to some patients. The study can be performed with a small (4 French) arterial catheter placed in the ascending aorta via the brachial or femoral artery, even in the outpatient setting. The advantages of arterial injections are improved contrast bolus, the need for a smaller volume of contrast material, and the ability to selectively catheterize an artery if necessary. This can help solve the other major limitation, which is simultaneous filling of all cerebral vessels and possible superimposition. Selectively catheterized arteries studied with DSA can often provide more than adequate information about the intracranial circulation as well.

Figure 10-23 is a left anterior oblique projection of the cervical cerebral arteries of the patient studied by DCS above (see Fig. 10-22B). Although a complete examination will include multiple projections from the aortic arch to the base of the brain, this projection best demonstrates in this patient both the normally patent right common carotid artery bifurcation and the markedly stenotic left internal carotid artery origin as predicted by DCS.

ARTERIOGRAPHY

Selective cerebral arteriography provides the greatest resolution of arterial (intraluminal) and venous anatomy. The procedure requires sophisticated radiographic equipment with the ability of providing serial images (one to three or more per second) usually with biplane capabilities. Although there are several options, usually the right femoral artery is punctured percutaneously at the groin. With the aid of a guide wire, the needle is exchanged for a preformed catheter which is then advanced to selectively catheterize the artery of interest, all under fluoroscopic control. Essentially all major and many minor arterial branches are accessible. The procedure requires considerable skill and knowledge of arterial anatomy and its many variations. More of the patient's medical history must be known by the radiologist, including blood pressure, coagulation status, the presence of systemic disease such as diabetes, and renal function. The examination is very specific and requires a detailed knowledge of the indication (e.g., study of the extracranial circulation for occlusive disease with general assessment of the intracranial circulation; study of intracranial lesions seen on CT or MRI; search for a site of subarachnoid hemorrhage, etc). The major risk of an

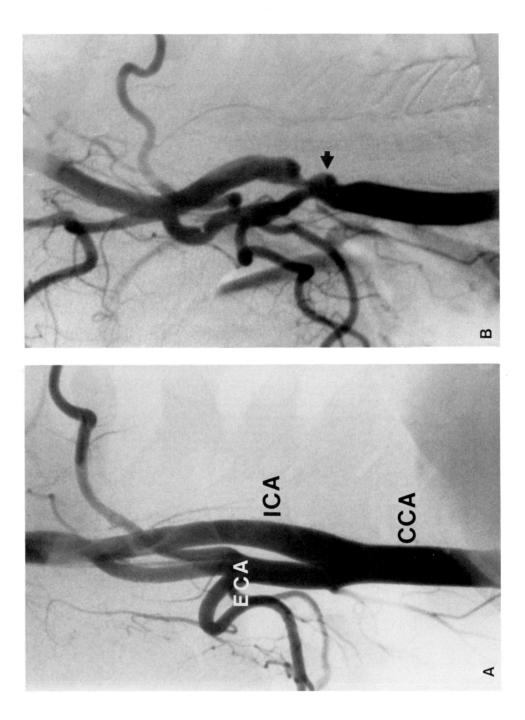

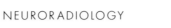

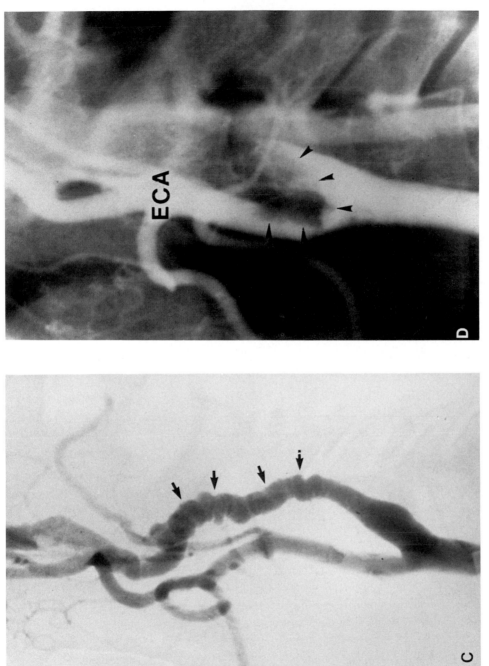

Figure 10-24. Arterial occlusive disease. Illustrations **A** through **D** are lateral projection arteriograms of the common carotid artery (CCA), cervical internal carotid (ICA), and external carotid (ECA) arteries. Figure A is normal; anterior is on the reader's left. Arteriosclerotic stenosis of the CCA, ECA, and ICA is seen in B with a smooth ulceration within a plaque (arrow). In C there is a "beaded" appearance to the midcervical ICA, characteristic of fibromuscular dysplasia (small arrows). A saddle embolus (arrowheads) occludes the ICA in D and partially occludes the ECA.

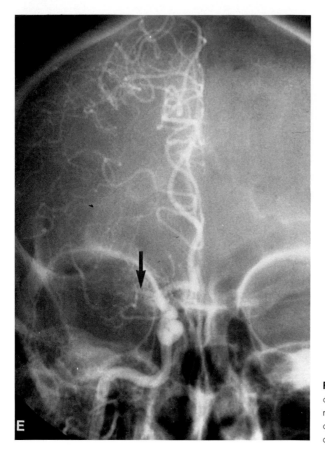

Figure 10-24 (cont.).   A frontal projection of the intracranial circulation in **E** shows the normally opacified anterior cerebral artery circulation and occlusion of the right middle cerebral artery at its origin (arrow).

intraarterial injection is stroke. Although the risk is small (less than 0.5 per cent permanent neurologic deficit), the indication for this study must be strong.

PATHOLOGY

Occlusive Disease

The focus of attention in the study of arterial occlusive disease will usually be clinically determined and guided by previous studies such as duplex carotid sonography. Although the carotid bifurcation is the most common site of surgically accessible arteriosclerotic disease, the aortic arch is usually included, as is the distal internal carotid artery to include its major intracranial branches. More than one radiographic projection is obtained. One must remember that we are imaging only the patent arterial lumen. While we are looking for intimal plaque and compromise of the lumen, we do not see the arterial wall itself, so we do not really know the thickness of the wall or plaque.

In practice, we measure the residual lumen at its narrowest point and compare this to the expected lumen by measuring a segment of more normal-appearing lumen. Although arteriosclerotic disease is diffuse, stenoses tend to be focal. The stenosis can be characterized as to its smoothness, irregularity, and the presence or absence of ulceration. Within a focal area of plaque, there may be a small focal excavation called an ulceration. Pathologically this represents slough of necrotic debris forming a potential site for fibrin-platelet aggregate to form, break off, and embolize.

Even though the angiographic diagnosis of stenosis or occlusion may be precise, the etiology is only presumptive. Some angiographic appearances, however, are quite specific and highly suggestive. *Fibromuscular dysplasia* tends to have a "beaded" appearance affecting the middle third of the cervical internal carotid artery. *Spontaneous dissections* are evidenced by their gradual tapering and frequently associated pseudoaneurysm. The contrast-capped intraluminal filling defect of an embolus is usually diagnostic, although emboli tend to be small enough to travel to more distal branches.

Examples of arterial occlusive disease demonstrable angiographically are illustrated in Figure 10-24, where A is a normal common carotid artery (CCA) bifurcation for comparison. Note the smooth regular margins. Figure 10-24B shows an arteriosclerotic plaque at the CCA bifurcation with mild stenosis of the external carotid artery (ECA), marked stenosis of the internal carotid artery (ICA), and a relatively smooth ulceration. The typical beaded appearance of fibromuscular dysplasia is seen in Figure 10-24C. Note the normal appearance of the CCA bifurcation. Figure 10-24D shows a large saddle embolus that has totally occluded the ICA. The thrombus is well outlined and is partially occluding the ECA as well. The necessity of visualizing the intracranial circulation is illustrated on the frontal projection cerebral arteriogram (Fig. 10-24E) in which the anterior cerebral artery is well opacified, while there is a sharp cut-off of the occluded right middle cerebral artery at its origin.

While the etiologies of arteritis are many, the angiographic appearance is nonspecific. A detailed study of the intracranial circulation is necessary to demonstrate the abrupt transitions in arterial diameters often with vessel occlusions seen to involve medium size and smaller arterial branches.

SUBARACHNOID HEMORRHAGE

Occasionally the CT scan will give a clue as to the site of hemorrhage. This may determine the starting point for the arteriographic study, although the entire intracranial circulation must be studied to exclude additional potential sites of hemorrhage. There is a 20 per cent incidence of multiple aneurysms and an approximately 10 per cent incidence of aneurysms in patients with arteriovenous malformations. Arteriography in the diagnosis of the etiology and site of subarachnoid hemorrhage requires the closest of monitoring. Routine angiographic projections are usually supplemented with less routine oblique projections. The ideal projection to demonstrate the size and site of origin or neck of an aneurysm is often determined only after review of the initial more routine projections.

Aneurysms tend to arise from the internal carotid system at bifurcations or origins of major branches. The aneurysm is usually named relative to the arterial branch to which it is most closely associated rather than the major artery from which it actually arises. A "P-Comm" aneurysm thus refers to an aneurysm arising from the internal carotid artery at

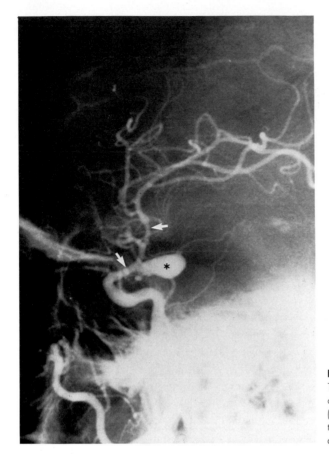

Figure 10-25. Cerebral berry aneurysm. The aneurysm (*) arises from the ICA at the origin of the posterior communicating artery (not opacified). There is narrowing (spasm) of the adjacent ICA and major branches (white arrows).

the origin of the posterior communicating artery. The most common sites of berry aneurysms are the anterior communicating and posterior communicating arteries (approximately 35 per cent each), followed by the middle cerebral trifurcation (20 per cent), and internal carotid artery bifurcation. The posterior circulation accounts for approximately 15 per cent of aneurysms, most related to the basilar artery.

Angiographically, aneurysms appear as outpouchings from the parent artery. They are usually smoothly rounded but may be lobulated or have a focal outpouching, frequently the site of the bleed. They vary in size from a few millimeters to several centimeters (giant aneurysms). Since rupture and bleeding had occurred only as a brief event, bleeding is not demonstrated angiographically. Blood free within the subarachnoid space is not well tolerated and adjacent arteries frequently respond by constricting, referred to as *spasm*. Spasm is recognized by focal or diffuse tapered narrowings. Aneurysms may thrombose partially or completely, but they may also excavate and renew their lumens. The slightly lobulated aneurysm in Figure 10-25 arises from the ICA at the site of origin of the posterior communicating artery (not seen). There is mild spasm of adjacent arteries.

Vascular malformations are usually at least in part on the brain surface being supplied by

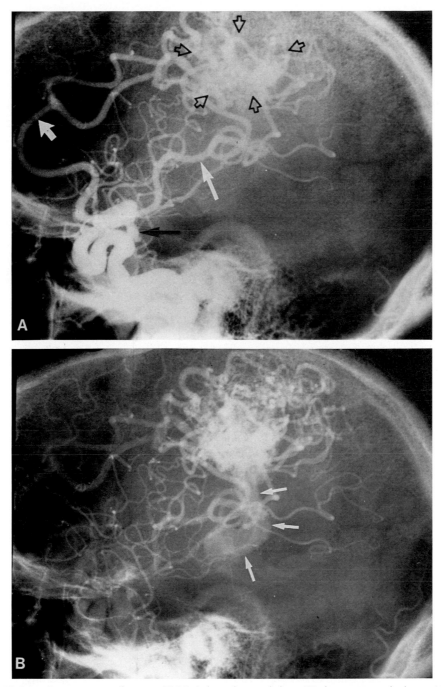

Figure 10-26. Arteriovenous malformation (AVM). In the early arterial phase **(A),** the anterior cerebral artery (short white arrow) and a branch of the middle cerebral artery (thin white arrow) are enlarged and supply the AVM, a cluster of vessels in the parietal lobe (black open arrows). Note the incidental aneurysm in (A) (solid black arrow). Immediate arteriovenous shunting **(B)** is evidenced by early opacification of a large draining vein (small white arrows) seen in the arterial phase.

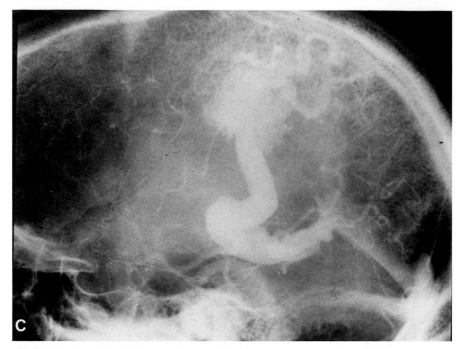

Figure 10-26 (cont.).   There is further opacification of this abnormally large vein on a later film **(C).**

pial arteries. Knowledge of the contribution from the external carotid and meningeal circulations is important in treatment planning. Such distinctions can best be made with selective internal and external carotid injections. Arteriovenous malformations are usually readily diagnosed angiographically. Although a few are quite small (and some cryptic), most are seen as a focus of markedly tortuous vessels that shunt directly into dilated veins. Differentiation of feeding arteries from overlying arteries often requires an especially rapid filming sequence, (for example four films per second) and multiple projections. A moderate size AVM is illustrated in Figure 10-26.

NEOPLASM

Arteriography for the study of tumor vasculature has become less important as tumor diagnosis has become more refined with CT and MRI. Only occasionally is angiography necessary for diagnosis, although preoperative knowledge of vascular anatomy may be an aid to the surgeon.

Meningiomas tend to have a predominant meningeal (external carotid) arterial supply consisting of radiating fine vasculature with a tumor "stain" that persists well into the late venous phase. The meningeal supply can be defined preoperatively and can occasionally be embolized to decrease bleeding during surgery. A selective ECA injection of the meningioma seen on CT in Figure 10-13 demonstrates a markedly enlarged posterior division of the middle meningeal artery providing sharply defined tumor vasculature and stain (Fig.

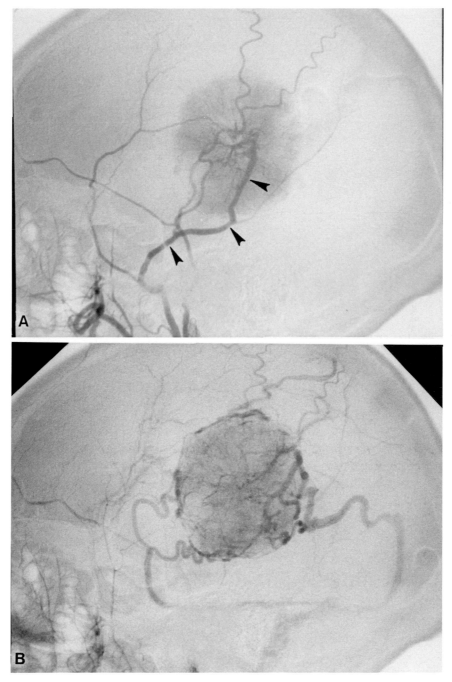

Figure 10-27. Meningioma. External carotid arteriogram of the patient whose CT scan appears in Figure 10-13. Anterior is on the reader's left. The arterial phase of a selective external carotid arteriogram **(A)** shows a markedly enlarged posterior division of the middle meningeal artery (arrowheads) as the primary supply to the meningioma. The tumor ''blush,'' which appears gray on this subtraction film, persists into the late venous phase **(B).** Although the draining veins are prominent, there is no arteriovenous shunting.

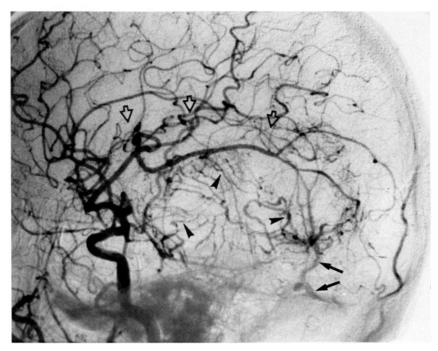

Figure 10-28.   Glioblastoma. A common carotid arteriogram of the patient whose CT scan is illustrated in Figure 10-11 demonstrates elevation and stretching of the sylvian branches of the middle cerebral artery (open arrows), pathologic vessels (arrow heads), and an early draining vein (solid arrows).

10-27A). The tumor stain persists well into the late venous phase (Fig. 10-27B). While venous drainage is prominent, arteriovenous shunting is not present.

Many malignant neoplasms will have characteristic pathologic vasculature consisting of abnormal, irregular vessels with "pooling," tumor stain, and arteriovenous shunting as evidenced by early appearing draining veins. A lateral right carotid arteriogram of the patient whose CT scan is illustrated in Figure 10-11 shows, in the early arterial phase, elevation and stretching of the middle cerebral artery sylvian branches, multiple pathologic tumor vessels, and arteriovenous shunting as evidenced by the appearance of an early draining vein (Fig. 10-28).

When the only angiographic findings consist of displacement of normal vessels from their normal position, one is left with the interpretation of "avascular mass." Such an impression is nonspecific, in that any space-occupying lesion will result in mass effect. The differential diagnosis might still range from hematoma to abscess to malignant neoplasm. Correlation with the clinical history and with other diagnostic studies then becomes essential.

THE SPINE

As with the skull and brain, several imaging modalities are available for the study of the spine and its contents. Communication between the physician who is most familiar with the patient's signs and symptoms and the neuroradiologist who is most familiar with the application and limitations of neurodiagnostic procedures will provide the most expeditious and accurate neurodiagnosis.

"Back pain" in itself is too general a term to dictate which imaging procedure should be used. Much more information is needed. The pain must be characterized as to site, duration, and radiation. Is there a history of trauma and, if so, how acute? Is there an associated neurologic deficit or reflex change and, if so, for how long? Is it progressive? Is there a history of malignancy or previous surgery?

TRAUMA

CASE NUMBER 8: ACUTE TRAUMA

A 40-year-old woman was involved in an auto accident and suffered minor injuries, with the exception of persistent neck pain and paresthesias in her left arm.

Acute trauma, especially with neurologic deficit, requires immediate radiologic evaluation. Assuming that the patient's general medical condition is appropriately stable, radiographic examination must be carried out with little or no patient movement. This usually requires immobilization of the patient's neck with sandbags, soft collar, or other device when applicable. Frontal and cross-table lateral projection radiographs can be obtained in the emergency room. If no abnormalities are found, one can proceed to a more complete examination.

One must look not only for the obvious fracture but also for the more subtle changes that may be indicators of more serious injury. Prespinous soft tissue swelling may accompany ligamentous injury. Similar clues may be provided by a widened disc space or interspinous space. Alignment of articular facets must be carefully defined to exclude subluxation, fracture, or dislocation. Suspicious findings or questionable abnormalities require further investigation. CT can be performed with minimal patient movement. The technique of examination is tailored to the specific question raised. For example, the plane of fracture might be parallel to the plane of the scan (routinely axial) and possibly overlooked. Thinner scans (e.g., 1.5mm) with sagittal or coronal reformations might then be necessary to help eliminate this potential error.

A lateral radiograph (Fig. 10-29A) of the cervical spine of the patient whose case is presented above demonstrates minimal anterior subluxation of the vertebral body of C5 on C6, widening of the C5–6 interspinous space, narrowing of the disc space, and widening of one of the articular facet joints posteriorly. The contralateral facet joints cannot be precisely outlined. Compare with the normal disc space, alignment, and facet joints at the C4–5 level. These findings alone are indicative of ligamentous injury and a potentially unstable condition. While maintaining the patient in a supine position with very little movement, a CT scan is able to demonstrate a fracture of the left superior articular facet of C6 extending to the pedicle (Fig. 10-29B).

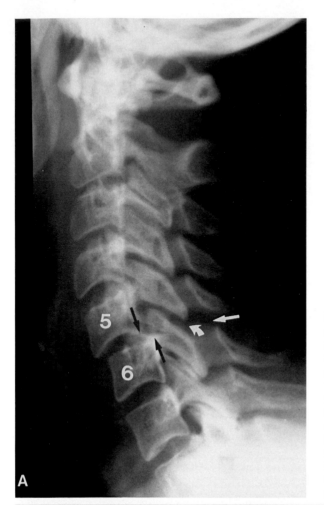

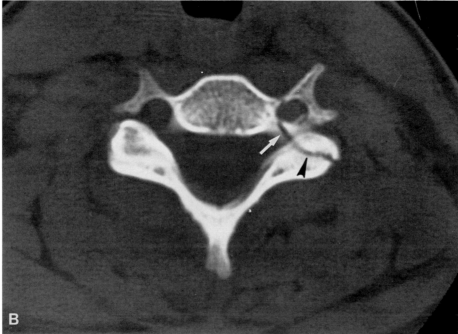

Figure 10-29. Cervical spine. Fracture/subluxation. A lateral radiograph (**A**) demonstrates anterior subluxation of C5 on C6, best appreciated by observing the posterior vertebral body margins (black arrows). Note the C5–6 disc space narrowing, widening of one of the apophyseal joints posteriorly (curved white arrow), as well as the interspinous space (straight white arrow). A single thin section axial CT scan through the body of C6 (**B**) demonstrates fracture of the left superior articular facet (arrowhead) extending into the pedicle (white arrow).

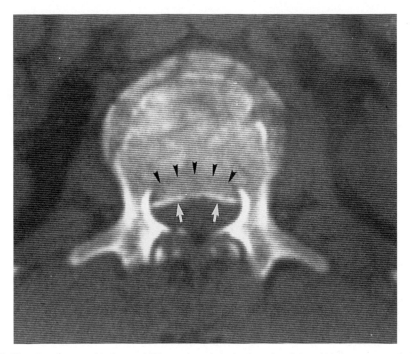

Figure 10-30. Burst fracture, L1. An axial CT scan through the body and pedicles of L1 demonstrates displacement of bone fragments circumferentially, the most significant of which is the large vertebral body fragment displaced posteriorly (white arrows) compromising the spinal canal. Black arrowheads designate the projected anterior margin of the spinal canal.

The need for myelographic or CT-myelographic information is usually made in joint consultation with neuroradiologist, orthopedist, and/or neurosurgeon. Surgical stabilization or reduction does not necessarily require exploration of the spinal canal, but the presence of a bone fragment within the canal might, especially if it is of sufficient size to cause cord compression or a block to the flow of contrast material in the subarachnoid space.

Treatment of a burst-type compression fracture is complicated by the presence of a fragment of the posterior vertebral body which has been displaced posteriorly to compromise the spinal canal. The full extent of such fractures is often best demonstrated by CT (Fig. 10-30).

ACUTE ONSET BACK PAIN (INCLUDING HERNIATED DISC)

One of the most common requests for the radiologic study of the low back (and less often the neck) is that of radicular pain. The onset is often relatively acute and the clinical localization of the root involved quite precise. The differentiation of disc herniation, spondylosis, spinal stenosis, and even unsuspected tumor requires radiologic evaluation.

Plain film examination is often the first step. The subtle changes of mild disc space narrowing or splinting to the painful side adds little information, but knowledge of the presence of scoliosis, spondylosis with hypertrophic spur formation, spondylolisthesis, or

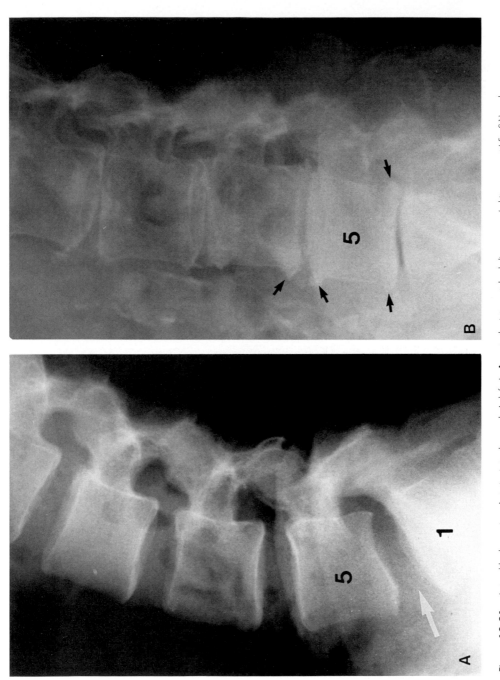

Figure 10-31. Lateral lumbar spine. Anterior is to the reader's left. In **A,** note the intervertebral disc spaces (white arrow at L5–S1) and vertebral body height and alignment in the normal spine. There is marked degenerative disc disease in **B** with disc space narrowing at L4–5 and L5–S1 and hypertrophic osteophyte formation at vertebral body margins (arrows).

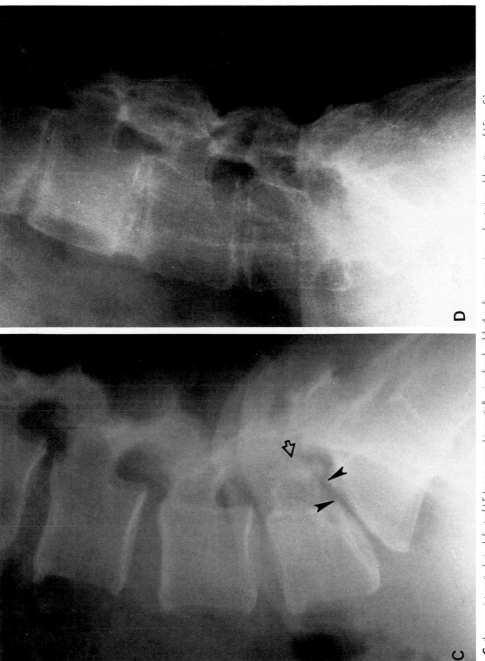

In **C,** the pars interarticularis defect of L5 (open arrow) is partially visualized, while the disc narrowing and anterior subluxation of L5 on S1 (spondylolisthesis) is quite apparent. Arrowheads point to the posterior vertebral body margins of L5 and S1. In ankylosing spondylitis **(D),** many landmarks are lost due to bony bridging of disc spaces and fusion of joints posteriorly.

unsuspected neoplasm is valuable. Traditionally, opacification of the CSF compartment with contrast material and visualization of nerve root sleeves and nerve roots themselves (myelography) has been the standard in the diagnosis of herniated nucleus pulposis. CT has in part replaced myelography in that the disc itself is visualized as is the spinal canal in cross section. MRI is becoming the procedure of choice, especially with its ability to readily study the spinal canal in the sagittal plane as well as the axial plane without contrast material or radiation exposure.

CASE NUMBER 9: ACUTE ONSET LOW BACK PAIN

A 33-year-old man complains of low back pain radiating down the side of his left leg since doing some unusually heavy lifting several weeks ago. He notes some tingling over his lateral lower leg, and on physical examination there is a diminished ankle jerk.

Lumbosacral Spine Radiographs

A plain film examination of the low back consists of frontal, lateral, right and left oblique projections, as well as a coned lateral film of the lumbosacral junction. Disc spaces and vertebral bodies are readily seen. Alignment of the posterior margins of the vertebral bodies is noted. On the lateral as well as oblique projections the pars interarticularis is examined for potential defect (spondylolysis) especially if subluxation is present (spondylolisthesis). The articular joints are usually best seen on the oblique views. Also noted is the presence of hypertrophic spurs and the sclerotic vertebral end-plates adjacent to a narrowed degenerated disc.

   Figure 10-31A is a lateral projection of a normal lumbar spine. This is contrasted with the markedly narrowed disc space at L4–5 and L5–S1 in Figure 10-31B. There is reactive bone (sclerosis) and hypertrophic spur formation as well as a "vacuum" phenomenon in this patient with severe degenerative disc disease. In another patient with only minimal spur formation shown in Figure 10-31C, there is anterior subluxation of the body of L5 on the body of S1. The bone defect seen is that of a bilateral pars interarticularis defect accounting for the spondylolisthesis. In Figure 10-31D, there is a relative "opacification" of disc spaces due to syndesmophyte formation and disc bridging. The apophyseal joints posteriorly are fused, appearing as one continuous bone in this case of ankylosing spondylitis.

Myelography

The introduction of contrast material into the subarachnoid space requires lumbar puncture usually at the L2–3 or L3–4 level, since the great majority of herniated discs are seen at L4–5 and L5–S1. Of course, a particular clinical situation may dictate otherwise. Usually with fluoroscopic assistance, a small gauge (22 or less) spinal needle can be used. Water soluble (and absorbable) contrast material is used almost exclusively. The concentration and amount used is determined by the specifics of the examination. Serious complications from myelography are quite rare although side effects are common. Headache and back pain may be seen with any lumbar puncture, although the incidence of headache is slightly higher with myelography, up to 30 per cent. Nausea occurs in less than 10 per cent of patients following the procedure. Seizures and, especially in the elderly, short term confusion are less common with newer contrast agents.

Multiple radiographic projections are obtained guided by fluoroscopy. Nerve roots are visualized and can be followed as they exit the spinal canal. Filling of the nerve root sleeve is variable. One looks for intradural filling defects as well as extradural impressions. In the case of disc herniation, as illustrated in Figure 10-32, the disc itself is not visualized, but seen instead is its effect of impressing the thecal sac, compressing and displacing a nerve root, and amputating or decreasing distal filling of a nerve root sleeve. The contrast material is allowed to flow cephalad to at least the lower thoracic spinal canal to include the conus medullaris.

Following a myelogram, patients may resume their normal preprocedure activity. However, they must avoid lying flat for the first eight to ten hours to keep at a minimum the concentration of contrast material that reaches their head, hopefully decreasing the likelihood of after-effects.

Computed Tomography

CT scans are targeted to the spine usually with slice thickness of approximately 5mm. One of several procedures may be used, the purpose of all of which in general is to scan through the disc space while at the same time including enough of the vertebral body to evaluate the bony canal and neural foramina. Once scanned, both soft tissue and bone windows are imaged. Intervertebral disc material has a higher density on CT than does the subarachnoid space and surrounding fat. A protrusion of disc beyond its normal confines with compression of the thecal sac and nerve root can be identified. Settings to emphasize bone allow evaluation of the apophyseal joints and the remainder of the osseous structures. An axial scan at the L4 – 5 disc space shown in Figure 10-33A demonstrates the normal intervertebral disc (averaged partially with the inferior end-plate of L4), thecal sac surrounded by fat, and exiting nerve roots. This is contrasted with that of a herniated disc at L5 – S1 seen in Figure 10-33B, the fragment of which impresses the thecal sac and displaces posteriorly the left S1 nerve root.

While the presentation of patients with spinal stenosis tends to be more chronic, they may present acutely with low back and radicular pain. A small spinal canal compromised by hypertrophied facets, thickened ligamentum flava, and bulging disc can be quite apparent on axial CT. A markedly constricted spinal canal is seen in Figure 10-33C. Facet hypertrophy is better appreciated with "bone window" settings as in Figure 10-33D.

Magnetic Resonance Imaging

The readily obtainable sagittal projection on MRI defines the disc and its relationship to the vertebral body and posterior longitudinal ligament. An extruded fragment compressing the thecal sac may be quite apparent. Neural foramina may be well seen in this projection in the lumbar area. The axial MR image may add additional or confirmatory information. MRI has the added advantage of imaging the level of the conus. This is becoming the procedure of choice, obviating the need for myelography or CT. The intermediate weighted sagittal image in Figure 10-34 readily shows a disc herniation at L5 – S1.

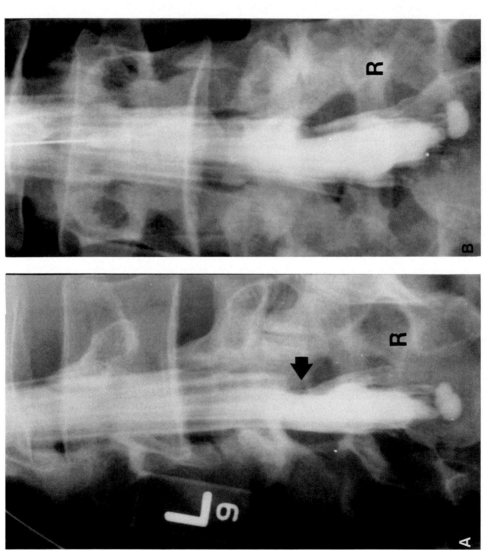

Figure 10-32. Herniated disc. Lumbar myelogram. Right posterior oblique (**A**), frontal (**B**), left posterior oblique (**C**), and lateral (**D**) radiographs.

Contrast material is opaque, appearing white and outlining the lucent (gray) linear nerve roots. Normal exiting nerve root sleeves on the left are seen in C. The arrow points to the S1 root sleeve. On the right in A, there is an extradural impression (wide arrow) obliterating the right S1 root sleeve, displacing and widening both the S1 and S2 nerve roots. The asymmetry and lack of root sleeve filling is less apparent in the frontal projection (B), and the lateral projection (D) is relatively insensitive to this lateral disc fragment.

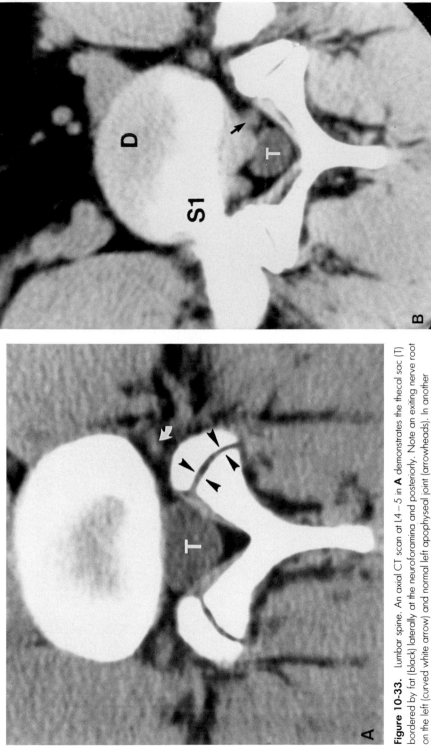

Figure 10-33. Lumbar spine. An axial CT scan at L4–5 in **A** demonstrates the thecal sac (T) bordered by fat (black) laterally at the neuroforamina and posteriorly. Note an exiting nerve root on the left (curved white arrow) and normal left apophyseal joint (arrowheads). In another patient shown in **B,** the intervertebral disc at L5–S1 is seen to be lighter than the thecal sac (T). The scan thickness partially includes the superior endplate of S1, especially on the right. The intervertebral disc (labeled D) is seen anteriorly and a large fragment is herniated posteriorly displacing the left nerve root posterolaterally (black arrow) and compressing the thecal sac.

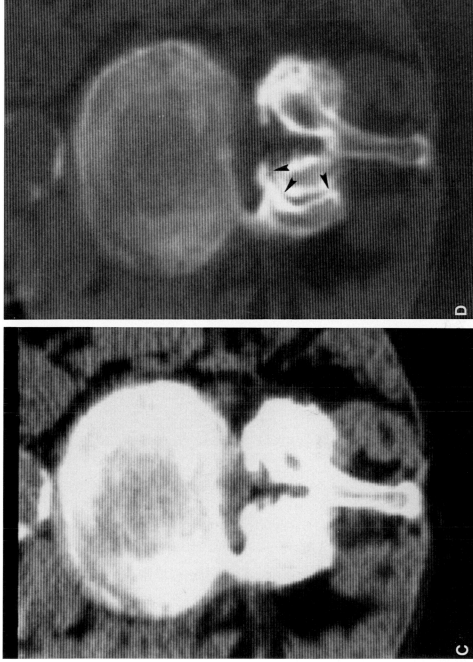

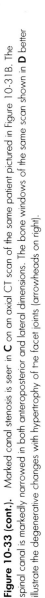

Figure 10-33 (cont.). Marked canal stenosis is seen in **C** on an axial CT scan of the same patient pictured in Figure 10-31B. The spinal canal is markedly narrowed in both anteroposterior and lateral dimensions. The bone windows of the same scan shown in **D** better illustrate the degenerative changes with hypertrophy of the facet joints (arrowheads on right).

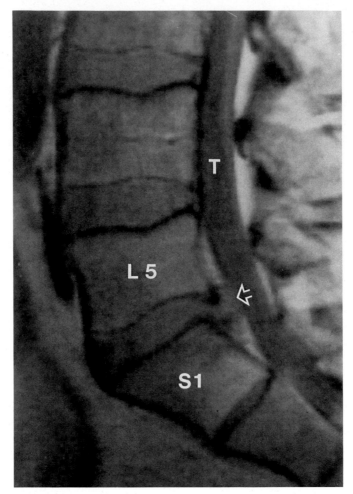

Figure 10-34. Lumbar herniated disc. An intermediate-weighted sagittal MR image demonstrates a herniated disc (open white arrow) as intermediate signal intensity material continuous with the L5–S1 intervertebral disc. The CSF-filled thecal sac (T) has a lower signal intensity, while epidural fat has a much higher intensity (whiteness).

CHRONIC OR PROGRESSIVE BACK PAIN WITH NEUROLOGIC DEFICIT

CASE NUMBER 10: PROGRESSIVE BACK PAIN AND NEUROLOGIC DEFICIT

A 55-year-old woman complains of persistent midthoracic back pain aggravated slightly with activity but not radiating. Over the past few days, she has noted increasing leg weakness and urinary bladder incontinence. Physical examination reveals bilateral lower extremity weakness, bilateral Babinski signs, and a sensory deficit to pin prick.

When the clinical presentation suggests a focal cord lesion, several possible mechanisms of cord involvement must be considered. The clinical history may provide clues such as known malignancy. Metastasis to bone with subsequent extradural spinal cord compression is common. The benign tumors meningioma and neurofibroma tend to occur in the extramedullary intradural space. Primary spinal cord tumors are rare. Arteriovenous malformations and syringomyelia may give a presentation not unlike that of tumor, and acute cord compression rarely will be secondary to epidural abscess or hematoma.

The diagnostic procedure of choice is determined by the most probable working diagnosis and the acuteness of the presentation. In some cases, MRI will be the only necessary and definitive study. Replacement of bone marrow by tumor with expansion beyond bony confines sufficient to compress the spinal canal and cord can be seen on sagittal images alone. This may be sufficient, in the case of known metastatic disease, for definitive radiation therapy or decompressive surgery. An example of vertebral body metastasis with spinal cord compression studied by MRI is illustrated in Figure 10-35.

Although CT delineates the osseous structures well, there is limited visualization of the thecal contents above the level of the conus without opacification of cerebrospinal fluid with contrast material. In such instances, if the exact level of the lesion is uncertain clinically,

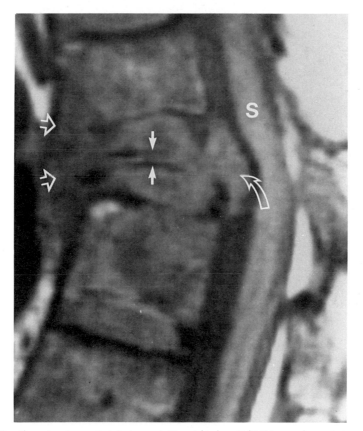

Figure 10-35. Thoracic spine, metastatic tumor. A T1-weighted sagittal MR image demonstrates variable signal from vertebral bodies involved with metastatic tumor. There is collapse of a vertebral body (small white arrows) with extension of tumor anteriorly (open arrows). The posterior extension (open curved arrow) compresses the spinal cord (S).

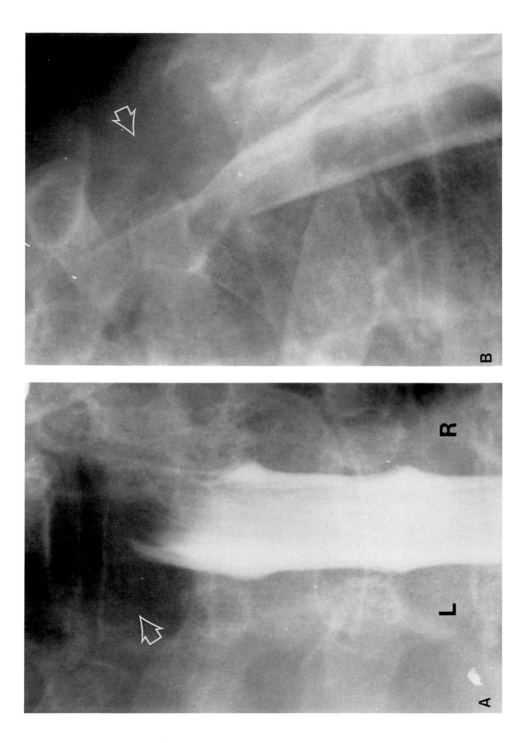

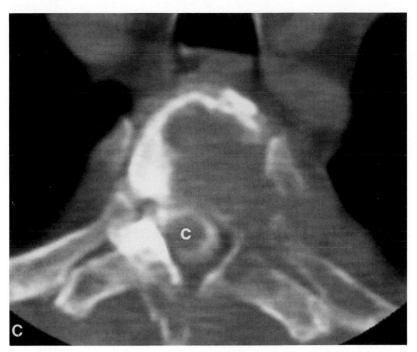

Figure 10-36. Thoracic spine. Metastatic tumor. Frontal **(A)** and lateral **(B)** projections of a myelogram demonstrate the thecal sac and cord (lighter gray within the opacified CSF) displaced to the right and anteriorly. There is destruction of a portion of the vertebral body and pedicle of T2 on the right (open arrow in A) and rib posteriorly (open arrow in B). The arrows point to a void or absence of bone. The extent of bone destruction is most evident on the axial CT scan in **C. C.** Normal bone has been replaced by tumor. Residual myelographic contrast material surrounds the spinal cord (c) which is displaced to the right.

myelography may be the first procedure of choice with CT to follow for additional cross-sectional delineation. When a block to the flow of cerebrospinal is suspected, a smaller amount of contrast is injected without first removing CSF. CSF removal in the presence of a complete block may accelerate the progression of a neurologic deficit and mandate more immediate surgical intervention.

A block to the cephalad flow of contrast material is seen in frontal (Fig. 10-36A) and lateral (Fig. 10-36B) projections at T3. Bone destruction is evident by the absence of the right pedicle of T2 and rib posteriorly. The full extent of bone involvement, however, is best delineated on axial CT (Fig. 10-36C).

Intradural extramedullary masses tend to be round and capped by contrast material. Multiple projections are necessary since the spinal cord may be flattened and therefore widened, giving the false impression of an intrinsic lesion in a single projection. Extradural masses compress the entire thecal sac from without, while intramedullary cord lesions will expand the cord in both dimensions.

An example of an intradural extramedullary tumor in a middle-aged woman is that of a meningioma seen in Figure 10-37A displacing the spinal cord to the left and blocking the cephalad flow of contrast material. A composite of four CT images (Fig. 10-37B) demonstrates the marked compression of the lower thoracic cord.

CT with residual myelographic contrast material still in place may add valuable additional information especially if the myelogram is not definitive. An infected disc space with epidural

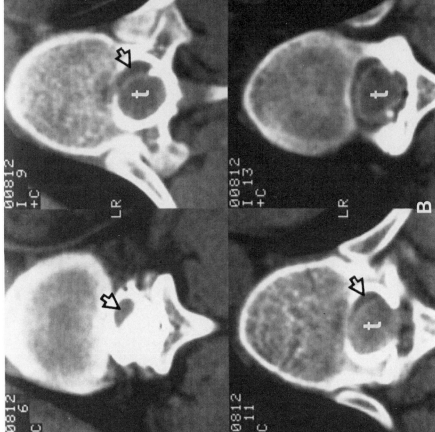

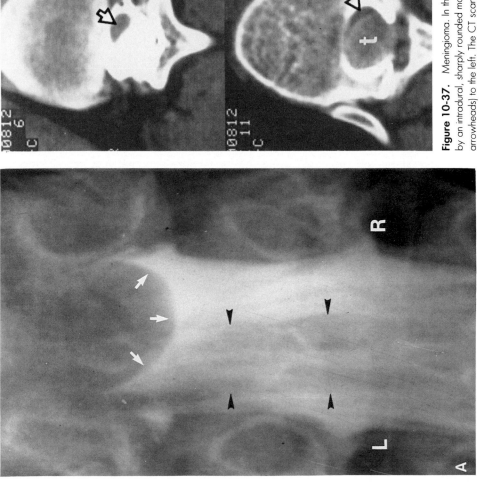

Figure 10-37.   Meningioma. In the myelogram in **A,** there is a block to the flow of contrast material by an intradural, sharply rounded mass (white arrows) which has displaced the spinal cord (black arrowheads) to the left. The CT scans in **B** with residual myelographic contrast material clearly show the intradural location of the meningioma (t) markedly compressing the spinal cord (open black arrows).

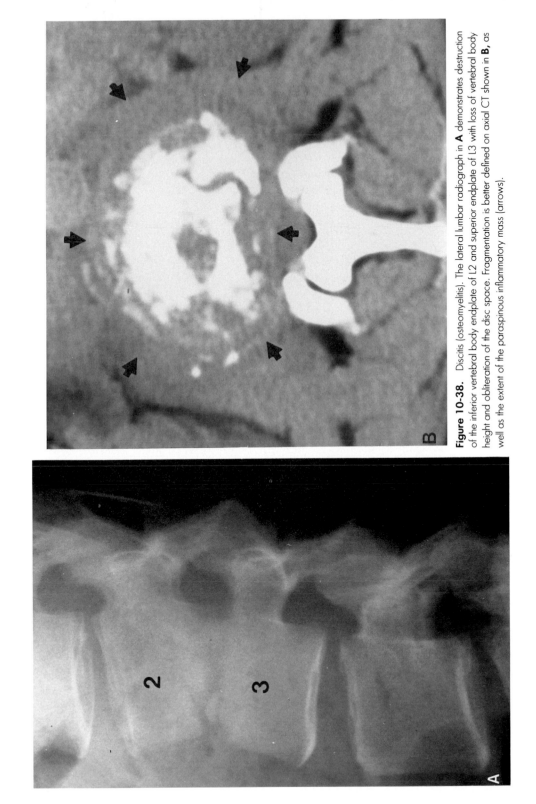

Figure 10-38. Discitis (osteomyelitis). The lateral lumbar radiograph in **A** demonstrates destruction of the inferior vertebral body endplate of L2 and superior endplate of L3 with loss of vertebral body height and obliteration of the disc space. Fragmentation is better defined on axial CT shown in **B**, as well as the extent of the paraspinous inflammatory mass (arrows).

extension might not have been appreciated on plain films for example. A syrinx may opacify with contrast material either immediately or after a several hour delay.

CHRONIC OR PROGRESSIVE NONRADIATING BACK PAIN

CASE NUMBER 11: PROGRESSIVE NONRADIATING BACK PAIN

A 23-year-old male complains of a several week history of progressive low back pain which is now debilitating. The pain is severe with any movement but without radiation. He is tender to palpation at L2–3 and has a low-grade fever. An important part of his history is that of intravenous drug abuse.

Early in the course of infectious diseases of the spine, plain films may be normal, but later reveal demineralization and loss of cortical bone at the vertebral body endplates, progressive disc space narrowing and endplate destruction (Fig. 10-38A). Hematogenous disc space infection actually begins within the vertebral body at the endplate. Bone destruction with loss of vertebral body height then occurs over weeks. CT will better define the paraspinous inflammatory mass component and vertebral end-plate fragmentation (Fig. 10-38B). MRI may prove to be the single most definitive procedure of choice. Fluoroscopic or CT-guided biopsy or aspiration is usually necessary to culture the pathogen when blood cultures are negative.

Determining the etiology of more chronic nonradiating low back pain is difficult. Especially in the elderly, it may be impossible to determine whether or not the changes of spondylosis and degenerative disc disease are actually pain-producing in a particular patient since such bony changes are so common. Spinal stenosis is not necessarily symptomatic; neither is a herniated disc for that matter. For example, detailed clinical information may be necessary if the radiologist is to know to search for ankylosing spondylitis in the sacroiliac joints and possibly recommend follow-up or appropriate further studies knowing the clinical suspicion. At what point does spondylolisthesis become symptomatic? Not all patients need all examinations, but certainly all examinations performed must be compared with one another in order to detect the earliest clues. Clinical history and previous examinations must be relayed to the radiologist. There is no substitute for personal communication.

C H A P T E R 1 1

INTERVENTIONAL RADIOLOGY

Edward M. Druy

Interventional radiology is the commonly accepted term used to define that subspecialty of radiology devoted to the use of invasive techniques for both the diagnosis and therapy of disease. Interventional radiology began as an outgrowth of angiography, the radiologic evaluation of blood vessels, and was conceived as early as 1967 with a simple but novel idea: The ability to gain percutaneous access to a blood vessel meant that the organ supplied by that vessel could be modified by the delivery of pharmacologic agents via catheter. Early applications of this technique were directed toward the control of gastrointestional hemorrhage through the delivery of agents such as Pitressin or Epinephrine. Following the demonstration of the validity of this concept, additional applications, both vascular and nonvascular were readily conceived.

This subspeciality of diagnostic radiology has now evolved to its modern definition: Percutaneous access to any structure implies a potential to diagnose, modify, or treat many of the disease processes affecting that particular structure. The primary tools of the interventional radiologist are needles, catheters, guidewires, and balloons, all of which can be directed under fluoroscopic, CT, or ultrasonic control. Thus, stenotic vessels can be dilated, and occluded vessels can be recanalized. Hemorrhage can often be controlled, and arteriovenous malformations and fistulas can be closed. Chemotherapeutic drugs can be delivered directly to tumor-containing organs, and lytic agents can be infused directly onto thrombus. Similarly, the biliary system and upper urinary tract can be percutaneously catheterized and, if obstructed, drained. Stones can be removed from these organs, strictures can be dilated, and certain malignancies palliated, often obviating the need for open surgical decompression or bypass.

The safe, percutaneous, and nonoperative biopsy of deep-seated lesions in virtually any portion of the body has been facilitated by advances in cross-sectional imaging. It is now the rare patient that needs to undergo exploratory laparotomy purely for diagnosis. Many of the disease processes that interventional radiologists now see, diagnose, and treat were once considered "surgical" lesions, best dealt with through a formal surgical approach. In the majority of instances, however, the usefulness of these new techniques opens new avenues of treatment to many patients who are not surgical candidates or whose underlying disease could not be successfully treated by surgery.

INTERVENTIONAL TECHNIQUES

The approach to most interventional procedures consists of variations on two basic techniques: (1) the Seldinger method of guidewire exchange for dealing with vessels and small tubular structures, and (2) the trocar puncture of larger viscera. The Seldinger exchange technique, devised in 1953, was initially designed to enable catheters to be placed into blood vessels percutaneously, eliminating the need for open arteriotomy with its attendant complications. The Seldinger technique allows catheters to be exchanged easily if a different shape or diameter catheter is necessary for a particular examination. Seldinger's technique can be easily modified to permit a similar percutaneous approach to tubular structures that were relatively close to the skin surface, such as the biliary or urinary system. The basic difference is the size of the initial puncture needle, usually an 18 gauge needle for blood vessels and a longer sheathed needle for puncturing bile ducts or renal collecting structures.

The attractiveness of the Seldinger technique for interventional procedures is its relative safety. The initial puncture may be made with a needle as small as 22-gauge, through which a .018-inch guidewire can be passed. Once the guidewire is in place, specialized catheters are available which will permit the initial puncture site to be dilated to any size desired, usually within the 8 to 12Fr range, but occasionally, depending on the application, up to 24 or 30Fr. The fact that the initial puncture is small is thought to be a chief safety factor of the technique, but is also one of its main disadvantages. A small tract must be dilated with successively larger dilators before the appropriate, final catheter is placed. This requires multiple exchanges of dilators, each dilator being 2Fr sizes larger than the previous one. The necessity for multiple dilations adds to the length of the procedure and may contribute to patient discomfort, as each exchange for a larger dilator entails additional manipulation through a newly created percutaneous tract.

The trocar technique of percutaneous entry is a tradeoff between the safety of the Seldinger technique and the speed and relative comfort of a one-stick approach, which permits the initial insertion of the desired size and shape catheter. The diameter of the trocar set is usually from 8 to 12Fr, although larger sets are available for specialized needs. The safety of the Seldinger technique stems from the fact that multiple puncture attempts may be made with small diameter needles with relative safety if the initial puncture is not successful in entering the desired structure. When attempting to place a 12Fr or larger trocar, a misdirected thrust of the trocar may mean a dangerous laceration of a normal structure, such as the aorta or colon. Trocars are used predominately for gaining entry into large fluid collections which are relatively close to a skin surface. Percutaneous abscess drainage is one technique where trocars are used to advantage, as the goal is to place a large multiholed catheter into the collection with as little manipulation as possible, thereby reducing the risk of pus spilling into noncontaminated body cavities.

PATIENT RISKS

By its very nature, interventional radiologic procedures carry a certain definable risk to the patient, over and above any risk inherent in the use of radiographic contrast media. Risks, side effects, and potential complications must be appreciated by clinician and patient prior to the recommendation of such a course. Although the interventional radiologist will explain potential risks and complications to the patient prior to a study, the clinician should inform the patient in a general way that the special procedure is not just another test, that the examination is being considered because there is no other way to obtain the necessary information or because no other reasonable therapeutic options are available. Thus prepared, most patients will not be unduly apprehensive when the radiologist arrives to discuss the procedure with the patient. Virtually all interventional radiologic procedures need to be coordinated and discussed with the radiologist prior to their performance. Indications, contraindications, and basic preparation for the patient should be discussed and ascertained at that time.

While most interventional procedures carry less risk and morbidity than general surgical procedures, potential for complications abound. Vascular interventional procedures carry the same general risks as arteriography (hematoma, local thrombosis, distal embolization, contrast toxicity, and pseudoaneurysm). Additionally, the risks specific to the particular procedure must be taken into account. Transcatheter infusions of pharmacologic or chemotherapeutic agents pose the risk of reactions to the specific drug infused. Particulate material or larger mechanical devices designed to occlude or embolize blood vessels may be misplaced or migrate, potentially resulting in ischemia or infarction of the accidentally embolized organ or extremity. Dilating balloons used in percutaneous transluminal angioplasty may burst inadvertently and rupture the vessel, potentially causing hemorrhage. The commonest complications of procedures performed on nonvascular structures such as the liver or kidney are hemorrhage and infection, usually amenable to nonsurgical control, but occasionally requiring a major surgical intervention for adequate repair.

A realistic appraisal of degree of discomfort, postprocedural pain, and length of recuperation should be discussed with the patient. It should be stressed that the proposed procedure may be an alternative to surgery, but the alternative procedure, with attendant complications, must be mentioned in order to comply with the legal requirements of informed consent.

PATIENT PREPARATION

For procedures that require the use of large amounts of intravascular radiographic contrast media, it is essential that the patient's renal function be known in advance. Coagulation studies must be obtained prior to any procedure which requires the percutaneous puncture of any viscus or solid organ. If percutaneous aspiration of a lung nodule is to be performed, the decision to admit a patient prior to the procedure should be based on evidence that even a small pneumothorax would not be tolerated.

An informed, well-prepared patient may be more important to the successful outcome of an interventional procedure than it is to traditional surgical procedures. Since most procedures are performed under a combination of local anesthesia and intravenous sedation, the patient will be awake and relatively aware of his surroundings. While an individual's tolerance of pain is highly variable, the operator should assume that most of these procedures will be uncomfortable at best and painful at worst. Anxiety will heighten whatever pain is present, and the combination of anxiety and pain will lead to an uncooperative patient. Therefore, adequate sedation and careful attention to pain control is mandatory. As the complexity of the procedure increases, there is a tendency to use more sophisticated types of anesthesia, ranging from epidural to general anesthesia. Just as no surgeon would consider performing certain procedures under local anesthesia, it would be totally unrealistic to think that all interventional procedures can be done under local anesthesia.

SCOPE OF INTERVENTIONAL RADIOLOGY

Interventional radiology can be divided into two broad categories: the vascular and the nonvascular. Each of these categories may be subdivided into diagnostic and therapeutic components (Table 11-1). Vascular, diagnostic studies include aortography, cavography, peripheral, pulmonary, renal, and visceral angiography. Some therapeutic counterparts would be percutaneous transluminal angioplasty of peripheral, renal, and visceral vessels; embolization of vessels supplying tumors and arteriovenous malformations; pharmacologic control of bleeding ulcers; and regional, intraarterial chemotherapy of neoplasms.

Nonvascular interventional procedures are usually directed toward the biliary and genitourinary system, and for convenience can also be divided into diagnostic and corresponding therapeutic modalities. Percutaneous transhepatic cholangiography has, as its therapeutic counterpart, percutaneous biliary drainage; percutaneous nephrostomy would be the therapeutic counterpart of antegrade pyelography; the diagnostic aspiration of tumors and fluid collections would lead to the percutaneous drainage of abscesses.

PULMONARY ANGIOGRAPHY

DEFINITION

Pulmonary angiography refers to the radiographic evaluation of the lung vasculature following the placement of a catheter into the pulmonary artery, usually by a percutaneous, transfemoral route, using the Seldinger technique.

Pulmonary angiography, to be most accurate, should only be undertaken after prior perfusion lung scanning coupled with ventilation scanning (V/Q scanning), since the highest

TABLE 11-1. SCOPE OF INTERVENTIONAL RADIOLOGY

ORGAN	DIAGNOSTIC	THERAPEUTIC
Lungs	Pulmonary arteriogram	Embolization of AVM
	Bronchial arteriogram	Embolization of bronchial artery for hemoptysis
Liver	Hepatic angiography	Tumor embolization
		Arterial infusion of chemotherapeutic drugs
	Percutaneous cholangiogram	Bilary drainage
		Stone basketing
Kidney	Renal angiography	Angioplasty
		Tumor embolization
		AVM embolization
	Antegrade pyelography	Percutaneous nephrostomy
		Ureteteral stents
		Stone removal
GI Tract	Angiography	Embolization of hemorrhage
		Infusion for ischemia
Extremities	Angiography	Angioplasty
		Fibrinolysis

quality and safest pulmonary arteriograms are obtained when selective injections are made into lung segments which the V/Q scan shows to be abnormal.

INDICATIONS

Pulmonary angiography remains the gold standard for diagnosing pulmonary embolism despite the many attempts to increase the certainty of diagnosis of pulmonary embolism by noninvasive means. V/Q scans, under the best of circumstances, can be placed into one of four categories: negative, high probability, low probability, and indeterminate. A negative V/Q scan effectively excludes the diagnosis of pulmonary embolism, while a high probability scan is greater than 85 per cent accurate in predicting pulmonary embolism. Patients with high probability or negative V/Q scans do not need to undergo angiography unless there is either contraindication to anticoagulation, in the case of the former, or an overwhelmingly strong clinical suspicion of the diagnosis, in case of the latter. If the scan is interpreted as low probability or indeterminate, pulmonary angiography may often be needed to confirm or exclude the diagnosis, as a host of other pulmonary diseases can mimic the same scan patterns.

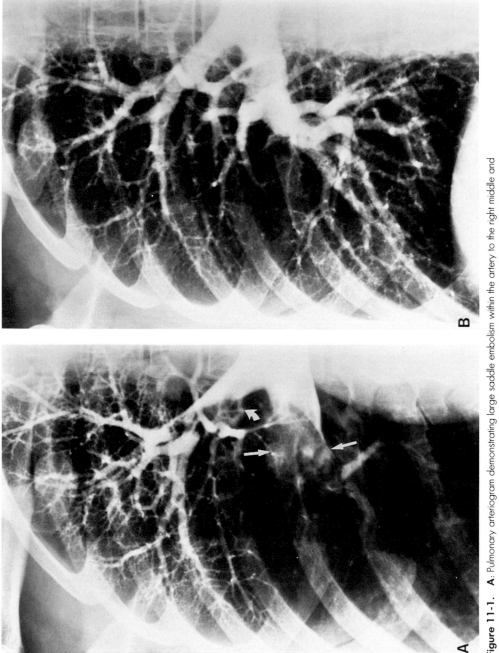

Figure 11-1. **A**: Pulmonary arteriogram demonstrating large saddle embolism within the artery to the right middle and lower lobes (arrows). Nonoccluding thrombus is present within the right upper lobe artery (curved arrow). **B**: Same patient following fibrinolytic therapy. There has been total resolution of all visible thrombus.

If pulmonary angiography is an indicated procedure, it is important that the examination be performed as soon after the onset of symptoms as possible. If the examination is performed later than 48 hours after the onset of symptoms, a false-negative study may result from lysis and fragmentation of larger thrombi. While small peripheral emboli may still be detected if the study is of the highest technical quality, it is much more difficult to document these smaller filling defects. Pulmonary angiography can usually be performed on a semi-elective basis if the patient is relatively stable. It is indicated as an emergency study when a patient is hemodynamically unstable and emergency procedures such as pulmonary embolectomy or systemic fibrinolysis are considered the therapeutic procedure of choice (Fig. 11-1).

PATIENT RISKS AND SAFETY

Morbidity and mortality associated with pulmonary angiography is low with modern techniques. While cardiac perforation and subsequent tamponade has been documented in the past, the use of soft pigtail catheters has reduced this risk virtually to zero. Cardiac arrhythmias may occur during passage of the catheter through the right ventricle, but these should be transient and not pose any clinical difficulty. The only exceptions are patients with left bundle branch block, who are at a high risk for cardiac arrest, should conduction disturbances result from catheter manipulation. If pulmonary angiography is indicated in these individuals, a right atrial pacemaker should be inserted prior to the examination.

Right ventricular end-diastolic pressure and pulmonary arterial pressures must be obtained prior to contrast injection. In the face of pulmonary hypertension (end-diastolic pressures greater than 20mm Hg), deaths have been reported from acute cor pulmonale when main pulmonary artery injections have been performed. In patients with pulmonary hypertension, this risk can be virtually eliminated by placing the catheter into a more selective position and by injecting less contrast at a slower rate.

PERIPHERAL ANGIOGRAPHY

DESCRIPTION

Peripheral angiography is most commonly performed to assess the anatomic status of the vessels to the arms or legs. Lower extremity angiography is a vital component in the evaluation of patients with atherosclerotic vascular disease. Determination of therapy is usually based on the angiographic findings. The relative benefits of conservative therapy, transluminal angioplasty, or surgery can only be determined after angiography has been performed.

PATIENT PREPARATION

Since these patients are often elderly and may have concommitant renal disease, dehydration must be avoided prior to the study. The amounts of contrast used should not pose any dangers to most individuals with satisfactory renal function. Should there be any question of adequacy of renal function prior to the procedure, the radiologist needs to be alerted prior to the study to help ensure that contrast loads be kept to a minimum. Newer imaging techniques, such as digital subtraction angiography make it feasible to evaluate fully even patients with markedly reduced renal function, as the process of computer enhancement allows the images to be made with much less contrast.

PERCUTANEOUS TRANSLUMINAL ANGIOPLASTY

DESCRIPTION

Percutaneous transluminal angioplasty (PTA) refers to the dilation of vascular stenoses with special catheters that are introduced in the same manner as are diagnostic angiographic catheters. Initially, transluminal angioplasty was performed with coaxially introduced vascular dilators, ranging in size from 6 to 10Fr. While this method was relatively successful, the high complication rate arising from the percutaneous introduction of 10Fr and larger catheters led to disillusionment on the part of referring physicians. Dissatisfaction with the coaxial dilating catheters stimulated the development of balloon dilatation catheters, which were introduced in the mid-1970s. These catheters are minimally larger than the diagnostic catheters, thus they avoid many of the complications of the earlier designs. The specialized balloon on the end of the catheter is designed to inflate to a specific diameter under constant inflation pressures; thus a 2.5mm catheter can have a balloon which, when inflated, will have a diameter of 10mm or larger.

The exact mechanism of transluminal angioplasty is not completely understood, however, histologic sections of vessels that have undergone angioplasty show evidence of intimal tearing with overdistension of the media. This results in an expansion of the total surface area of the lumen of the vessel. Despite the potential for distal embolization or vessel disruption, these complications are unusual. Compression of the plaque, once thought to be the primary result of angioplasty, contributes very little to the overall increase in lumen diameter (Fig. 11-2, 3).

INDICATIONS

Percutaneous transluminal angioplasty is indicated whenever symptoms of vascular insufficiency are referable to vascular stenosis. Lifestyle-limiting or progressive claudication, pain at rest, nonhealing ulcerations, or ischemic gangrene may be partially or definitively treated by angioplasty when the arteriogram demonstrates stenoses of the iliac, femoral, or popliteal arteries. Stenoses will respond more favorably to angioplasty than will occlusions. However, if the patient is not a surgical candidate, it is still worthwhile to attempt angioplasty, particularly if the only alternative is amputation of the affected limb.

The larger the vessel and the shorter the stenosis, the better the results. Success will be optimal in those patients who have a short stenosis, good run-off distal to the stenosis, with major disease limited to the site of the stenosis. For instance, iliac angioplasty has cure rates

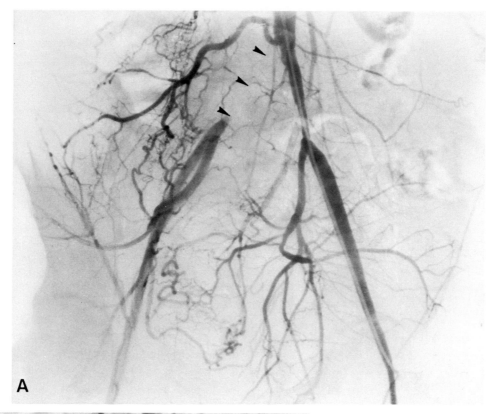

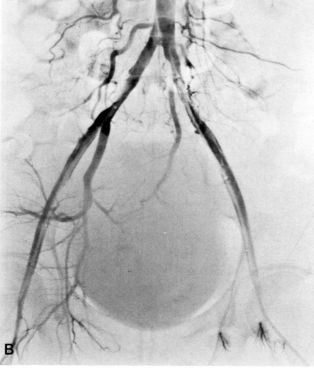

Figure 11-2. **A**: Arteriography demonstrates a total occlusion of the right common iliac artery extending from the aortic bifurcation (arrowheads). **B**: Following percutaneous balloon angioplasty, the lumen of the right common iliac artery is widely patent. The patient's claudication was no longer present.

331

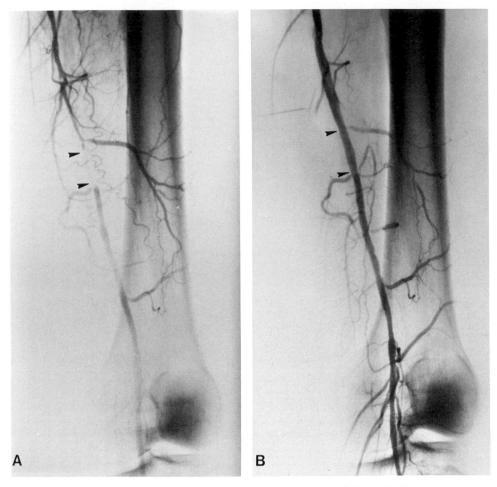

Figure 11-3. **A**: Femoral arteriogram demonstrating a short segment occlusion of the superficial femoral artery (arrowheads). **B**: Same patient following balloon angioplasty. The site of the angioplasty is demonstrated by the arrowheads. There is nothing to indicate that this segment had been previously occluded.

approaching those of aortofemoral bypass, with considerably less morbidity, fewer hospital days, and a recuperative period measured in days rather than weeks. A particular advantage of angioplasty is that even should the stenosis recur several years later, the procedure can be repeated without any increase in morbidity.

RESULTS

Clinical success rates approximate 90 per cent or better for angioplasty of the iliac vessels at one year, dropping to 85 per cent at three years. Success rates for the femoral and popliteal arteries are 80 to 90 per cent at one year, dropping to 60 to 75 per cent at three years. These rates are similar to bypass surgery of the comparable sites.

COMPLICATIONS

Up to 10 per cent of patients undergoing angioplasty via the transfemoral route may develop hematomata at the puncture site. Distal embolization may develop in 5 per cent of individuals, with the majority of these emboli not clinically significant. Rarely, vessels have ruptured during the dilation. If the iliac artery is ruptured, life-threatening hemorrhage can result, and immediate surgical repair is the only therapy. Surgical intervention is required in 2 to 3 per cent of those individuals who develop complications, with thrombosis at the angioplasty site the most common event necessitating subsequent surgery. Distal embolization is a rare occurrence, but surgery is usually mandatory if the embolization results in severe ischemia.

COST-EFFECTIVENESS

Patients who have undergone successful, uncomplicated angioplasty are often discharged from 1 to 3 days following the procedure, without limitation on subsequent activity. Under favorable circumstances, angioplasty can be performed on an outpatient basis, further reducing the cost of hospitalization. Time away from work is reduced, utilization of scarce resources is reduced, and total charges for the procedure should be less than for surgical bypass. Angioplasty, when an indicated procedure, is an attractive and economic alternative to traditional surgical bypass.

ANGIOGRAPHY OF GASTROINTESTINAL BLEEDING

ACUTE HEMORRHAGE

Studies have shown that the morbidity and mortality of gastrointestinal hemorrhage is reduced when there is accurate localization of the source and determination of the etiology of the hemorrhage. Barium studies, endoscopy, nuclear tracer studies, and angiography are the principle diagnostic tools available. No single method is 100 per cent accurate for both of these goals, but a combination of several methods will often provide a maximum yield. The angiographic evaluation of acute GI bleeding will often demonstrate the source, but is less likely to identify the cause. Endoscopy or barium studies are more likely to identify the etiology of hemorrhage, but in an emergency situation where bleeding is rapid, determination of the source is more important than determination of the etiology. If the bleeding can be stopped and the patient stabilized, a more elaborate diagnostic workup can be undertaken to determine etiology and to plan the ultimate treatment.

Identifying the source of hemorrhage angiographically requires that the patient be bleeding at a rate rapid enough so that extravasation of contrast from a vessel into the bowel lumen can be recognized. Empiric observation suggests this minimum rate of blood loss to be on the order of 2cc/min or 5 to 6 units/day. One of the great frustrations in determining the source of blood loss is that even active hemorrhage may be intermittent. Even with brisk bleeding, the source will not be recognized if the patient is not bleeding *at the time of the arteriogram.*

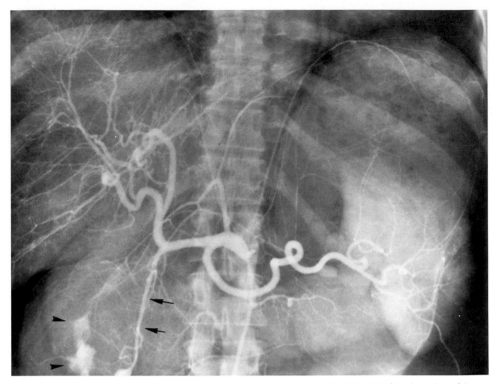

Figure 11-4. Celiac arteriogram demonstrating extravascular contrast (arrowheads) arising from branches of the gastroduodenal artery (arrows). This is the typical appearance of hemorrhage from a duodenal ulcer.

Active bleeding is usually easier to determine when the patient is bleeding from the upper GI tract than from the lower GI tract, as continuous aspiration of fresh blood from the stomach via a nasogastric tube is reliable evidence of active bleeding from the lower esophagus, stomach, or duodenum. However, passage of a bloody stool implies only that the patient has recently bled somewhere distal to the ligament of Treitz. For this reason, the success of angiography in determining the site of bleeding is usually greater for upper than for lower GI hemorrhage (Fig. 11-4, 5).

Endoscopy and angiography are complementary procedures for the localization of GI hemorrhage. If possible, endoscopy should be performed prior to angiography, as it may demonstrate both the source and the etiology of the bleeding. The presence or absence of esophageal varices must be noted, as variceal bleeding cannot be directly diagnosed by angiography. Even if nondiagnostic, endoscopy may facilitate the subsequent angiographic examination by demonstrating that certain portions of the bowel are normal, thereby reducing the number of vessels that need to be catheterized. Without prior endoscopy, selective injections into the left gastric, splenic, hepatic, gastroduodenal, inferior phrenic, and superior mesenteric arteries must often be performed to evaluate the entire upper gastrointestinal tract (from the distal esophagus through the duodenum). If endoscopy demonstrates that no blood is present in the esophagus or proximal portion of the stomach, the number of vessels to be catheterized is reduced.

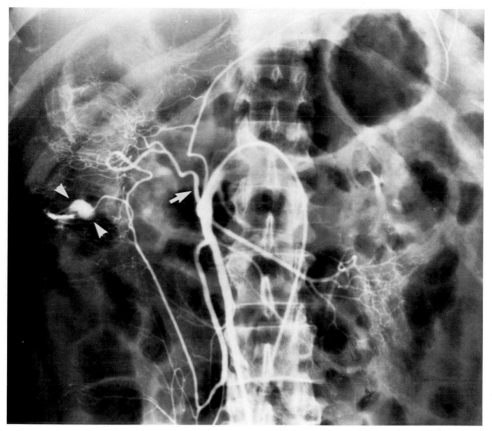

Figure 11-5. Superior mesenteric arteriogram demonstrating extravasated contrast (arrowheads) arising from a branch of the right colic artery (arrow). This is the appearance of a bleeding diverticulum of the colon.

The timing of angiography in the evaluation of active GI hemorrhage is critical. As most bleeding will stop spontaneously, it is prudent not to rush into angiography without a trial of conservative, supportive measures. However, if bleeding shows no evidence of abating, angiography should be performed before coagulation defects arise from the rapid administration of stored blood products. As a rule, if the patient loses more than several units of blood in a 6-hour period, angiography should be performed for attempted localization and subsequent transcatheter therapy.

CHRONIC HEMORRHAGE

Patients with unexplained chronic or recurrent gastrointestinal hemorrhage may benefit from angiographic examination even though active bleeding is not present at the time of the study. In this clinical setting the goal of the examination is to demonstrate a possible etiology, rather than a source. Angiodysplasias, vascular malformations, vascular tumors, malignancies, and inflammatory or ischemic changes of the bowel can be recognized by angiography. Angiographic examination is usually the last examination to be performed for the evaluation of chronic recurrent bleeding. Endoscopy and barium studies are the first order diagnostic studies.

TRANSCATHETER THERAPY OF GASTROINTESTINAL BLEEDING

DESCRIPTION

Once the source of bleeding has been identified angiographically, the angiographer should next attempt to control the blood loss. The method used depends on the location of hemorrhage, the underlying diagnosis, and the patient's medical condition. Generally, there are two options: the infusion of vasopressin or the transcatheter delivery of occlusive agents to the bleeding vessel.

INDICATIONS

Vasopressin (Pitressin), a posterior pituitary extract, exerts a vasoconstrictive action on splanchnic blood vessels. Infused into an artery via a percutaneously placed catheter, it is most successful in controlling the bleeding from diffuse gastritis and diverticular hemorrhage of the colon. It will have less of an effect on the bleeding from Mallory-Weiss tears of the esophagus, peptic ulcer disease, anastamotic ulcers, or the malignant erosion of blood vessels. It will have no effect on bleeding from mycotic or pseudoaneurysms secondary to infection or pancreatitis. For those conditions where vasopressin has little or no effect, transcatheter embolization is the procedure of choice. Gelfoam, an absorbable gelatin sponge, is a temporary occluding agent, effective in controlling the bleeding from peptic ulcer disease. The sponge will be resorbed over a period of weeks, and flow through the occluded vessel will usually be restored. In those conditions where it is desirable to achieve a permanent vascular occlusion, polyvinyl alcohol can be used instead of Gelfoam. Pseudoaneurysms secondary to pancreatitis or infection, tumor vessels, or arteriovenous malformations are best embolized with permanent occlusive agents.

COMPLICATIONS

Complications arising from either vasopressin infusion or transcatheter embolization occur but are relatively infrequent. The cardiovascular effects of vasopressin are well known and patients need to be carefully observed for arrhythmias, myocardial ischemia, and hypertension. Vasopressin can also lead to bowel ischemia and skin necrosis, particularly with high doses over long periods of time. Once bleeding has been controlled, infusions should be tapered slowly and discontinued after 48 hours to minimize these risks.

Complications arising from transcatheter embolization usually result from either inadvertant occlusion of the wrong vessel or organ, or dislodgement of the occluding device with distal migration of the device into a more peripheral vessel. These occurrences may lead to ischemia of an organ or extremity of sufficient magnitude that surgery will be required.

EMBOLOTHERAPY

DEFINITION

The transcatheter occlusion of vessels or vascular beds refers to the deliberate injection of particulate matter or mechanical devices through a percutaneously placed catheter. The ultimate goal of the procedure is to cause a cessation of blood flow through a vessel or to an organ to achieve a desired therapeutic effect. The underlying disorders and diseases that can be treated by transcatheter therapy can be divided into several classifications: soft tissue hemorrhage, gastrointestinal hemorrhage, neoplasm, and primary vascular abnormalities such as arteriovenous malformations or varicoceles of the spermatic vein (Table 11-2).

METHODS

A wide variety of inert materials can be delivered via a percutaneously introduced vascular catheter. The choice of agent to use is a function of the disorder being treated, materials available, experience of the angiographer, and desirability of achieving a temporary or permanent occlusion. Gelfoam, an absorbable gelatin sponge, is the most commonly used embolic material. Widely available, easy to cut into small particles, and easy to deliver without specialized catheters or devices, Gelfoam will cause rapid clot formation and vascular obstruction which will last for up to 3 months.

Steel coils (often called "wooley worms") were developed in 1975 as devices for long-lasting occlusion. They are available in various sizes for placement in vessels of varying diameter and are effective whenever proximal occlusion of a vessel is desired.

Polyvinyl alcohol (Ivalon) is prepared in a fashion similar to Gelfoam, but has the advantage of producing a permanent occlusion because of the inflammatory response it

TABLE 11-2. INDICATIONS FOR EMBOLOTHERAPY

SOFT TISSUE	GASTROINTESTINAL
Trauma	Peptic ulcer disease
Hemoptysis	Mallory-Weiss bleeding
Neoplastic	Pseudoaneurysm
Postpartum	
VASCULAR MALFORMATIONS	**NEOPLASIA**
AV fistulae	Preoperative embolization
Arteriovenous malformations	Palliation for pain
Varicoceles	Palliation for local control
Aneurysm	

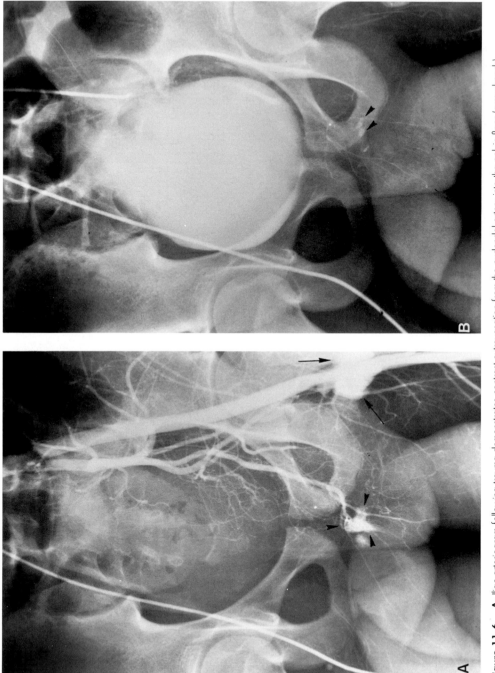

Figure 11-6. **A:** Iliac arteriogram following trauma demonstrates contrast extravasation from the pudendal artery into the pelvic floor (arrowheads). Arrow demonstrates a traumatic pseudoaneurysm of the left femoral artery. **B:** Same patient following Gelfoam embolization of the pudendal artery. The hemorrhage has been totally controlled. Small puddles of contrast (arrowheads) demonstrate stasis of contrast within the embolized vessels.

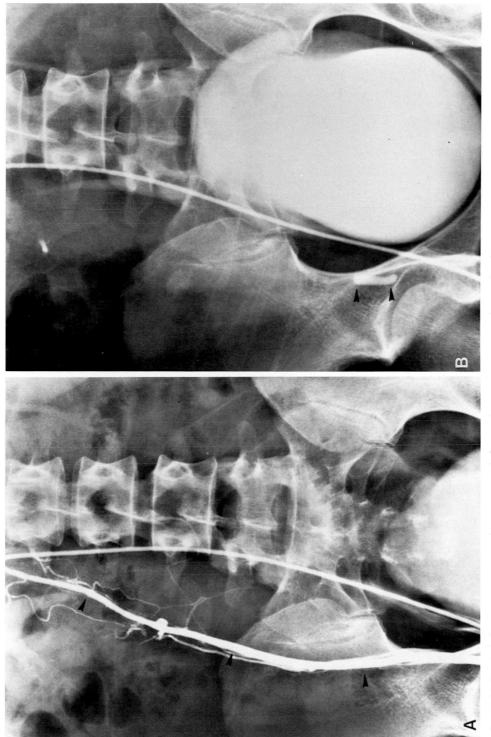

Figure 11-7. A: Right spermatic venogram showing retrograde flow into large spermatic varicocele (arrowheads). **B:** Inflated detachable balloon (arrowheads) in place within the spermatic vein.

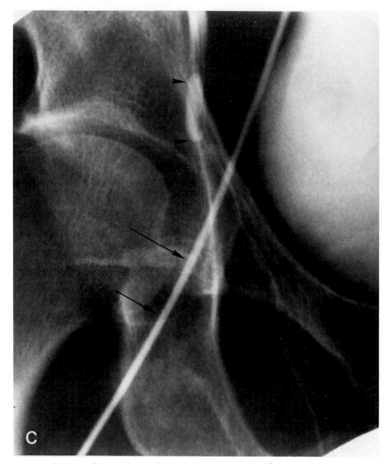

Figure 11-7 (cont.).   C: View of inguinal area during spermatic venogram following balloon inflation. Contrast is no longer seen within the spermatic vein distal to the balloon. The balloon is indicated by the arrowheads. The arrows are pointing to the catheter used for the venogram.

incites. Particles ranging in size from 250 microns to 1mm can be produced, making this substance ideal for producing long-term occlusion of vessels of varying diameter.

Detachable balloons are the "high-tech" devices of the interventional radiologist. They are introduced coaxially through an outer introducer catheter and can be flow directed to the desired place. Because of their propensity to follow the bloodstream, they will tend to flow in the direction of highest flow, making them ideal for the occlusion of arteriovenous fistulae. When filled with an isoosmotic solution and detached from their delivery catheter, they will remain inflated for long periods of time, in effect causing a permanent occlusion at the site of placement.

Embolotherapy of gastrointestinal hemorrhage has been discussed in the previous section. Gelfoam embolization of the left gastric artery is effective for the control of gastric hemorrhage secondary to gastritis, Mallory-Weiss tears, or gastric ulcerations. Injected into the gastroduodenal artery, Gelfoam can effectively control bleeding from peptic ulcer disease. Embolotherapy of gastrointestinal hemorrhage should be considered in individuals who are not surgical candidates or whose condition is too precarious for emergency surgery. While embolotherapy is efficacious in controlling hemorrhage, it does not alter the course of the underlying disorder, which must continue to be managed aggressively.

Soft tissue hemorrhage of various etiologies can be effectively controlled by embolotherapy. Traumatic hemorrhage into the pelvic or retroperitoneal soft tissues following blunt trauma may be a life-threatening complication, not readily amenable to surgical control. Ligation of the hypogastric artery is an ineffective means of dealing with this problem, and if the bleeding shows no evidence of stopping spontaneously, emergency arteriography to demonstrate the site of bleeding, followed by selective injection of Gelfoam into the bleeding branch vessel should be undertaken without delay (Fig. 11-6).

There are numerous indications for embolotherapy of neoplasms. Preoperative embolization of vascular tumors such as hypernephromas may reduce the need for blood replacement during surgery. Embolization can also be performed for palliation of symptoms such as bone pain or recurrent hemorrhage. There is also evidence that embolization of certain tumors metastatic to the liver may result in longer survival rates than would otherwise occur.

Embolotherapy for vascular abnormalities such as arteriovenous fistulae and malformations has become widely accepted as primary treatment modalities. The use of detachable balloons filled with isoosmotic fluids has revolutionized the treatment of posttraumatic carotid artery – cavernous sinus fistulae. Spermatic varicoceles are routinely occluded with detachable balloons or coil springs (Fig. 11-7).

PERCUTANEOUS ASPIRATION BIOPSY (PAB)

DEFINITION

One of the most significant advances that interventional radiology has brought to medicine is the capability of making specific tissue diagnoses of abnormal structures without the necessity of resorting to open surgical biopsy. This diagnostic ability is a direct result of innovations in imaging technology that have occurred over the past 10 years. Gray scale ultrasound, followed soon after by computed tomography, provided the radiologist with detailed cross-sectional images of the body. The ability to view anatomy in a cross-sectional plane carried important implications: the spatial anatomical interrelationships between various organs and surrounding structures could be evaluated for the first time in a live patient without surgery.

With the development of flexible 22-gauge needles (the "skinny" or Chiba needle) it was possible to obtain percutaneous aspiration biopsies from virtually any part of the body under direct imaging guidance. As the skill of both the cytopathologist and radiologist increased, it became possible to make positive diagnoses from lesions as small as 2 to 3cm in organs that were 10 or more centimeters deep to the skin surface. The safety and accuracy of the skinny needle biopsy has practically eliminated the exploratory laparotomy as a diagnostic procedure, and has enabled the tissue diagnosis of deep-seated lesions to become an office procedure.

INDICATIONS

Any mass which can be palpated or identified on an imaging study is a candidate for PAB. A definitive diagnosis of a benign lesion will spare the patient further exploratory surgery. If a patient presents with metastatic disease, PAB of one of the metastases may demonstrate the tissue type of the malignancy and the organ of origin, thus helping to determine the future course of therapy. If the patient has a history of a previous malignancy and a new lesion is subsequently identified, percutaneous aspiration biopsy may demonstrate whether the second lesion is a metastasis of the original tumor or a second primary neoplasm. Finally, the diagnosis of type of malignancy in a patient without a prior history of malignancy will help determine the therapy that should be undertaken.

METHODOLOGY

The way in which PAB is performed is often a reflection of the individual institution or expertise of its physicians. Ultrasound localization of a mass prior to biopsy is faster than localization by CT, but ultrasound suffers from two disadvantages: (1) some lesions may be "hidden" behind air or bone densities, making their identification difficult, and (2) it is difficult to image the tip of the needle within a mass under ultrasound. CT, on the other hand, easily demonstrates the position of the biopsy needle within a mass, thus increasing the accuracy of localization (Fig. 11-8). Balanced against this exquisite accuracy is the need for patient throughput in a heavily utilized radiology department. To locate a mass accurately and perform the biopsy under CT guidance may take over one hour, during which time two or more general diagnostic CT studies may be performed. In order to increase the efficiency of utilization of the CT scanner, it is not uncommon for a diagnostic study to be performed on one occasion, and if a lesion is found, to reschedule the patient for biopsy under CT control on a second occasion.

Cross-sectional imaging is not the only type of guidance for PAB. If a mass is identified on any type of study, that study can serve as the localizing examination for subsequent biopsy. If percutaneous cholangiography or endoscopic retrograde pancreatography demonstrate a stricture of the common bile duct or pancreatic duct which can be identified fluoroscopically, then biopsy can be performed under fluoroscopic guidance with the same precision as CT or ultrasound control (Fig. 11-9). Similarly, lymphangiography, duodenography, and angiography can all serve as points of reference for biopsy.

PATIENT PREPARATION

Virtually no patient preparation is necessary prior to PAB other than common sense precautions. The patient should avoid solid food prior to any procedure. The radiologist must

Figure 11-8.   **A**: CT scan through the pelvis demonstrating a destructive process involving the transverse process of S-1. An expansile soft tissue mass is arising from the transverse process (curved arrow). **B**: Under CT guidance, a biopsy needle has been introduced into the soft tissue mass. The tip of the needle is demonstrated lying within the center of the mass (arrowheads).

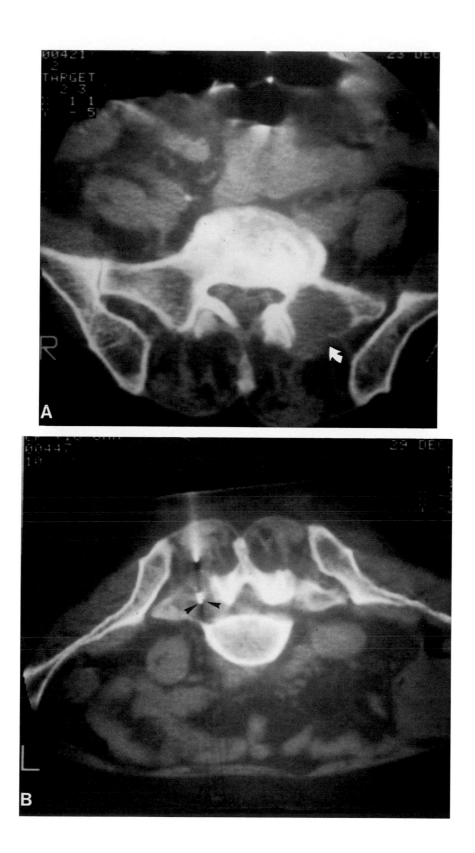

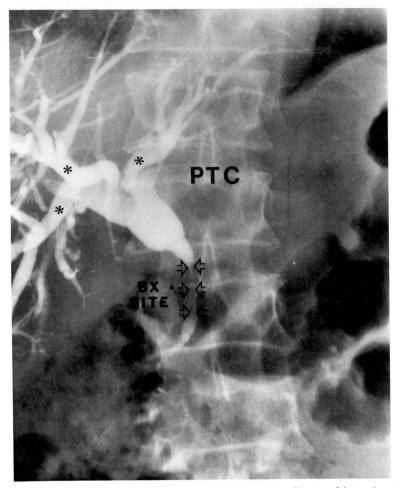

Figure 11-9. Percutaneous transhepatic cholangiogram (PTC) demonstrating dilatation of the intrahepatic biliary radicals (asterisks). Using fluoroscopic guidance, biopsy can be performed at the site indicated by the arrows.

have knowledge of coagulation studies. The only time that special precautions need be taken is when there is a possibility that the lesion may be a cavernous hemangioma of the liver. Under this circumstance it may be wise to observe the patient for up to several hours after the procedure, as bleeding can occur when such a vascular lesion is biopsied. Frequently, the procedure is performed on an outpatient basis under minimal or no sedation. Following xylocaine infiltration of the skin, there is usually no discomfort associated with the procedure.

RESULTS

The overall accuracy of PAB depends on the size of the lesion, the type of lesion, the location of the lesion, and the skill of both the radiologist and the cytopathologist. For large epithelial tumors, located fairly superficially, the diagnostic accuracy is close to 90 per cent. For tumors of the lymphoma series, cytologic accuracy is as low as 40 per cent. The overall accuracy of all lesions biopsied, regardless of cell type or location is on the order of 85 per cent, a high enough figure to make PAB a first choice procedure for the positive diagnosis of occult malignancy following identification of an abnormal mass or structure within the body.

PERCUTANEOUS ABSCESS DRAINAGE

DEFINITION

The same cross-sectional imaging technology that stimulated the development of percutaneous aspiration biopsy served as the impetus for the development of percutaneous drainage of intraabdominal and retroperitoneal abscesses. Prior to the advent of cross-sectional imaging, there was no capability of either recognizing the fluid-filled nature of a mass or of demonstrating contiguous or adjacent structures. Both ultrasound and CT made the recognition of a fluid-filled mass relatively simple, and with the precise localizing information provided by CT, it became possible to diagnose the presence of an abscess and to demonstrate what tissue structures or organs surrounded the abscess.

Initially, these masses were punctured with the same type of skinny needles that were used for aspiration biopsy, and the procedure was limited to the diagnostic aspiration of pus for culture and Gram's stain. Within a relatively short time it was realized that larger catheters, introduced into the cavity by catheter-guidewire exchange techniques, could facilitate evacuation of the abscess cavity and forestall the necessity of surgical intervention. Even though surgery is thus avoided, the principles of surgical drainage apply to the percutaneous drainage of abscesses: uncontaminated spaces are not violated, retroperitoneal abscesses are approached retroperitoneally, and intraabdominal abscesses are approached transperitoneally. Catheters remain in place until subsequent imaging studies demonstrate that the cavities are empty, and the drain is then backed out over the course of the next several days.

INDICATIONS

Any abscess that develops in an accessible part of the abdominal or retroperitoneal space should be considered suitable for percutaneous drainage. The demonstration of a safe, percutaneous route is critical, and CT guidance is virtually mandatory to demonstrate the route that the catheter must take to avoid interposed organs, vessels, or structures. Percutaneous drainage is only the first stage of the therapeutic process, however. It must be kept in mind that there is usually an underlying cause behind the development of an abdominal or retroperitoneal abscess and all efforts must be directed toward the identification and correction of such causes. Crohn's disease, diverticulitis, appendicitis, and pelvic inflammatory disease are only a few of the underlying diseases which may present as an intraabdominal abscess. Drainage of the abscess without correction of the underlying process will only result in recurrent infection, poor healing, and delayed diagnosis. The underlying disease

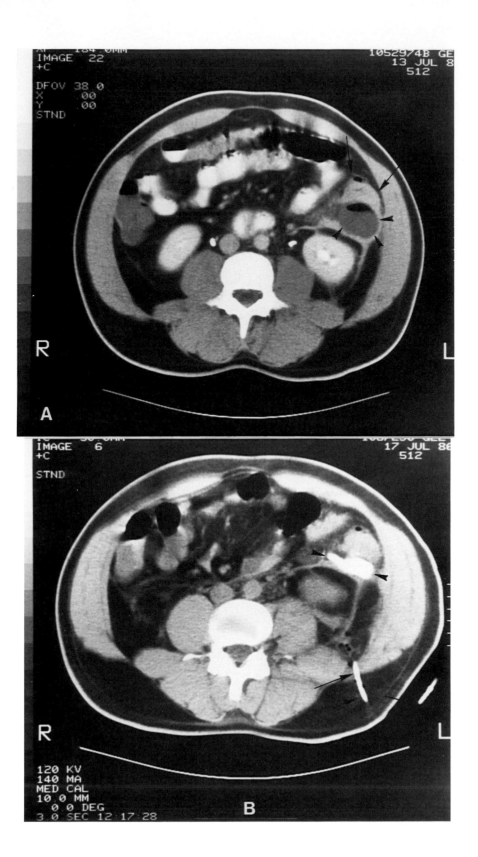

may be treated medically, as in Crohn's disease, but often surgery will still be necessary for correction of the underlying disorder, as in diverticulitis. The prior percutaneous drainage of a peridiverticular abscess, however, markedly decreases the morbidity of a bowel resection (Fig. 11-10).

METHODOLOGY

Depending on the size and location of the abscess, either the trocar technique or the Seldinger technique may be used. Smaller catheters, introduced via catheter-guidewire exchanges are usually used for deeper abscesses, while trocar techniques are used for large, superficially situated abscesses. Once the catheter is secured in place, the abscess is evacuated as completely as possible and irrigated with small aliquots of sterile saline. A repeat CT scan should be performed 24 to 48 hours following the initial drainage to assess the resolution of the abscess and to look for undrained locules. The patient's clinical course should show a significant change within 48 hours, with rapid decline of fever and return to a normal white blood count. Should neither of these occur, continued infection must be suspected and aggressive diagnostic evaluation be continued.

INTERVENTIONAL BILIARY RADIOLOGY

DEFINITION

Those procedures which relate to the direct percutaneous opacification, instrumentation, and drainage of the biliary system comprise a large and important segment of interventional radiology. Access to the bile ducts can be obtained either through a newly created percutaneous, transhepatic tract at the time of the procedure or via a previously created surgical tract. The goals of biliary interventional procedures are to delineate biliary anatomy, to determine the site and etiology of biliary tract pathology, and to obviate either the need for surgery or to facilitate and make safer any indicated surgery.

Percutaneous transhepatic cholangiography (PTC) is the basic procedure from which all interventional biliary procedures arise. This procedure provides the initial access to the biliary system, and, depending on the demonstrated pathology, serves as the framework for the palliation or definitive treatment of both benign and malignant mechanical abnormalities of the intra- or extrahepatic biliary system.

INDICATIONS

Despite advances in imaging technology, direct opacification of the biliary system by percutaneous transhepatic cholangiography remains a key procedure in the evaluation of

Figure 11-10. **A**: CT scan through the abdomen demonstrates an abscess cavity (arrowheads) related to the undersurface of the descending colon (arrows). **B**: Following percutaneous drainage of the abscess, contrast media has been injected through the catheter to determine the degree of involution of the abscess (arrowheads). The drainage catheter is shown by the arrows.

jaundice. Two important questions must be answered when evaluating the patient presenting with jaundice: (1) is there a mechanical basis for the jaundice, and (2) if mechanical obstruction if present, how can it best be relieved? PTC should be able to predict with 100 per cent accuracy the level of the biliary obstruction, and should be able to predict with over 90 per cent accuracy whether the obstruction is secondary to a benign or malignant process. Once obstructive jaundice is diagnosed, the mode of therapy needs to be ascertained. Surgical, endoscopic, or transhepatic intervention all have a role in the treatment of mechanical obstruction.

METHODOLOGY

Percutaneous transhepatic cholangiography is the direct opacification of the biliary ducts via a percutaneous, transhepatic approach. The 22-gauge Chiba needle, the same type of needle as used for aspiration biopsies, is relatively atraumatic, and has little associated morbidity with its use. Following xylocaine infiltration of the skin, the needle is advanced through the liver capsule into the substance of the liver. Small amounts of contrast are injected through the needle as it is withdrawn toward the periphery. In the presence of biliary obstruction, PTC should have a greater than 90 per cent success rate of ductal opacification. While PTC is usually performed following the CT or ultrasonic demonstration of biliary dilatation, it may be performed in the presence of normal caliber ducts if obstruction is suspected clinically. If the ducts are not dilated, the success rate will fall to approximately 70 per cent. Once ductal opacification has been achieved, fluoroscopic spot films are obtained to delineate the ductal anatomy (Fig. 11-11).

There are numerous indications for percutaneous transhepatic biliary catheterization and drainage. It is indicated to permit decompression of the biliary tract in cases of neoplastic obstruction of the common hepatic or common bile duct, either as a preoperative measure or as a definitive palliative procedure. These tumors may be primary biliary, primary pancreatic, or metastatic. In patients with ascending cholangitis, percutaneous drainage, along with appropriate antibiotics, will lessen the morbidity and mortality of the disorder, and should enable the patient to have elective, rather than emergency surgery for relief of the mechanical obstruction. Benign posttraumatic or postsurgical strictures of the common bile duct may be definitively treated with percutaneous drainage, followed by transluminal angioplasty of the stricture, using similar balloon catheters as those used in the vascular system. Inoperable primary tumors of the extrahepatic bile duct may be treated with percutaneous drainage and temporary implantation of Iridium[192] seeds into the drainage catheter to deliver high levels of radiation directly to the tumor without compromising normal structures. Percutaneous access to the biliary system allows retained common duct stones to be removed without resorting to reexploration. Following percutaneous access, cytologic samples can be obtained from the lumen of the duct at the exact site of the obstruction. Percutaneous choledochoscopy may be performed for direct visual inspection of the biliary system.

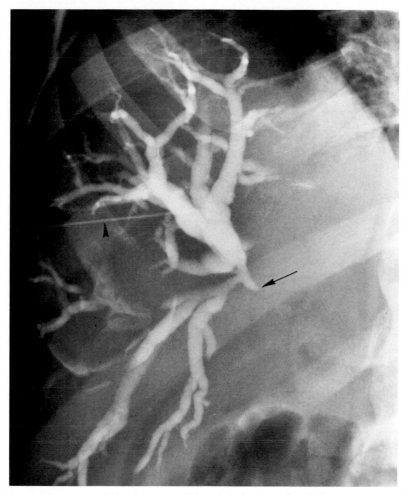

Figure 11-11. A 22-gauge needle has been inserted through the liver (arrowhead). Contrast injection results in delineation of the intrahepatic biliary structures. There is a high grade obstruction involving the right hepatic duct (arrow).

COMPLICATIONS

Percutaneous transhepatic biliary drainage is associated with a higher risk and greater morbidity when compared to other interventional procedures. The primary complications are infection and hemorrhage, both of which can occur acutely after the procedure or months after effective drainage has been established. Bleeding which occurs shortly after the procedure will usually be self-limited, although it might be sufficient to require blood replacement. Late hemorrhage is almost always secondary to a fistula between the bile duct and a large blood vessel. Transcatheter embolization techniques have been successful in controlling this complication (Fig. 11-12). Cholangitis following the procedure is not un-

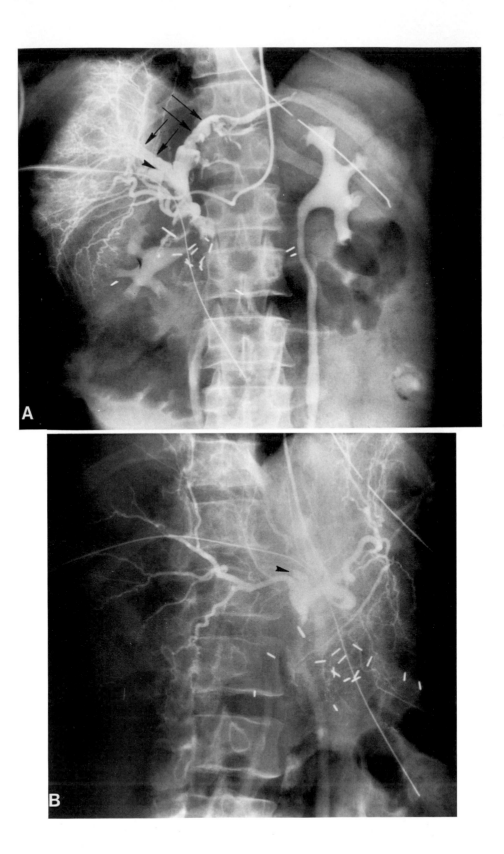

common, particularly in patients with malignant obstruction. Ironically, while percutaneous drainage is part of the management of cholangitis, the long-term use of indwelling catheters for permanent biliary drainage is associated with a 10 to 20 per cent infection rate.

ENDOUROLOGY

DEFINITION

The traditional practice of urology, sparked by innovations in technology and instrumentation, has undergone dramatic changes in the past ten years. This is graphically demonstrated in interventions of the upper urinary tract, where radiology and urology have focused their energies toward a common goal of developing methods which have reduced the morbidity and increased the efficacy of renal stone surgery, renal and ureteral decompression, stenting, and biopsy techniques. With little modification, the basic instruments of the interventional radiologist, the catheter and guidewire, have enabled the radiologist to gain entry into every portion of the renal collecting system, from calyx to urethra. Once the radiologist has gained entry, the entire armamentarium of the urologist can be used to remove, cut, biopsy, drain, and dilate. As catheters became larger, it became possible to introduce endoscopes through these percutaneous tracts, allowing the urologist to perform the same type of endoscopic surgery on the upper urinary tracts that for years he had been performing on the bladder.

Multiple imaging techniques may often be required, not only for diagnosis, but also for providing sufficient information for planning an appropriate intervention. While hydronephrosis may be diagnosed by intravenous urography, CT and antegrade pyelography will provide additional information concerning the exact location and possibly the cause of the obstruction (Fig. 11-13).

INDICATIONS

The primary indication for antegrade pyelography is the direct opacification of the upper urinary tract and ureter. While retrograde urography has long been considered the imaging technique of choice when direct opacification is desired, antegrade pyelography offers significant advantages and should be considered when retrograde studies have failed to provide sufficient diagnostic information. When tight strictures are present, retrograde techniques may fail to opacify the ureter proximal to the obstruction. Severe bladder deformity or recent bladder surgery may prevent retrograde catheterization of the ureter. Thus, antegrade pyelography is a necessity if intravenous urography has failed to produce adequate opacification because of poor renal function or obstruction, or when retrograde

---

Figure 11-12.   **A**: Hepatic arteriogram demonstrates extravasation of contrast from a branch of the hepatic artery directly into the common hepatic duct (arrowhead). Contrast is outlining the entire right and left hepatic ducts (arrows). **B**: Gelfoam embolization has been performed with occlusion of the hepatic artery branch that was previously shown to be the site of extravasation (arrowhead).

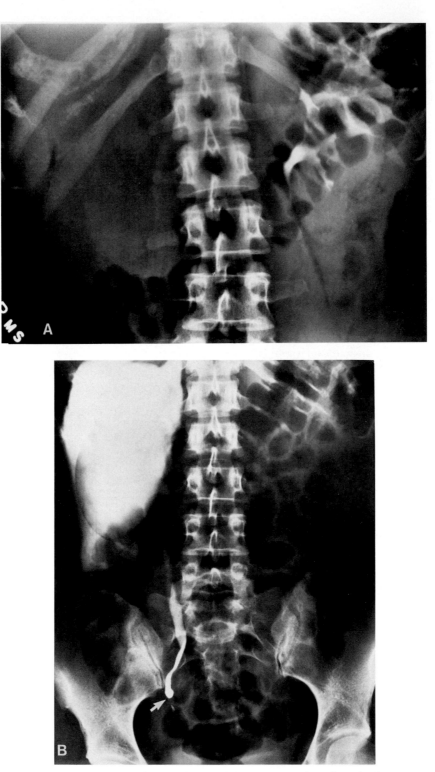

Figure 11-13. **A**: IVP demonstrates no function of the right kidney. **B**: Antegrade pyelography demonstrates marked hydronephrosis of the right kidney. The ureter ends in a blind-ending pouch within the pelvis (arrow).

urography is impossible to perform, is contraindicated, or is of little diagnostic value. Urinary fistulae following surgery and recent renal transplantation are primary indications for percutaneous nephrostomy and stenting techniques. Antegrade pyelography will of necessity be performed prior to establishment of a nephrostomy, as this may be the only study which can demonstrate the origin of leaks, fistulae, or sites of obstruction (Fig. 11-14).

Percutaneous nephrostomy and antegrade placement of indwelling ureteral stents are the two most frequently performed interventional therapeutic procedures in the urinary tract. Percutaneous nephrostomy is indicated for benign or malignant obstruction, and is often performed in conjunction with extracorporeal shock wave lithotrypsy (ESWL), which is a nonsurgical technique for reducing kidney stones to a dust-like material which can then be passed spontaneously. Percutaneous nephrostomy also serves as the method of access to the collecting system of the kidney, permitting the instillation of various solvents into the collecting system for the dissolution of stones which are insufficiently calcified to permit their fluoroscopic visualization. This is mandatory if ESWL is to be used. Endourologic surgery, which requires the introduction of a endoscope into the renal pelvis, is performed following establishment of a percutaneous nephrostomy tract and dilatation of the tract from 8 to 24Fr with special dilators or balloon catheters.

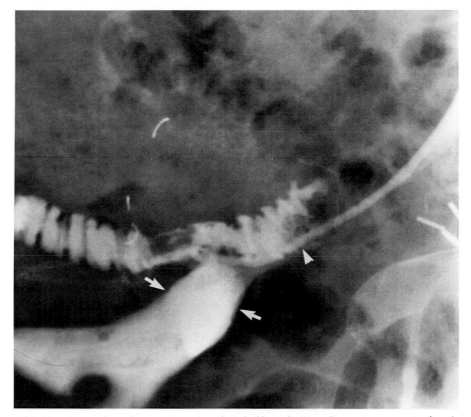

Figure 11-14.   Antegrade pyelogram in a patient with an ileal-loop diversion. Contrast is extravasating from the ureteral-ileal anastomosis (arrows). The anastomosis is demonstrated by the arrowheads.

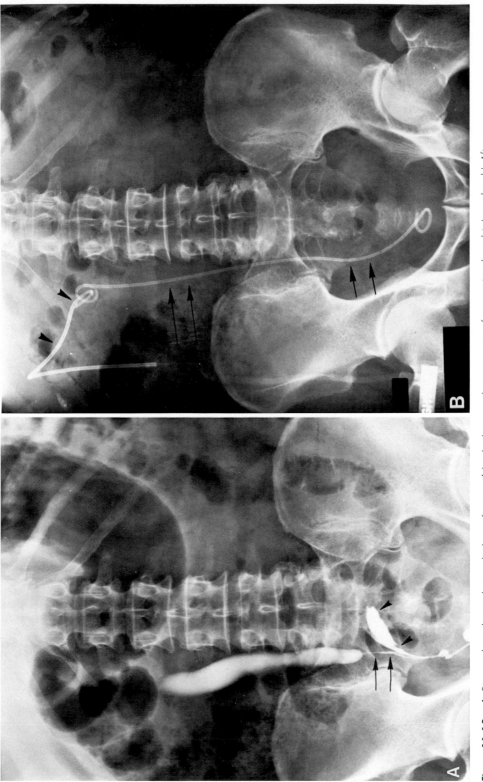

Figure 11-15. **A:** Retrograde pyelogram has resulted in perforation of the distal ureter with extravasation of contrast into the pelvis (arrowheads). After perforation occurred, the urologist was not able to pass a ureteral stent through the stenosis (arrows). **B:** Ureteral stent (arrows) has been placed by the radiologist in an antegrade, transrenal manner. A nephrostomy catheter is temporarily in place (arrowheads).

Ureteral stents are often placed cystoscopically by urologists whenever a ureteral stricture or obstruction is present which cannot be relieved surgically, or if the patient is not a surgical candidate. Most commonly, ureteral stents are placed to palliate renal failure secondary to malignant ureteral obstruction. There are circumstances when the retrograde cystoscopic technique cannot be used, and, in these instances, interventional radiologists can place ureteral stents in an antegrade transrenal fashion (Fig. 11-15).

METHODOLOGY

The placement of catheters and drains into the renal collecting system via a pertcutaneous, transrenal approach requires a sophisticated team approach by radiologist and urologist. Prior to placing nephrostomy catheters, there must be adequate visualization of the collecting structures, either by antegrade pyelography, retrograde pyelography, ultrasound, or CT. Most of the actual placement of the appropriate catheters is done under fluroscopic control. If the nephrostomy catheter placement is a prelude to further instrumentation by either the radiologist or urologist, it must be decided in advance where the point of entry of the catheter will be, which calyx it will enter, and how large a tract should be created.

PATIENT PREPARATION

As with other major interventional procedures, knowledge of coagulation studies is mandatory, as the gravest complication of percutaneous transrenal interventions is uncontrolled hemorrhage. If the patient's urine is infected prior to a percutaneous procedure, and the patient is found to be obstructed, as little manipulation of catheters and drains as possible should take place until nephrostomy drainage has been established and kidney function has stabilized.

COMPLICATIONS

Bleeding and infection are the two most common complications. Risk of hemorrhage is reduced by accurate placement of the nephrostomy catheter from the start. A posterolateral approach to the kidney carries less risk of hemorrhage than does a straight posterior approach, as the diameter and number of vessels coursing over the posterolateral aspect are less than those over the direct posterior aspect. The risk of infection can be reduced by careful attention to technique, maintaining adequate urinary drainage, and judicious use of appropriate antibiotics if the patient has a preexisting urinary infection.

NUCLEAR MEDICINE STUDIES

Richard C. Reba, M.D.
Eduard V. Kotlyarov, M.D.

INTRODUCTION

Nuclear medicine is primarily a diagnostic discipline that uses radioactive tracers, called radiopharmaceuticals, for the detection and localization of disease and for the functional assessment of *in vivo* biochemical processes. The tracer methodology depends on the unique properties of radiopharmaceuticals to localize in a target organ or system or to participate in a specific process. Radiopharmaceuticals are commonly introduced into the body by intravenous injection or by mouth. The mass of the radiopharmaceuticals introduced is small, i.e., subphysiologic and subpharmacologic, and does not alter the physicologic and biochemical reactions into which they are incorporated.

It is possible to record the rate of movement of the radiopharmaceuticals and their spatial distribution within the body because the radionuclides selected decay with the emission of suitable x-ray, gamma, or annihilation radiations. The most commonly used detection device, a scintillation camera, is a single large sodium iodide crystal which interacts with and absorbs the emitted gamma ray or photon, and converts the energy into light. Photomultiplier tubes are positioned over the crystal to collect and multiply the light, which is converted to an electric charge, amplified, and sorted by a pulse height analyzer. The origin of the radioactivity is positioned in space by analyzing the pattern of activation of the phototube array. Finally, the record is displayed using an image recording device. A lead collimator, usually with multiple apertures, is placed on the front of the crystal to decrease radiation scatter and increase the overall spatial resolution of the system. The size and sensitivity of the scintillation camera allow recording of the time course of rapid dynamic processes, such as blood flow through specific parts of the body.

THYROID NUCLEAR MEDICINE STUDIES

Thyroid nuclear medicine studies can be divided into *in vivo* and *in vitro* procedures. *In vitro* procedures involve the determination of serum concentration of thyroid hormones such as T3 and T4, as well as thyroid stimulating hormone, TSH. These measurements are important for the complete evaluation of thyroid function. Determination of TSH is the most important step for the confirmation of hypothyroidism. Occasionally, and for specific indications, such as equivocal basal TSH, secondary and tertiary hypothyroidism, it is necessary to measure TSH after stimulation with thyroid releasing hormone.

In vivo thyroid procedures include thyroid scanning with technetium-99m (Tc-99m) pertechnetate or sodium iodide-123 or -131 (I-123, I-131) and the determination of the percent thyroid uptake. Thyroid scanning is performed 20 minutes after the intravenous injection of Tc-99m pertechnetate, usually 10m Ci. Technetium is actively trapped by the thyroid follicles but is not organified. When radioactive iodine is used, the scans are performed 24 hours after oral administration of 25 to 50m Ci NaI-131 (T$\frac{1}{2}$ = 8.1 days) or as early as 6 hours when 100 to 200m Ci NaI-123 (T$\frac{1}{2}$ = 13.6 hours) is used. Iodide is actively trapped and organified by the thyroid.

The major indications for thyroid imaging are to determine thyroid size, detect and evaluate thyroid nodules, determine the cause of hyperthyroidism (diffuse hyperplasia versus multiple toxic nodules versus solitary toxic nodule), locate ectopic or functioning metastatic thyroid tissue, evaluate acute or subacute thyroiditis, and evaluate thyroid cancer patients following thyroidectomy.

Routinely, thyroid scans are performed using Tc-99m, because it is less expensive and there is a lower radiation dose compared to I-123 or I-131. The nodule that is suspicious for thyroid cancer is the "cold" nodule, that is, nonfunctioning. This strategy of risk stratification for thyroid nodules was developed when only radioiodine was used and, therefore, is based on evaluating organification. It is known that some small number of thyroid cancers, perhaps 1 to 3 per cent, retain the trapping function and, therefore, may appear as a warm or "hot" nodule on an early thyroid scan (20 minutes to 2 hours). Therefore, if a nodule is functioning on a Tc-99m scan, the study should be repeated using radioactive iodide because 30 to 40 per cent of discordant nodules are malignant. After identification of a hypofunctioning or cold nodule that might be malignant, needle aspiration is usually recommended. After careful clinical, ultrasound, and nuclear medicine scan assessment, the vast majority of solitary nodules removed (about 70 per cent) are pathologically benign follicular adenomas.

Another use of thyroid scanning is in the evaluation of autonomous function, usually of a nodule and associated with some suppression of the remainder of the thyroid tissue. For complete evaluation of this condition, it is necessary to repeat the scans after adequate suppression following cytomel (T3) or thyroxine (T4) administration and TSH stimulation.

A diffuse decrease in technetium and iodine concentration on the thyroid scan occurs in patients with hypothyroidism and in patients with acute or subacute thyroiditis. It is important to be aware of the relatively common condition called subacute thyroiditis, which may be painless in one third to one half of the patients. Clinically, the patient appears thyrotoxic, with increased serum T3 and T4 concentrations, the thyroid gland may or may not be enlarged, but the uptake is markedly depressed. The same condition is seen in postpartum thyrotoxicosis. This condition is transient and does not require antithyroid treatment.

Iodine-131 is used to scan patients with substernal goiter and for screening of metastases of follicular and papillary carcinoma. The long physical halflife (8.1 days) and high gamma ray energy (365keV) of I-131 allow scanning 48 to 72 hours after oral administration of 2 to 10m Ci of the radiopharmaceutical. Screening for thyroid metastases should be performed only when the patient is clinically and biochemically hypothyroid, with elevated serum TSH. Rarely exogenous TSH must be administered if sufficient endogenous TSH elevation does not occur.

CARDIAC NUCLEAR MEDICINE STUDIES

Simple, noninvasive cardiac nuclear medicine studies are widely applied in the practice of cardiology. Using one of several available radiopharmaceuticals, a gamma camera coupled to a digital computer and electrocardiographic gating, nuclear medicine tests can now rapidly provide quantitative information about ventricular volumes, global and regional wall motion, regional myocardial blood flow, myocardial glucose and fatty acid metabolism, and a number of physiological indices, such as cardiac output, stroke volume, systolic and diastolic time intervals, and ejection fraction.

For many of the function and wall motion studies, the cardiac blood pool is outlined using Tc-99m labeled red blood cells, similar to that used in any blood pool study. The usual dose of radiopharmaceutical is between 20 and 30m Ci of Tc-99m.

Since cardiac function is frequently normal when a patient is in a resting state, in selected instances it is important to repeat the study using maximum stress, usually physical exercise or the administration of a cardiac vasodilator drug. The heart is positioned to maximize separation of the right and left ventricles, usually 45° LAO, but anterior, left lateral, and different oblique views may be necessary to evaluate different cardiac walls.

The detected radioactivity is sorted in the temporal domain into a minimum of 24 memories of a computer which is controlled by ECG gating. This allows the acquisition of the cardiac blood pool in each of 24 temporal segments of a R-R ECG interval. It is necessary to continue the collection of counts during several minutes so that statistical reliability is achieved in each of the brief time intervals. Counts from each segment are then viewed in a real-time cine presentation which results in the production of a high resolution image of left and right ventricular wall motion and reconstruction of the time/activity curves. The counts from each ventricle are proportional to volume. Ejection fraction is calculated as the counts at end-diastole minus the counts at end-systole, divided by the counts at end-distole. When supine, the normal left ventricular ejection fraction (LVEF) is greater than 45 per cent. When compared to the resting LVEF, a normal person will increase the EF at least 5 per cent during maximum stress. Cinematic display of ventricular contraction allows evaluation of segmental wall motion, and areas of hypokinesia, akinesia, and dyskinesia, or paradoxical movement are readily recognized (Figs. 12-1, 12-2, 12-3).

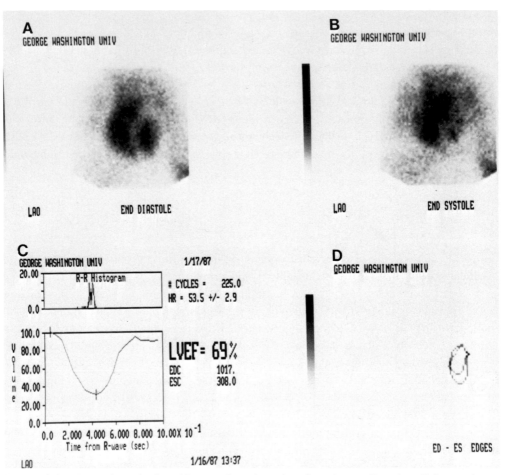

Figure 12-1. A normal gated radionuclide ventriculography study performed at rest. The right and left ventricular blood pools (RV and LV) are identified, as well as the blood in the aorta (AO), pulmonary artery (PA) and spleen (SPLN). The space between the RV and LV is the intraventricular septum. **A:** Images at end-diastole (ED). **B:** Images at end-systole (ES). **C:** This image displays the left ventricular time/activity curve, equivalent to time/volume, of an average single LV contraction. The left ventricular ejection fraction (LVEF) is 69 per cent, normal being greater than 45 per cent. A plot of the frequency distribution of the R-R time intervals is also displayed. **D:** The edges of ED and ES volumes are superimposed so that the extent of regional contraction may be immediately evaluated.

Another test, thallium-201 (Tl-201) stress test, is used in the evaluation of myocardial perfusion. Thallium is a potassium analogue and is injected as thallous chloride. When injected during maximum tolerated physical exercise, approximately 5 per cent of the radiopharmaceutical is concentrated in the heart muscle. The concentration is proportional to myocardial blood flow.

The study consists of the injection of 2m Ci of Tl-201 chloride during a treadmill stress test. The radiopharmaceutical is injected at the peak of exercise and the patient is asked to continue exercising for another minute. When the stress test is completed, the patient is immediately scanned, obtaining left anterior oblique, anterior, and left lateral images. The

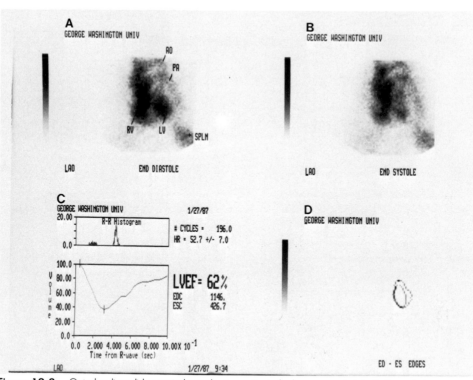

Figure 12-2. Gated radionuclide ventriculography in a patient who has a normal global left ventricular ejection fraction at rest, 62 per cent, but akinesia of the septal wall is present. The patient has a history of previous myocardial infarction. The free left ventricular wall is contracting normally. **A, B, C, D** and labels are the same as in Fig 12-1.

study is repeated 2 to 4 hours later, after allowing for myocardial reperfusion, a condition almost equivalent to the resting state.

Segmental areas of myocardial hypoperfusion are recognized as a focal decrease in Tl-201 within the ventricular wall. If a hypoperfusion defect is present in the immediate stress images, but is reperfused and appears homogeneous on the delayed resting study, myocardial ischemia is present. A study which shows a perfusion defect which persists at rest represents cardiomyopathy with a transmural myocardial infarction. Knowledge of the coronary artery anatomy allows localization of specific involved vessels. Although a symmetrical "free vessel" is occasionally difficult to diagnose because all myocardial segments are equally involved, measuring the kinetics of Tl-201 influx and efflux from the myocardial wall will overcome this possibility.

A new method of computer processing of multiangular scanning acquisition, single photon emission computed tomography, or SPECT, has resulted in high sensitivity and specificity of test results in patients with coronary artery disease.

The tests described, available in the stress test laboratory and the coronary care unit, can readily answer these clinical questions: What is the cause of a patient's chest pain? What is the significance of the electrocardiographic changes? Has the patient had a myocardial infarction; if so, how large and how recent? What is the ventricular function and is there a

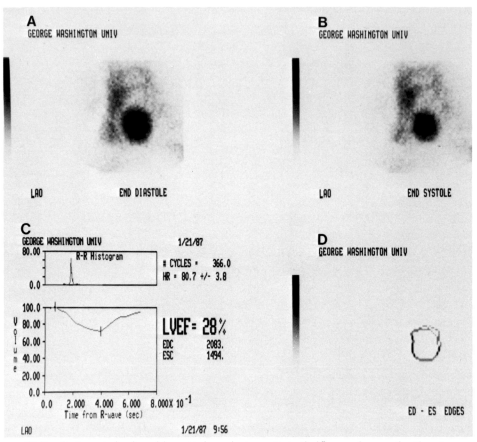

Figure 12-3. Resting gated radionuclide ventriculography in a patient with diffuse cardiomyopathy. There is a marked increase of end-diastolic and end-systolic volumes. There is a significant reduction of left ventricular function. The left ventricular ejection fraction is 28 per cent, indicating a marked reduction in LV function, with diffuse global hypokinesia. **A, B, C, D** and labels are the same as in Fig 12-1.

ventricular aneurysm? What is the patient's risk category and the overall prognosis? How does ventricular function respond to exercise or drug administration? In a practical setting, the answers to these questions may be used in the admission criteria for the coronary care unit, to evaluate the asymptomatic patient with a positive ECG stress test or a symptomatic patient with a negative ECG stress test; to determine if cardiac catheterization or surgery should be performed; in the preoperative and postoperative evaluation of the status of myocardial function and to document the effect of coronary artery bypass graft surgery.

VENTILATION/PERFUSION LUNG SCANS

A ventilation/perfusion lung scan can be employed as an effective noninvasive test for the diagnosis of pulmonary embolism. The study is based on detection of segmental or multiple subsegmental perfusion defects which are accompanied by normal regional ventilation. Those defects in the appropriate clinical setting are highly suggestive of a block in pulmonary arterial blood flow, with occlusion due to pulmonary venous thromboembolism. In most clinical institutions, a ventilation study is performed first. Between 15 to 30m Ci of xenon-133 (Xe-133) gas is injected into the spirometer system which delivers the xenon/air mixture and allows single breaths and rebreathing of the gas mixture. The total body radiation dose is between 0.005 and 0.0015 rad. The absorbed dose in the lung is between .5 and 1.5 rads.

Airway resistance and alveolar compliance are major factors in determining the distribution of radioactive xenon. Xenon is distributed in the apices to a lesser degree than in the bases, reflecting normal alveolar compliance. A wide field of view gamma camera is used so that the entire lung can be included on each image.

The study consists of single breath, equilibrium, and washout phases. With the patient sitting or supine, all of the radiopharmaceutical is deposited into the mask at the time the patient takes a deep breath. The patient is asked to hold his breath and an image of the initial distribution of the gas in the alveolae is recorded.

Then the patient breathes at tidal ventilation in a closed O_2 enriched system for at least three minutes. This length of time is important to allow radioactive gas to reach all parts of the lungs, even those which are poorly ventilated or not ventilated through the bronchial system, but through the collaterals of alveolar pores of Kohn and bronchial alveolar channels of Lampert. The image obtained is one equivalent to total lung volume.

After 4 minutes the washout phase begins. The inlet valve is maneuvered so the patient is breathing in room air and exhaling into the spirometer system where radioactive gas is trapped by the charcoal filter. Several images are obtained for at least 6 minutes (one image per minute). Posterior and oblique projections are obtained. The washout images are evaluated for the presence of gas trapping and regional obstructive airways disease.

The perfusion study is performed after an intravenous injection of 3m Ci of Tc-99m macroaggregated albumin (MAA). The radiation dose to the whole body is approximately 0.2 rad and the radiation dose to the lungs is approximately 0.5 rad. The minimal number of radioactive particles injected is approximately 100,000. The average particle size is approximately 50 microns (range 10 to 100 microns). The particles are temporarily lodged in the first capillary bed distal to the injection site, which is the pulmonary arterial capillary distribution.

The radioactive particles undergo degradation in the capillary bed and are removed from the blood by the reticuloendothelial system. The effective half-life of Tc-99m macroaggregated albumin is approximately 3.5 hours in the lung. At least six projections — anterior, posterior, both oblique, and both laterals — are obtained. Since most lung scans are obtained to evaluate a patient suspected of having pulmonary embolism, it is important to make the injection with the patient supine so that as even an apical-to-base distribution of pulmonary blood flow as possible is achieved.

There are multiple causes of perfusion abnormalities. The most common is chronic obstructive airways disease. Of course, all of the causes which produce opacification on the chest x-ray will result in perfusion abnormalities. These include inflammatory infiltrates, infarction, hemorrhage, pleural effusion, and atelectasis. Mucous plug, bulla formation, vascular compression by tumor, as well as vasculitis may present as common causes for single or multiple perfusion abnormalities.

Interpretation of ventilation/perfusion studies of the lungs should always be accompanied by the evaluation of a recent chest x-ray. Pulmonary embolism does not have specific x-ray changes and a significant proportion of patients have a normal chest x-ray. Atelectasis, infiltrate, pleural effusion, dilatation of a main pulmonary artery, a pleural based density, and regional paucity of vessels are some of the manifestations of pulmonary emboli on the chest x-ray. However, these radiographic signs have a low degree of specificity.

A normal perfusion study is a practical method of excluding pulmonary embolism. Multiple segmental perfusion defects in a patient with normal ventilation, V/Q mismatch, and a normal chest x-ray are 90 to 95 per cent sensitive and specific for pulmonary embolism.

Low Probability of Embolism (less than 7 per cent)

1. Normal chest x-ray, normal ventilation study, and a single or multiple nonsegmental, or single subsegmental (size less than one anatomic segment) perfusion defects.
2. Normal chest x-ray, normal ventilation study, and several small subsegmental defects, the combined size of which is equivalent to less than one anatomic segment.
3. Normal chest x-ray, single or multiple segmental or nonsegmental perfusion defects with matched ventilation abnormalities; that is, the ventilation defect occurs with the same anatomic pattern as the perfusion defect.

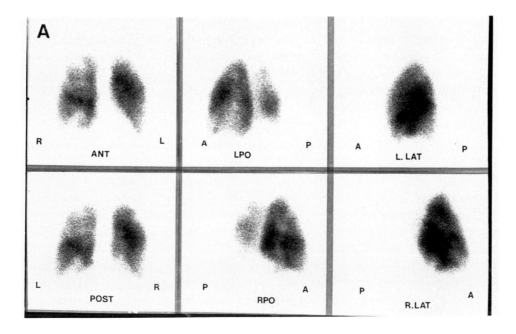

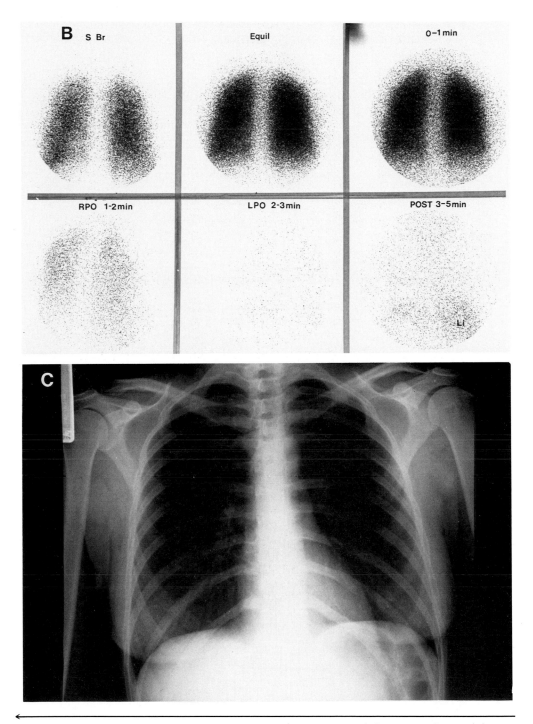

Figure 12-4. Ventilation and perfusion lung scans in a patient with pulmonary embolism, proven subsequently by angiography. The perfusion lung scan (**A**) is obtained in six projections and shows two segmental defects, the posterior basal segment of the right lower lobe and lateral segment of the left lower lobe plus defects in the upper lobes bilaterally. Single equilibrium and washout ventilation studies (**B**) and the chest x-ray (**C**) are normal. This is an example of ventilation/perfusion mismatch.

4. Opacification on the chest x-ray, the presence of any perfusion defect which is definitely smaller than an opacification on the chest x-ray in the same area.

High Probability of Embolism (over 85 per cent)

1. Normal chest x-ray, normal ventilation, and single or multiple segmental perfusion defects (Fig. 12-4).
2. Normal chest x-ray, normal ventilation study, and single lobar perfusion defect with accompanying single or multiple subsegmental or segmental defects.
3. Opacification of the chest x-ray and a segmental, lobar, or nonsegmental perfusion defect which is significantly larger than an opacification of the chest x-ray.

Moderate Probability of Embolism (20 to 30 per cent)

1. Normal chest x-ray, normal ventilation study, and several subsegmental perfusion defects the sum of which is equivalent to one to two segments; approximately 30 per cent.
2. Severe chronic obstructive airways disease, no opacification on the chest x-ray, and matched or partially unmatched perfusion defects; approximately 20 per cent.
3. Opacification of the chest x-ray and nonsegmental perfusion defect which is approximately equal in size to the area of x-ray opacification; approximately 30 per cent.

It should be emphasized that the single breath phase of the ventilation study is significantly less sensitive than is the retention of radioactive xenon in washout phase for the detection of obstructive airways disease. The washout phase of the ventilation study is considered abnormal if retention of radioactive xenon is seen on the fourth minute of washout. When ventilation abnormalities are seen only on one of those two phases, it is considered abnormal regardless of whether it is seen on the single breath or washout phase. Because of anatomic overlap of segments, oblique washout images are of significant help in matching ventilation and perfusion abnormalities.

The presence of an area of perfused lung tissue on the periphery of a segmental or lobar perfusion defect, the so called "stripe" sign, is rarely present in pulmonary embolism. This is usually seen in a patient with chronic obstructive pulmonary disease but may be present in a patient with pulmonary embolism and partial reperfusion. However, the presence of the "stripe" sign allows exclusion of pulmonary embolism in more than 90 per cent of patients (Figs. 12-5).

If it is not apparent that the ventilation abnormality matches the perfusion defect, a repeat so-called "second look" ventilation study, single breath and washout, is obtained following the perfusion study. The image is obtained in the projection where the perfusion defect is best defined. It is important to emphasize that ventilation/perfusion mismatch is not specific

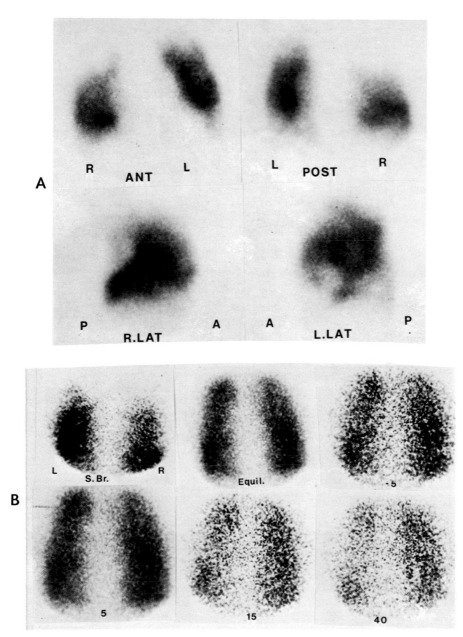

Figure 12-5. Perfusion ventilation scans in a patient with severe obstructive airways disease. **A:** Perfusion scan reveals multiple nonsegmental and subsegmental perfusion defects. **B:** Ventilation scans. Although the lower portions of the lungs were excluded from the image obtained during single breath holding (S.Br.), when compared to the posterior perfusion scan, there is bilateral decrease in apical ventilation, and matched ventilation/perfusion abnormalities. After rebreathing, the equilibrium image (Equil.) reveals a normal, but probably expanded, distribution of inhaled gas, representing intact alveoli in the total lung volume. There is uneven washout of Xe-133 gas with areas of retention (trapping) in the areas of abnormal perfusion. There was a 35 pk/yr history of cigarette smoking. The FEV$_1$ was 50 per cent and the chest x-ray was unremarkable. (Courtesy of W.B. Saunders Co.)

for pulmonary embolism. Mismatch may be seen in patients with previous pulmonary embolism and bronchogenic carcinoma, which compresses a branch of the pulmonary artery but does not significantly compress the adjacent bronchus. It is also seen in patients with congenital hypoplasia of a branch of the pulmonary artery, angiitis, and postradiation vasculitis.

The clinical history and the intensity of clinical suspicion of pulmonary embolism is extremely important for correct interpretation of ventilation/perfusion test results. The mentioned criteria are obtained in an inhomogeneous group of patients whose clinical *a priori* probability of pulmonary embolism was 40 to 50 per cent. A significant increase or decrease of the probability of pulmonary embolism prior to the lung scan test can significantly influence the posttest probability of the ventilation/perfusion studies. In instances where the interpretation of the lung scan does not agree with the clinical evaluation, and where interventional procedures are planned, e.g., inferior vena cava umbrella interruption, thrombectomy or local thrombolytic agent administration, or where the clinical probability of pulmonary embolism remains in a moderate range, a selective angiogram with placement of the catheter in the areas of perfusion abnormalities should be considered.

Interpretation of ventilation/perfusion studies of the lungs can be a difficult task even for an experienced nuclear medicine physician. Integration of the clinical details, complete knowledge of bronchopulmonary segmental anatomy, and interpretation of current x-rays are all necessary to arrive at a correct diagnosis.

Other uses of lung scanning include pre- and postoperative quantification of regional lung function in patients with cancer or obstructive pulmonary disease, especially for the prediction of postoperative pulmonary function.

LIVER/SPLEEN SCANS

The major indications for obtaining a liver/spleen scan in contemporary clinical practice is in evaluation of the size, shape, and position of the organs, detection of metastatic deposits, diagnosis of primary malignant and benign hepatic lesions, and evaluation of diffuse hepatocellular disease, such as cirrhosis. Technetium-99m sulfur colloid is injected intravenously in the average dose of 4m Ci. The whole body dose is approximately 0.07 rad and the dose to the liver is approximately 1.3 rads and to the spleen is 1 rad. Particle size is between 0.1 and 1 micron in diameter. The colloidal particles are extracted by reticuloendothelial cells. In the normal adult, 85 to 90 per cent of particles are trapped by Kupffer cells of the liver, 5 to 10 per cent by the reticuloendothelial system (RES) of the spleen, and the remainder is accumulated in smaller quantities in the RES of the lymph nodes, bone marrow, and lungs. The extraction fraction of colloid particles by the RES is very high, more than 95 per cent, and accumulation is accomplished within 15 minutes. Multiple planar images are obtained from various projections, so that each surface is examined. Emission computed tomography, spect, which produces reconstructed "slices" through the liver, is being used with increasing frequency (Fig. 12-6).

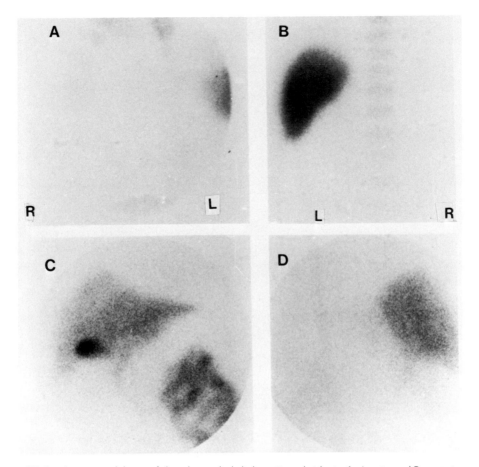

Figure 12-6. A patient with hepatic failure due to alcoholic hepatitis and cirrhosis. **A:** Anterior and **B:** posterior Tc-99m sulfur colloid scans reveal little or no liver phagocytic localization, an enlarged spleen with intense colloid concentration, and increased colloid in all of the visible bone marrow. **C:** Anterior and **D:** posterior scans in the same patient 60 minutes after injection of Tc-99m DSIDA reveal delayed but adequate parenchymal cell localization and biliary excretion. Neither spleen nor bone marrow is seen.

There are methods to estimate liver and spleen volume, but these are tedious, and simple measurements often suffice to evaluate organ size. Although absolute size varies with sex, age, height, and weight, the upper limits of normal for adult liver size are 16cm in the right midclavicular line, and 12cm for the long axis of the spleen. Normal liver scans may have decreased activity corresponding to the fissure separating the right and left lobes of the liver, porta hepatis, and gallbladder fossa. Decreased radioactivity also might be seen on the superior surface because of attenuation of radioactivity by hepatic veins.

Defects in the liver scan are due to absence of RES cells and are nonspecific. That is, intrahepatic primary and metastatic malignant growths, abscess, adenoma, hemangioma, or cyst all may have a similar liver scan appearance. Hepatoma may appear as a single defect,

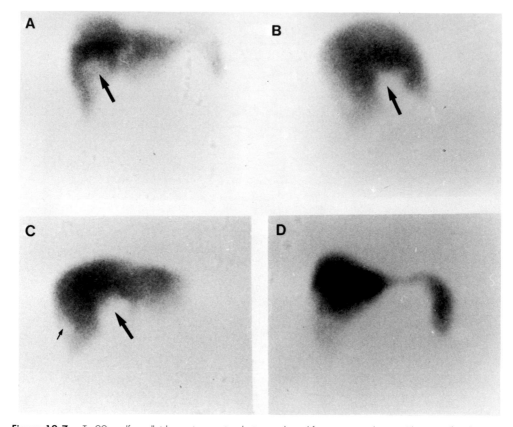

Figure 12-7. Tc-99m sulfur colloid scan in a patient being evaluated for metastatic disease. There is a focal area of decreased activity in the anterior segment of the right lobe extending to the quadrate lobe (arrow). **A:** Anterior. **B:** Right lateral. **C:** Right anterior oblique. **D:** Left anterior oblique.

as multiple defects, or as a nonhomogeneous pattern. Metastases of colon carcinoma are usually multiple and discrete. Approximately 40 per cent of focal nodular hyperplasia lesions maintain a normal hepatic architecture and, therefore, normal uptake of the radiopharmaceutical. On rare occasions, increased activity is present due to a high concentration of Kupffer cells. A "hot" spot in the quadrate lobe or central portion of the liver is the result of superior vena cava obstruction and diversion of colloid via the umbilical vein. A focal increase has also been described in patients with hepatic vein thrombosis and in cirrhosis.

When a hemangioma is suspected by an ultrasound, CT, or colloid liver scan defect, injection of radiolabeled red blood cells, converting the abnormality to a "hot" defect is a specific test for hepatic cavernous hemangioma. The patient with moderate hepatocellular disease from cirrhosis has enlarged right and left lobes of the liver, loss of the normal gradient of radiopharmaceutical between the right and left lobes of the liver, an inhomoge-

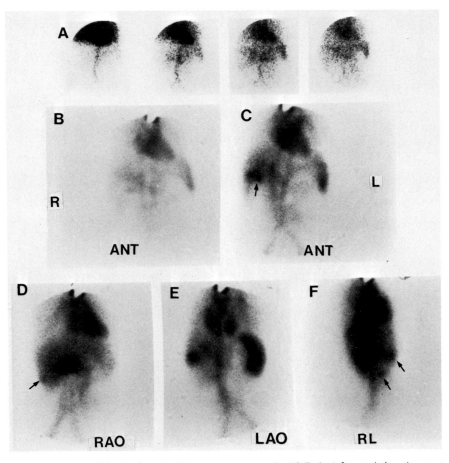

Figure 12-8. Tc-99m red blood cell study of the same patient as in Fig 12-7. **A:** A flow study from the anterior upper abdomen at 5-second intervals shows no increased activity in the early arterial phase and normal distribution in the venous phase. Note the cardiac blood pool above the liver. **B:** A normal immediate blood pool image. **C:** Anterior. **D:** Right anterior oblique. **E:** Left anterior oblique. **F:** Right lateral image one hour later demonstrates several focal areas of increased blood pool within the liver, indicating multiple cavernous hemangiomas of various sizes. This is the most common benign hepatic tumor.

neous distribution of radiopharmaceutical in the liver parenchyma, and a shift of sulfur colloid to the spleen, and in the later stages to the bone marrow. The spleen is enlarged late in the course. Hepatocellular disease secondary to uncomplicated viral hepatitis rarely produces a liver/spleen scan abnormality. In patients with chronic anemia and reactivation of bone marrow, visualization of bone marrow is seen without significant inhomogeneity of radiopharmaceutical uptake in the liver and without shift of sulfur colloid to the spleen (Figs. 12-6, 12-7, 12-8, 12-9).

The liver scan is more sensitive but less specific than ultrasound for detection of liver metastases and has almost the same diagnostic accuracy as a CT scan with contrast.

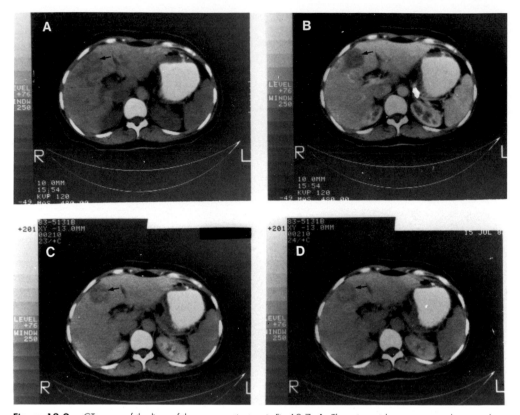

Figure 12-9. CT scans of the liver of the same patient as in Fig 12-7. **A:** There is an inhomogeneous decreased density noted within the liver in the same region described in Figure 12-7. Oral contrast is in the stomach. **B:** The same slice immediately following bolus intravenous injection of contrast material demonstrates increased enhancement of the liver, accentuating a well-circumscribed lesion that is not enhanced. **C:** The same slice at 5 minutes. **D:** The same slice 10 minutes later shows contrast enhancement of the lesion with decreasing contrast from the liver parenchyma, typical of a cavernous hemangioma and strengthening the conclusions derived from the Tc-99m red cell study in Figure 12-8.

GALLBLADDER SCANS

The differential dianosis of right upper quadrant or epigastric pain is complicated. A major cause of this symptom is cholecystitis, with or without gallstones. The number of people in the U.S. estimated to have gallstones exceeds 16,000,000 and the incidence increases with increasing age. Annually, more than 400,000 patients have gallbladder surgery each year at a total cost of 1 to 1.5 billion dollars. The recommended treatment for acute cholecystitis is to remove the gallbladder. The most sensitive, specific, and accurate test to diagnose cholecystitis is the hepatobiliary scan.

At the present time, the preferred radiopharmaceutical for hepatobiliary scintigraphy is DISIDA which is a diisopropyl derivative of iminodiacetic acid. This compound has a high ratio of liver to renal excretion and allows visualization of the hepatobiliary system even at serum bilirubin concentrations of 20mg/dl. An injection of 3 to 5m Ci of Tc-99m labeled DISIDA is administered to the patient who has been fasting for at least 4 hours. Within 5 to

10 minutes, there is rapid and efficient extraction from the blood by the hepatic parenchymal cells.

Normally, during the subsequent 60 minutes, the radiotracer is excreted into the hepatic ducts and is transported through the bile ducts into the small intestine. During this interval, and at various times, sequential images are obtained. Since the *sine qua non* of acute cholecystitis is cystic duct obstruction, the study may be terminated as soon as the gallbladder is visualized and contraction is evident. However, delayed views for up to 4 hours are important in selected instances, e.g., a distended gallbladder that has never filled (photon-deficient, Rule Out (R/O) hydrops), a distended and filled gallbladder that doesn't contract (R/O acalculous cholecystitis), a nonvisualized gallbladder (R/O chronic cholecystitis), and a normal parenchymal phase but no transit from the liver (R/O common duct obstruction).

The diagnosis of *cholecystitis* is made on hepatobiliary scintigraphy by nonvisualization of the gallbladder. Acute cholecystitis is differentiated from chronic on clinical grounds. If the gallbladder is visualized after only 1 hour, the diagnosis of chronic cholecystitis is made. In the appropriate clinical setting, nonvisualization of the gallbladder within 4 hours in a patient with adequate fasting prior to the study (at least 2 hours) is generally an accurate indication of acute cholecystitis in 95 to 97 per cent of patients. Visualization of the gallbladder within the first hour is 99 per cent accurate in excluding the diagnosis of acute cholecystitis. This percentage of diagnostic accuracy decreases to about 93 to 95 per cent if visualization takes up to 4 hours. Negative causes for visualization of the gallbladder within the first 4 hours include acalculus cholecystitis, duodenal diverticulum, and accessory cystic duct. Dilatation of the cystic duct proximal to obstruction may simulate gallbladder activity. False positive results are significantly more common than false negative results and include food intake less than 2 hours before the test, severe hepatic dysfunction, prolonged fasting, and hyperalimentation. Several techniques have been employed to improve the diagnostic accuracy of the test, including the use of cholecystokinin or its synthetic derivatives to ensure that gallbladder emptying is complete, and intravenous injection of morphine to contract the sphincter of Oddi, increase common duct pressure, and enhance retrograde flow into the gallbladder.

Partial or nonvisualization of the common biliary duct and gall bladder, and lack of appearance of the radiotracer in the intestine after 4 hours is usually quite specific for *biliary duct obstruction*. With normal hepatic extraction, the specificity of this sign is approximately 93 per cent, significantly better than the results of ultrasound. However, ultrasound is the preferred technique to evaluate chronic cholecystitis, especially for the detection of gallstones. It is the lack of normal transit from liver to the intestines that is the basis for the reliability of this test in the differential diagnosis of neonatal hepatitis and the detection of *biliary atresia*. *Choledochal cyst* is also readily diagnosed.

DETECTION OF GASTROINTESTINAL BLEEDING

The mortality from upper gastrointestinal tract bleeding has remained constant at approximately 10 per cent over the past 40 years. The diagnosis of gastrointestinal bleeding is especially difficult when bleeding originates distal to the ligament of Treitz. Identification of

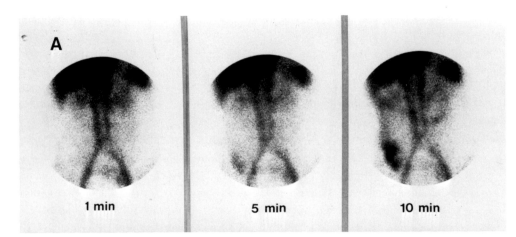

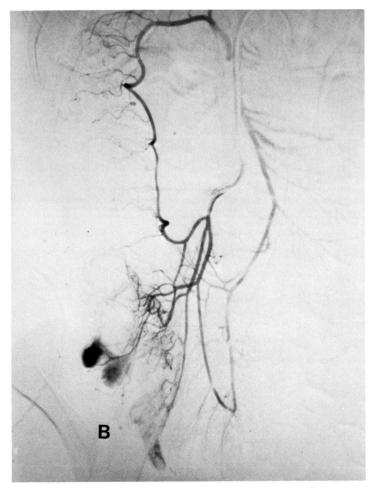

Figure 12-10. **A:** Tc-99m red blood cell study images obtained 5 and 10 minutes after injection show active bleeding in the cecum with subsequent extension of radiolabeled red cells to the ascending and transverse colon. **B:** Contrast angiography reveals bleeding in the cecal branches of the superior mesenteric artery.

the responsible artery is important because of the availability of interventional treatment, but the major problem with establishing the site of bleeding is the intermittent pattern of most bleeding.

The rationale of the nuclear medicine test is to introduce a radioactive label in the blood pool and then look for radioactivity in the gastrointestinal tract. Two such labels are available. The Tc-99m sulfur colloid method is an accurate and sensitive method for active bleeding and can detect bleeding as small as 0.1 ml per minute. However, in the patient with intermittent bleeding who does not bleed within the 15 to 20 minutes after the intravenous injection of the radiopharmaceutical, detection of the bleeding is not possible. Also because of intense uptake of the sulfur colloid by the liver and spleen, application of the technique to upper GI bleeding is limited. Labeled red blood cells remain in the blood pool and even with the 6-hour Tc-99m, scans can be repeated for 24 hours and intermittent bleeding can be detected during this period. The technique requires a large field of view camera so that the abdomen and pelvis can be examined in a single image.

Multiple images are obtained frequently during the first hour after the injection of 15m Ci of Tc-99m red blood cells. If no bleeding site is detected, images are repeated at 2 to 4 hours and if still negative, continued as long as 24 hours. The interpretation of the bleeding scan is based on the appearance of labeled red blood cells in the small intestine or colon. If increased activity is not seen on early images and only detected in the distal descending and sigmoid colon on delayed images, the actual bleeding site can not be identified (Fig. 12-10).

The important pitfalls in interpretation of GI bleeding include recognition of free pertechnetate in the gastric mucosa, excreted radioactivity in the urinary bladder or in a ptotic or fused kidney, and hyperemia or increased vascularity. Gastritis, neoplasm, varices, and aneurysm have all been known to lead to an erroneous diagnosis.

It is important to emphasize that imaging with labeled red blood cells should continue at least for 24 hours. Within the first 6 hours, approximately 55 to 75 percent of bleeding sites are visualized; within 24 hours, 90 to 100 per cent are visualized. The technique is so sensitive and has such a high degree of reliability that most angiographers will not study a patient who has not had or who has a negative nuclear medicine GI bleed study.

BONE SCAN

Bone scanning is one of the most frequently performed nuclear medicine studies in the hospital and in outpatient practice. The major indications for bone scanning include detection of occult metastatic disease, differentiation of osteomyelitis from cellulitis, detection of early aseptic necrosis, and differentiation of a stress fracture from shin splints and nonspecific physical stress related bone changes. The acquisition technique used depends upon the particular clinical indication, but in general, it consists of intravenous injection of 20m Ci of Tc-99m labeled methylene diphosphonate (MDP).

The three-phase bone scan technique is usually employed in evaluation of inflammatory and traumatic lesions. The dynamic flow study, the first or perfusion phase, is obtained immediately after intravenous injection of 20 mCi of radiopharmaceutical with the scintillation camera over the area of interest. Acquisition of radioactivity of 2 to 4 seconds in duration is recorded. After 1 or 2 minutes, the second phase is recorded and reflects the regional blood pool in the area of interest. The third phase is obtained 2 to 3 hours later, usually as part of a scan of the entire skeleton, and will reflect active bone metabolism. Except for patients being evaluated for osteomyelitis, or a sport injury, usually only the third phase, the typical whole body scan, is obtained.

The absorbed radiation dose to the skeleton is approximately 0.7 rad. The radiation dose to the kidney is approximately 1.5 rads and the whole body dose approximates 2 rads. The critical organ is the urinary bladder mucosa, which may receive a radiation dose in excess of 10 rads per study if the patient is not encouraged to urinate frequently. The kidneys excrete 55 to 60 per cent of the radiopharmaceutical within 2 hours and 80 per cent with 24 hours. The retention of radiopharmaceutical in the skeleton is markedly increased in primary hyperparathyroidism and in patients with renal osteodystrophy.

The vast majority of bone abnormalities appear on the bone scan as solitary or multiple focal areas of increased activity. Technetium-99m MDP accumulation depends on delivery, i.e., blood flow, and on the response of the biological activity of the surrounding normal bone tissue, and very little, if at all, on the pathologic process itself. Technetium-99m MDP is accumulated in precollagen and, to a lesser degree, in collagen and hydroxyapatite. An abnormality in the bone stimulates the normal physiologic processes of bone formation and bone resorption. Even though the net effect may be more bone resorption, such as from a metastatic malignancy or osteomyelitis, the "hot" spot is an indication that some new bone formation is taking place. Except for those primary bone tumors that have a predilection for joints and for fractures that involve a joint, the clinically significant focal areas of intense uptake rarely involve a joint. Ill-defined, diffuse, minimal to moderate uptake is frequently seen on both sides of many large and small joints, including the vertebral joints, and is symmetrical and characteristic of degenerative joint or synovial disease.

Most of the time, interpretation of the bone scan is based on the asymmetrical appearance of single or multiple "hot" spots, which are pathologically nonspecific. A traumatic fracture, osteomyelitis, primary and metastatic malignant tumors all will produce similar focal areas of increased activity. Therefore, only by careful and complete integration of the clinical history, physical examination, and laboratory and radiographic data will interpretation of the bone scan contribute useful information. For example, two or more rib lesions, aligned vertically, even in a patient with a malignancy known to metastasize to bone, are almost certainly due to traumatic fractures. Likewise, one or more intense focal lesions in the anterior costochondral joint, Tietze's disease, even in the absence of tenderness, should never be considered to be due to metastatic disease without x-ray confirmation of metastasis.

Bone scanning has a most important role in the management of the patient with cancer: for staging, evaluating bone pain with a normal x-ray, monitoring response to therapy, and determining prognosis. Bone scanning is now the preferred test for the detection of skeletal metastases because it is the most sensitive technique available for this purpose. This is so because it takes approximately 40 to 50 per cent replacement of bone (decalcification) by tumor before the regular x-ray becomes abnormal, while only 10 to 15 per cent decalcification by tumor is required to produce a scan abnormality.

Approximately 80 per cent of all skeletal metastases are localized in the axial skeleton. Lung, breast, prostate, thyroid, kidney, and skin melanoma are the most common primary cancers metastasizing to the appendicular skeleton. For this reason it is important to obtain a complete whole body bone scan including hands and feet. It has been reported on many occasions that an isolated metastatsis of oat cell carcinoma can occur in a finger or toe. It is unusual but not rare to see a solitary metastatic lesion in the sternum, especially in a patient with breast cancer. This should not be confused with the occasional hot manubrial-clavicular joint, a benign finding.

A literature review of the results of the bone scans in patients at the time of the diagnosis of Stage I and II breast carcinoma reveals a low percentage of abnormalities but a disturbing number of false positive results. In spite of the lack of evidence of metastatic disease on a baseline scan of patients with Stage I and II breast carcinoma, 7 per cent of patients in Stage I and 25 per cent of patients in Stage II will develop bone metastases, usually within 2 years of surgery. Half of the patients will complain of no bone pain. These results are not unexpected, given the 5- and 10-year survival of these patients. An abnormal bone scan is seen in approximately 35 to 40 per cent of patients with clinical Stage III breast cancer. The bone scan in 7 per cent of patients with Stage I and II prostatic carcinoma and 18 per cent of patients with Stage III will demonstrate metastases. The bone scan is significantly more sensitive than radiographs or elevated serum alkaline and acid phosphatase activities for the detection of bone metastases in early prostatic carcinoma. In patients with a history of prostrate cancer and bone pain, approximately 80 per cent will have a true positive bone scan; however, 40 per cent of patients with metastases, and therefore a positive bone scan, will not have bone pain.

Although the bone scan is quite accurate and used widely to detect metastatic disease and the need for therapy, such as x-ray therapy in patients found to have unsuspected metastases to a weight-bearing bone, false negative scans do occur in 3 to 4 per cent of proven metastases. These false negative scans are usually in predominantly lytic lesions. Therefore, palliative radiation therapy should be considered seriously in any patient complaining of focal bone pain with a normal bone scan and a cancer known to metastasize frequently to bone, even if the skeletal x-rays are also normal.

There is an entity described as "super scan" or "beautiful bone scan." This is when there is diffuse homogeneous intense radiopharmaceutical uptake throughout the entire skeleton with decreased renal uptake and high bone to soft tissue ratio of radioactivity. This pattern is most frequently seen in patients with widespread prostatic metastases but has been described also in patients with a number of disorders, e.g., carcinoma of the breast, lung, bladder, and lymphoma, primary and secondary hyperparathyroidism, and renal osteodystrophy (Fig. 12-11).

Patients with Paget's disease usually exhibit very intense diffuse or focal increased radiopharmaceutical uptake in the affected bone with increased size and deformity of the bone. Typically, there is involvement of the epiphysis and metaphysis of the long bones. The pelvis is most commonly involved followed by vertebrae, femur, and skull. The radiopharmaceutical is usually uniformly distributed within the lesion which is different from metastasis and fibrous dysplasia. Fibrous dysplasia does not usually involve the epiphysis of the long bones.

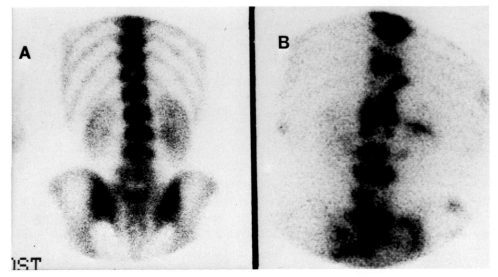

Figure 12-11. **A:** An image selected from a normal total body bone scan demonstrating the lower thoracic and lumbar vertebral bodies and pelvis. Normal symmetrical kidney activity is seen, the kidneys being the route of excretion. **B:** An image selected from a patient who had a transurethral prostatectomy three years earlier. There are multiple focal areas of abnormal activity in the vertebral bodies and pelvis typical of skeletal metastases. Such abnormal areas were widespread throughout the remainder of the skeleton. Kidney activity is not seen because so much of the radiotracer was deposited in the skeleton that renal excretion was markedly diminished, characteristic of a "super-scan."

Both benign and malignant primary bone tumors exhibit increased uptake of radiopharmaceutical. It is more typical for a malignant primary tumor to have increased flow and blood pool, which can be demonstrated on a three-phase bone scan study, as well as intense uptake of radiopharmaceutical in the tumor site on delayed images.

Osteochondromas (exostoses) constitute approximately 10 per cent of benign bone tumors. They exhibit variable uptake of Tc-99m MDP, and sometimes the degree of radiopharmaceutical uptake is as intense as that seen with a chondrosarcoma. Radiopharmaceutical uptake itself is not a reliable criterion for distinguishing a benign exostosis from a chondrosarcoma. It is particularly difficult to distinguish a benign exostosis from a low-grade sarcoma. Clinical history of recent growth or increased pain at the site of a previous benign exostosis are the important signs.

Osteoid osteoma comprises 10 to 12 per cent of all benign bone tumors and so represents a fairly common abnormality. A typical radiographic and clinical pattern does not always occur with this tumor, and a young patient with bone pain will often present a diagnostic dilemma. Immediate and delayed images usually show a well circumscribed focal area of increased activity, the so called "double density" sign. The double density sign may be useful in differentiation of osteoid osteoma from osteomyelitis.

Bone scans have limited application in patients with benign and primary malignant bone tumors. Scintigraphy is used mostly to exclude unsuspected skeletal lesions. Scintigraphic demonstration of multiple skeletal lesions in a patient who was originally thought to have a solitary lesion suggests metastatic disease. However, it should be remembered that multiple skeletal lesions are seen in benign bone lesions such as histiocytosis X, fibrous dysplasia, and enchondroma, all of which are often multifocal.

Photopenic areas, so called "cold" defects, are an uncommon finding in patients with multiple myeloma and are also rarely present with lesions of the lung, breast, prostate, and urinary bladder. Except for lesions of multiple myeloma, the photopenic abnormality is subtle and may go undetected. These and real false negative areas on the bone scan are not a major clinical problem because enough other metastatic deposits are present and multiple areas of focal increased activity occur. So even though a lesion or two may not be detected, the extent of bone involvement is relatively established.

Specifically with regard to multiple myeloma, the bone scan adds little to routine x-ray studies which are quite sensitive for the detection of bone involvement in this disease. Although the bone scan occasionally will detect a lesion not seen on x-ray, and disappearance of an area of uptake following chemotherapy can be considered as a therapeutic response and a sign of remission, the traditional x-ray examination is the preferred imaging study to evaluate skeletal involvement in patients with multiple myeloma.

Cold areas are most commonly seen in *early* avascular necrosis, aseptic necrosis of the femoral head before remodeling begins, spontaneous osteonecrosis of the femoral condyle, posttraumatic necrosis, and sickle cell disease. Osteomyelitis in an infant may show a photopenic defect in the very early stage because of pus subperiostally producing pressure which occludes the blood supply. On occasion, a benign tumor, e.g., hemangioma or bone cyst, produces a "cold" bone defect. The causes of an apparent "cold" bone defect include prosthesis, barium in the colon, and radiation therapy.

The three-phase bone scan has a special role in the differentiation of osteomyelitis and cellulitis. In osteomyelitis, the blood flow and immediate blood pool images show well-localized focal relative increased activity. On the delayed images the focal area of increased activity is localized in the bone. This characteristic appearance can be demonstrated within hours to a few days after the onset of clinical symptoms. Early during the first 2 weeks after the onset of clinical symptoms, the skeletal radiographs are usually normal or show only nonspecific soft tissue swelling (Fig. 12-12).

Cellulitis has a different and very specific appearance. The flow study, stage I, and the immediate static image, stage II, show a diffuse or focal increased activity in the involved area. The delayed image may have minimal diffuse soft tissue activity but no evidence of increased focal bone activity. An overlapping pattern may be encountered in patients with a neuropathic joint or diabetic ulcer. However, even in those conditions, compulsive attention to proper technique and the addition of a 24-hour image will help resolve the issue in most cases.

Sequential three-phase Tc-99m MDP bone scans and gallium-67 citrate scans have been widely used in the patient with pain in a joint prosthesis to differentiate loosening from infection. This is not a trivial problem since the consequence of each diagnosis results in divergent management, 6 weeks of intravenous antibiotics versus surgical revision. The interpretation of these studies also is not trivial because of the overlapping scan patterns of the two tests in the two conditions. The most reliable analysis is based on comparison of the

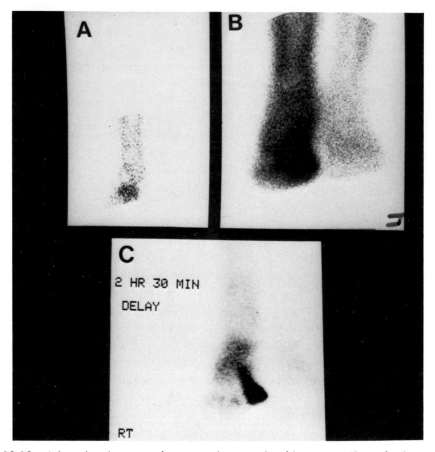

Figure 12-12. A three-phase bone scan of a patient with osteomyelitis of the great toe. There is focal increase of blood flow (**A**), focal increase of the blood pool (**B**), and localization of the radiopharmaceutical in the bones of the right great toe on the delayed image (**C**).

relative concentrations of the two radiotracers. That is, if the relative distributions are symmetrical to each other and congruent, the findings most likely reflect the increased bone activity of the prosthetic insertion or loosening of the orthopedic device and not necessarily osteomyelitis. Increased uptake at the distal tip of the device in the shaft of the femur is also commonly seen in patients with loosening. Indium-III labeled polymorphonuclear leukocytes, a technique that is being used with increased frequency for abscess detection, is not as sensitive as Ga-67 or Tc-99m MDP in the detection of chronic osteomyelitis (greater than 4 weeks duration). The combination of Tc-99m MDP and Ga-67 citrate scanning has also been used to distinguish osteomyelitis from infarction in patients with bone pain from sickle cell crisis; there is absent or relatively low Ga-67 uptake in infarction and an increase in osteomyelitis.

Bone scanning plays a special role in the evaluation of trauma, beginning with the recognition of unsuspected abuse of children, the battered child syndrome. The minimum time necessary for the bone scan to become abnormal following a traumatic fracture is dependent on the status of the mobile calcium pool. Normally, a fracture will always produce a focal abnormality in the scan within 24 hours. However, with increasing age, and especially in a patient with osteoporosis, it may take a week, or even longer, for the scan to become abnormal. This is important because scans are used frequently to confirm the clinical impression that a fracture did occur even though a fracture line is not demonstrated on x-ray.

The bone scan is quite useful for the detection of a fracture or metastases in bones that are difficult to evaluate radiographically, such as the scapula, sternum, sacrum, or the pubic symphyses, especially in an osteoporotic individual. The fractures seen in elderly osteopenic patients are frequently seen in women who give a history of minimal or no injury.

Disability from low back pain results in a high loss of personal and work time. Because radiographic findings are so common in asymptomatic adults, a "positive" x-ray exam is of limited diagnostic value in patients being evaluated for herniated nucleus pulposus, discitis, degenerative joint disease, lumbosacral muscle strain, or osteomyelitis and metastases. In such patients, the bone scan may be a useful adjunct to the x-ray examination, as it is in athletes with low back pain with or without spondylolisthesis. Early in the evolution of these processes, radiographs are frequently abnormal, but the age and activity of the radiographic lesion cannot be determined accurately while the bone scan results provide information useful in planning and monitoring therapy. For example, when spondylolysis or spondylolisthesis is the cause of low back pain, the defect in the pars interarticularis is frequently associated with increased scintigraphic activity.

The three-phase bone scan is capable of making significant contributions to the solutions of problems arising in sports medicine. This study allows simple and rapid differentiation of stress fracture from shin splints and from nonspecific so-called "undetermined bone lesions" in physically active adults. Most of the sports-related lesions are diagnosed on the bone scan in patients with persistent pain and when comparative radiographs are normal. A normal bone scan essentially excludes any underlying osseous pathologic condition.

Typically, a stress fracture of the lower leg has an abnormal, relatively increased initial radionuclide angiogram and a markedly abnormal blood pool image. Abnormalities of the first and second phases of the bone scan are focal. On the phase III delayed image, the stress fracture appears as a focal, fusiform, or longitudinal lesion of high intensity which more often localizes in the posterior tibial cortex. In about a quarter of patients, stress fracture is bilateral. Although distasteful and difficult for the jogger to accept, the only treatment for a stress fracture is to stop running. Continued exercise may produce a complete fracture and result in prolonged convalescence (Figs. 12-13A, B).

The specific scintigraphic pattern in patients with shin splints contrasts sharply with that seen with a stress fracture. With shin splints, the phase I radionuclide angiogram and phase II immediate blood pool images are normal, and the phase III delayed images show inhomogeneous longitudinal involvement of approximately one-third of the length of the shaft of the tibia, most often in both legs.

Abnormal extraskeletal localization of Tc-99m MDP has been described in various soft tissues associated with electric shock, crush injury, myositis ossificans, dermato-or polymyositis contusion, scars, rhabdomyolysis, and ectopic sites of any soft tissue calcium deposition.

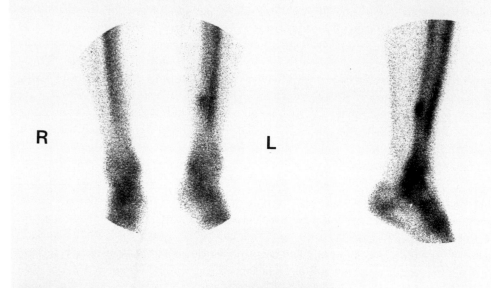

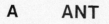

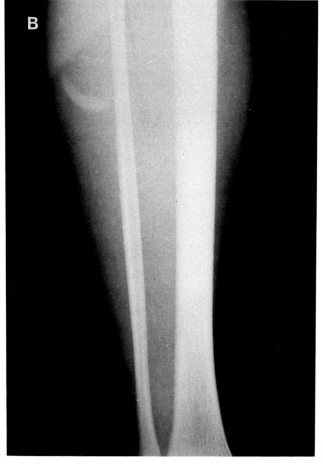

Figure 12-13. A 46-year-old man who ran 30 to 35 miles per week was referred because of focal pain in the left distal tibia. He had a stress fracture of the right distal tibia 2 years ago. There is a segment of increased activity on the delayed 3-hour bone scan (**A**). Corresponding x-ray of the lower extremity (**B**) shows no evidence of abnormality in the left tibia. The findings are characteristic of a stress fracture of the distal third of the left tibia.

In summary, it is important to emphasize that the bone scan is not specific and false negative results are encountered in approximately 3 per cent of all pathologic lesions. In certain false negative circumstances, multiple myeloma for example, sensitivity may only be 50 per cent for individual lesions. Considering the cost of imaging modalities, plain radiography is probably the best imaging technique for the differential diagnosis of primary bone tumors, and bone scintigraphy is the best for evaluating metastatic disease. At the present time the cost of a bone scan is approximately $450.00.

KIDNEY STUDIES

Nuclear medicine tests are used to measure differential right and left renal function and to evaluate the renal transplant recipient. The radiopharmaceuticals used are Tc-99m DTPA, a soluble chelate cleared from the body by glomerular filtration, or radioiodinated iodohippuric acid, cleared by tubular secretion. These agents are also used widely in pediatric patients to monitor safely and efficiently congenital abnormalities of the urinary outflow tract. The test results in a significant reduction in radiation dose to the gonads compared to the radiographic tests that have been utilized in the past.

OTHER NUCLEAR MEDICINE TESTS

Although the use of nuclear medicine procedures in diagnostic medicine for diseases of the thyroid, heart, lung, liver, spleen, gallbladder, G.I. bleed, bone, and kidney have been discussed, several other commonly used tests will be briefly mentioned here.

The clinical diagnosis of deep venous thrombosis is notoriously unreliable. Contrast venography is tedious, time consuming, and uncomfortable for the patient and radiologist. The areas that can be assessed are limited, as with Doppler ultrasound. Indium-111 (In-111) oxine, a lipophilic compound, has been used to label platelets which are readily incorporated into active clots. The labeling technique takes approximately 2 hours and scans are obtained 12 to 20 hours following the injection. The whole body may be surveyed and active clots are readily detected. Autologous and donor platelets are equally effective.

Abscess detection in a patient without lateralizing or localizing signs is difficult by any of the traditional imaging techniques. Using simple gradient sedimentation, the polymorphonuclear leukocytes can be concentrated and labeled with In-111 as the oxine. When injected, the PMN's retain their biologic integrity and accumulate at the site of an abscess. This technique has found particular utility for the detection of abdominal and pelvic abscess, but it has been used for abscess localization throughout the body. The technique is less sensitive for the detection of chronic osteomyelitis but otherwise has found wide application, even in patients who are leukopenic. Donor white cell labeling provides the same results. The 2.7-day physical half-life of the In-111 allows imaging to be repeated over several days.

Gallium-67 (Ga-67), injected intravenously as the citrate, is bound to plasma proteins, primarily transferrin, and is known to localize in malignant tumors and in inflammatory

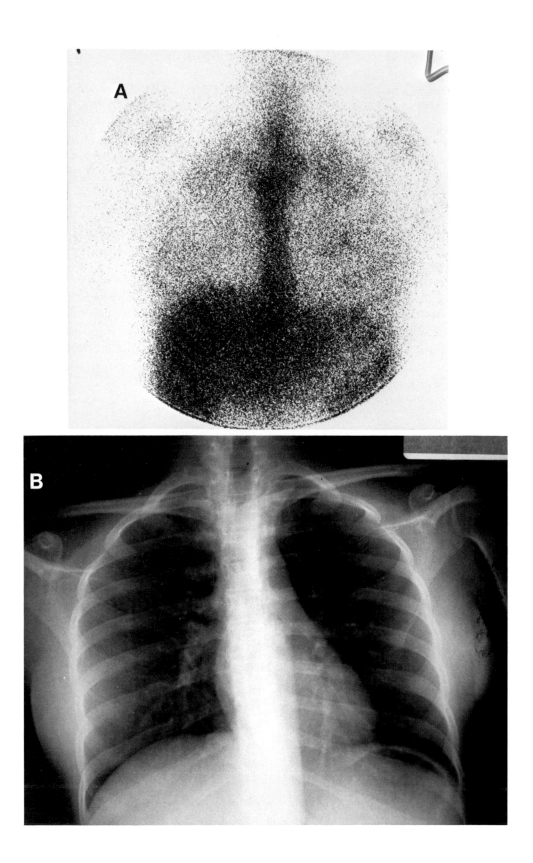

lesions, particularly abscesses. The specific mechanism of localization is unknown. Uptake in an abscess is rapid but clearance from blood and the interstitial space is slow so imaging must be delayed for 24 to 72 hours. Gallium localization is nonspecific and is now rarely used for diagnosis and staging of malignancy but is widely used in the assessment of a patient with a questionable lesion and in the evaluation of response to therapy, particularly in acute and chronic osteomyelitis.

Since Ga-67 is known to concentrate nonspecifically in any area of inflammation, this radiopharmaceutical has found wide use to monitor the activity of patients with sarcoidosis and their response to steroids or other treatment. Currently, Ga-67 citrate is the most sensitive method to detect pulmonary inflammatory disease, such as *pneumocystis carinii*, in immunosuppressed patients, even before the chest x-ray becomes abnormal (Figs. 12-14A, B).

Figure 12-14. **A:** Scan obtained from the thorax 48 hours after intravenous injection of Ga-67 citrate. There is diffuse increased activity in the upper lobes of both lungs in a patient with AIDS. **B:** The corresponding chest x-ray reveals only minimally diffuse increased interstitial markings bilaterally which are nonspecific. The diagnosis of pneumocystis carinii was suggested and confirmed by cytology of a bronchial aspirate. A chest x-ray obtained 2 weeks later showed interstitial and alveolar infiltrates in both upper lobes.

WHERE ARE WE GOING TOMORROW

Eugene R. Jacobs

When I first envisioned this book, I put down some preliminary thoughts about tomorrow. As I review them today, I am further convinced that our hindsight is far better than our ability to see into the future. I feel fortunate that last year's projections are not in print and I will therefore shorten the number of pages of "prediction" here. However, there are two areas I wish to specifically address. I am sure that these areas will be with us in the future, although I cannot predict precisely when, how, or how much.

TELERADIOLOGY

PHOTOELECTRONIC DIGITAL IMAGING, PROCESSING, ARCHIVING, AND TRANSMISSION

Currently digital images are routinely obtained in CT, MRI, ultrasound, nuclear medicine, and digital subtraction angiography. These images can be easily electronically transmitted, processed, stored, and presented for evaluation on a TV screen or transmitted to remote locations by telephone lines or other means of electronic communication. In addition, conventional radiographs may be converted to digitalized photoelectronic images for storage, transmission, and viewing on TV screens. Alternately, charged plates can be substituted for films or photoelectronic imaging devices can be used to provide digital images capable of rapid, cost-effective processing, storage, and transmission.

The viewer of the TV screen can often control not only brightness, but contrast and magnification. With the aid of teleradiology, one can transmit images to monitors anywhere in a medical complex or anywhere reachable by telephone without the risk of losing, misplacing or permanently borrowing, the images. One can recall old studies and compare them on the same or adjacent monitors.

I predict that such systems will become progressively better and cheaper and progressively more user-friendly as well as cost-effective. I would suspect that the utilization of such systems on a wide scale, and the interaction of such systems with each other for comparison of studies done at different institutions, may someday be quite commonplace. First, however, these systems must become more cost-effective compared to the cost of silver and the cost of conventional film archiving. Looking at medical images in the future may involve more gazing at TV monitors than shuffling of films at viewboxes. No predictions on when, how, or how much.

MAGNETIC RESONANCE IMAGING

MRI is definitely with us. It appears to be the gold standard of neuroradiology. It has definite promise in musculoskeletal radiology and in cardiac imaging. It has definite promise as a research tool. Cost remains a serious factor as does the shielding of the magnetic field so that the MRI unit is not interfered with by external sources and so that the MRI unit does not interfere with other electronic equipment. Again, no predictions on when, how, and how much.

INDEX